HISTOCHEMICAL TECHNIQUES

HISTOCHEMICAL TECHNIQUES

2nd Edition

J. D. BANCROFT

Senior Chief Technician
Nottingham University Medical School
part time course tutor and lecturer in Histopathology (MLS),
Trent Polytechnic, Nottingham

Introductory Chapter by

A. STEVENS, M.B., B.S., M.R.C.Path.,

Senior Lecturer
Nottingham University Medical School
Honorary Consultant Pathologist,
Trent Health Authority (T)

With a Foreword by

A. G. E. PEARSE, M.A., M.D., F.R.C.Path.,

Professor of Histochemistry
University of London

BUTTERWORTHS
LONDON AND BOSTON

THE BUTTERWORTH GROUP

ENGLAND
Butterworth & Co (Publishers) Ltd,
London: 88 Kingsway, WC2B 6AB

AUSTRALIA
Butterworths Pty Ltd
Sydney: 586 Pacific Highway, NSW 2067
Melbourne: 343 Little Collins Street, 3000
Brisbane: Commonwealth Bank Building,
King George Square, 4000

CANADA
Butterworth & Co (Canada) Ltd
Toronto: 2265 Midland Avenue,
Scarborough, Ontario, M1P 4S1

NEW ZEALAND
Butterworths of New Zealand Ltd
Wellington: 26–28 Waring Taylor Street, 1

SOUTH AFRICA
Butterworth & Co (South Africa) (Pty) Ltd
Durban: 152–154 Gale Street

USA
Butterworths (Publishers) Inc
161 Ash Street,
Reading, Mass. 01867

First published 1975

ISBN 0 407 00033 X

Library of Congress Cataloging in Publication Data

Bancroft, John D
Histochemical techniques.
First ed. published in 1967 under title: An introduction to histochemical techniques.
Includes bibliographies and index.
1. Histochemistry—Technique. I. Title.
[DNLM: 1. Histocytochemistry—Laboratory manuals.
2. Histological Technics. QS525 B213i]
QH613.B36 1975 574.8'2'028 75–23430
ISBN 0–407–00033–X

Printed and bound in Great Britain by R. J. Acford Ltd, Industrial Estate, Chichester, Sussex

CONTENTS

FOREWORD

Histochemistry continues to play an increasingly important role in its application to the Biological Sciences. Its technology, increasing in volume and to some extent in complexity, is handled in this volume essentially in the light of practicability.

The author has had long experience of the techniques of which he writes and he speaks with the authority conferred by this experience.

I have no doubt that this worthy successor to the first edition, will be equally acceptable and, as is proper, of greatly enhanced value to its users.

A. G. Everson Pearse

PREFACE

In the time since the First Edition of this book was published, the field of histochemistry has expanded considerably and many more reliable histochemical methods are now available. The best and most useful of these methods I have included in this Second Edition, and I have omitted a few methods which I included in the First Edition in a rush of youthful enthusiasm, but which I have subsequently found unreliable or technically difficult.

Dr Alan Stevens has written an introductory chapter discussing the problems and values of histochemistry, and the chapter on carbohydrates has been increased in size to incorporate new concepts and methods in carbohydrate histochemistry. New chapters include a separate and distinct chapter on amyloid, in which there has been a considerable increase in knowledge in the last seven years, and a new chapter in which the theoretical concepts in enyzme histochemistry are discussed. The final chapter is an introduction to a fast-expanding facet of histochemistry, namely ultra-histochemistry, the application of histochemistry to electron microscopy.

In the production of this edition I am indebted to Alan Stevens who read the entire manuscript and played an important role in its revision; to Professor A. G. E. Pearse for his Foreword; and to Professor I. M. P. Dawson for his encouragement and tolerance. For secretarial assistance thanks are due to Miss Colleen Peel and to my wife Stella.

J. D. Bancroft

1

Introduction

by A. Stevens

Histochemical techniques enable the identification and localization of specific substances within tissues. The methods depend on chemical reactions between the substance to be identified and localized in a tissue section, and one or more reagents in which the tissue section is incubated. The histochemist tries to arrange matters so that the end product of the chemical reaction is both coloured and insoluble, and therefore easily visible on microscopy. Histochemical methods such as the PAS reaction and the Perls' Prussian Blue reaction are well known to histopathologists, but until recently the scope of histochemistry has been limited by one big problem. To cut thin sections of tissue it is necessary for it to be made rigid and to be embedded in a firm supporting medium; the embedding medium used in routine histopathology is paraffin wax. The process of embedding the tissue is a violent one, involving the immersion of the tissue in hot molten wax; it is essential, to minimize the distortion and disruption of the tissue during processing, that the tissue is adequately fixed beforehand. Furthermore the tissue must be completely dehydrated with alcohol and finally infiltrated with an organic solvent (usually toluene) with which the embedding wax is totally miscible. The major limiting factor in histochemistry is that all these processes, so essential for the successful cutting of thin sections, inevitably chemically modify or completely destroy or remove the very substances we are attempting to demonstrate. Lipids in the tissue are dissolved out by the alcohols and xylene used in dehydration and clearing of the tissue. Many tissue enzymes are destroyed by the fixative and by the heat necessary in the embedding of the tissue in wax, and the accurate intracytoplasmic localization of soluble substances such as glycogen is impossible in tissue exposed to aqueous fixatives.

TABLE 1.1

Different methods of tissue processing and their application to histochemical procedures

Processing method	*Histochemical method*
(1) Routine paraffin processing	Carbohydrates Proteins Pigments
(2) Special paraffin processing	Proteins Hydrolytic enzymes (if no other method available)
(3) Freeze drying	Carbohydrates Proteins
(4) Freeze drying formol-vapour fixation	Carbohydrates Proteins Fluorescence techniques
(5) Freeze drying with double embedding	Hydrolytic enzymes Proteins Carbohydrates
(6) Frozen sections formalin-fixed	Fat stains Amyloid stains
(7) Cryostat sections fresh unfixed	Oxidative enzymes Hydrolytic enzymes Almost all techniques after suitable fixation
(8) Cryostat sections from fixed block	Hydrolytic enzymes

Histochemical techniques in some cases may be applied to sections produced by different methods than recommended above. The above Table is included as a guide.

Tissue to be investigated histochemically must therefore be processed in an entirely different manner to tissue for normal histological stains, although certain very stable substances can be demonstrated by histochemical means in paraffin sections. These are discussed in Chapter 2. For the majority of histochemical reactions, however, an entirely new method of tissue processing and section cutting has had to be devised, and most of the improvements in histochemistry have only emerged in recent years after the development of satisfactory methods of tissue preparation. The most important problem to overcome was that of producing high quality thin sections of tissue without the use of a supporting medium such as paraffin wax, and without having to subject the tissue to the necessary pre-treatment with organic solvents and heat implicit in normal tissue embedding. In normal histology the tissue is partly protected from the ill-effects of such treatment by the process known as fixation. For a histochemist's purposes however the protection offered by fixing the tissue is totally inadequate. As we have seen, the very process of fixing the tissue, while it preserves to a certain extent the architectural integrity of the tissue, inevitably destroys many of the substances which the histochemist wishes to demonstrate.

The solution to this problem lay in the development of techniques for producing thin sections from a piece of tissue which has been frozen hard. The intrinsic water content of the tissue, when frozen, acts as a very suitable supporting medium for the tissue and renders the tissue rigid enough for thin sections to be cut from it using specialized microtomes such as the freezing microtome and cryostat. Although the formation of ice within the tissue when it is frozen, and the subsequent dissolution of the ice when the section is thawed, may lead to some architectural distortion and other artefact, the substances in which the histochemist is interested remain largely unaltered and are capable of being demonstrated by histochemical reactions. Sections produced in this way contain the full complement of substances, and the tissue has been exposed to no damaging agent other than a low temperature; this seems to matter very little from a practical point ot view. The ability to consistently produce high quality thin frozen sections, using both a freezing microtome and a cryostat, is the first requirement of a technologist involved in histochemical work; the procedures are dealt with in the relevant chapters later in this book.

It can be seen that the tissues sectioned in this way do not need the protection offered by preceding fixation. However this protective effect is not the only function of fixatives; they are also important in fixing the chemical substances in place within the cell cytoplasm and preventing diffusion (therefore facilitating accurate localization), and also may act as mordants, enhancing the staining characteristics of certain substances and structures. In certain circumstances fixation has an important part to play in histochemistry, although it is avoided completely if any of the oxidative enzymes are to be demonstrated. Paradoxically, accurate localization of sites of hydrolytic enzyme activity is considerably enhanced if the tissue has been properly fixed; fixation reduces the amount of diffusion of the enzyme which inevitably occurs when the frozen section thaws. Although the process of fixation reduces by a small amount the quantity of demonstrable hydrolytic enzyme present, this is of no consequence practically and the improved localization makes fixation well worthwhile. The most widely used fixative for histochemical purposes is formol calcium, fixation usually being carried out at 4°C. Although fixation is valuable in the demonstration of hydrolytic enzymes, it must be for a limited time only (usually about 12 hours). The longer the tissue is kept in fixative, the more appreciable will be the loss of demonstrable enzyme activity.

Two more sophisticated methods based on the freezing of tissue are *freeze drying* and *freeze substitution*. In freeze drying, the tissue is frozen, and the water (in the form of ice) is completely removed in conditions of partial vacuum and at sub-zero temperatures. In freeze substitution the water in the tissue is replaced by an organic solvent, again at sub-zero temperatures, but at normal atmospheric pressure. These two techniques, although they require special equipment and some expertise, are most valuable in the histochemical identification and localization of carbohydrates and proteins. Freeze-dried tissue blocks are best fixed in formalin vapour before embedding and sectioning; in freeze substitution fixation can be effected by incorporating a fixative such as picric acid in the substituting fluid.

Now that the histochemist is equipped with adequate tools for his job, the number of substances for which histochemical methods have been devised is increasing rapidly. Adequate histochemical methods now exist for the demonstration of carbohydrates, proteins, lipids, nucleic acids, pigments, amines and a very wide range of enzymes. However, we must accept that most of the histochemical reactions which we use are embarrassingly non-specific and that we are unable to identify substances with the accuracy of the biochemist with the reagents at our disposal. At this juncture it is perhaps relevant to mention the very important part which the chemical manufacturing industry, and a handful of firms in particular, have played in the development of histochemistry. They have continually striven to produce reagents, and particularly enzyme substrates, of such purity and specificity that there is now some hope of increasing the specificity of our histochemical reactions. Histochemists have used considerable ingenuity in devising methods to increase the specificity of their reactions, and the use of such techniques as specific enzyme inhibition has led to more accurate identification of certain enzymes. A good example of this is in the elucidation of the various types of 'esterase'.

A very recent development in histochemistry has been the application of a limited number of histochemical methods (mainly involving the demonstration of enzymes) to blocks of tissue which are subsequently to be processed for electron microscopy. In this way we can study the ultrastructural localization of enzyme activity within cell organelles.

Histochemistry is fast gaining respectability; it has long been used as a research tool in all branches of the biological sciences, and is now being increasingly used in diagnostic histopathology. If we wish this to continue we must ensure that any new methods are simple enough to be performed in a routine laboratory and that they are consistently reproducible.

2

Fixation

The requirements of a fixative vary, depending upon whether the tissue is to be used for the demonstration of enzymes, or for other purposes. The main functions of a fixative are:—

(1) to preserve the tissue
(2) to prevent diffusion
(3) to protect the tissue from subsequent treatment.

For tissue that is processed for paraffin wax embedding the following factors are also relevant.

(1) The hardening of the tissue by the fixative
(2) The rate of penetration of the fixative
(3) The conversion of semi-liquids—gels—to semi-solids
(4) The effect on staining reactions.

PRESERVATION OF THE TISSUE

The first consideration of fixation must be to preserve the tissue as near as possible as it was in life, whilst at the same time not altering the chemical composition or localization of the constituents of the tissue. This with present day fixatives is not wholly possible; however, thought must be given to what is required of the tissue before a means of fixation is chosen.

Tissue on removal from the body, if left in the air, will dry, shrink and undergo bacteriological changes and autolysis (chemical reactions taking place by the enzymes within the tissue cells). If the tissue is placed in water, the tissue swells rapidly and is unrecognizable. Upon death, autolysis and putrefaction (the tissue being affected by bacteria from an outside source) take place. To avoid these changes, fixation must be carried out as rapidly as possible if the tissue is to be preserved in a state comparable with that in life. The preserving fluid (fixative) must not cause swelling of the tissue, it must stop chemical reactions taking place with the autolytic enzymes, whilst not removing all other enzymes from the tissue. The preservative must also cause as little shrinkage of the tissue as possible.

Preservation by freezing

Tissues frozen rapidly to temperatures of −70°C and below are well preserved. There is no major loss of enzyme activity and diffusion is prevented. The chemically reactive constituents remain unaltered until the tissue is thawed.

Prevention of diffusion or loss of substance

For the majority of histochemical procedures, it is necessary that the substances to be demonstrated are in their true position. Despite all the fixatives to hand today, this is not always possible. In some instances, the substances are affected and moved by the fixative itself, e.g. the diffusion artefact shown in glycogen. It is possible to avoid this effect with glycogen by using freeze drying, followed by formalin vapour fixation. In other cases, the fixative by its action on cell constituents will render the substances insoluble to other reagents and hence demonstrable by histochemical techniques. The correct choice of a fixative is vital. Formaldehyde does not act upon lipids, and is therefore ideal for their demonstration, whereas any of the many alcohol-containing fixatives cannot be used, because of the extraction of lipid material by the alcohol.

Protecting the tissue from subsequent treatments

After suitable fixation, the tissue is generally processed either through to paraffin wax or as an alternative, it is quenched and frozen sections are cut. In both of these procedures, the tissue is subjected to fluids or actions (thawing) which will cause loss of substances in the first technique, or diffusion of substances in both techniques. These can be overcome to a certain degree by the correct fixation at the start of the process for paraffin-embedded material, and by fixation before freezing when demonstrating lysosomal enzymes.

Hardening of material for paraffin processing

To obtain a suitable consistency for cutting paraffin sections, the tissue must be hardened by the fixative. All the fixatives in routine use will harden the tissue. The problem is that some will overharden the material, if it is left in too long. Hardening also allows very soft and friable tissues to be handled without undue damage during the treatment before embedding.

Rate of penetration of fixative

Before a tissue can be considered fixed, the fixative must have fully penetrated it. The rate of penetration varies with different fixatives; formaldehyde, for instance, has a rapid rate of penetration compared with picric acid, which penetrates at a moderate rate. Osmium tetroxide has a slower rate than either. The faster the rate of penetration of a fixative the better, as autolytic changes may still occur in the centre of a specimen despite it being in a fixative. The question of penetration is more complicated in the case of compound fixatives. Here, if one agent causes swelling, another usually causes shrinkage, so that uneven fixation sometimes results.

Effect of fixation on staining reactions

The choice of fixative usually depends upon three factors: (1) which stain or reaction is to be applied to the section; (2) whether there is any urgency; and (3) the size of the piece of tissue.

If the reason for processing the tissue is to demonstrate glycogen, then cold Bouin's or Gendre's would be used. However, if the Feulgen reaction was to be applied, Bouin's would not be used, as it causes overhydrolysis (see Feulgen reaction).

Some fixatives act as a mordant, a constituent of the fixative making a chemical linkage between the dye and the tissue. When this type of fixative is used, more specific staining occurs. An example of this is the use of mercury in a fixative, which gives the tissue an affinity for trichrome stains.

Freezing instead of fixing

For some histochemical procedures, it is necessary to use unfixed material. When this is required, the tissue is rapidly frozen on removal from the body. The freezing of the tissue preserves it by stopping the autolytic enzymes from reacting and, whilst the tissue remains frozen, it remains preserved. On thawing, the tissue must be placed in a fixative. As well as stopping the chemical reactions, freezing also brings the tissue to a solid state, the ice in the tissue acting as the embedding medium when the sections are cut.

The preservation of enzymes is difficult. The optimal method for hydrolytic enzymes is fixation in formol calcium or formol saline at 4°C. The enzymes are less affected by the fixatives at low temperatures, and little loss of enzyme activity occurs. After this fixation, the tissue is placed in gum sucrose for 24 hours. The blocks are then blotted dry and frozen. Sections are cut in a cryostat and the histochemical method applied. The prefixation of the block stops the diffusion of the enzymes from their true localization when the section is thawed before incubating.

GENERAL CONSIDERATIONS

The fixation of proteins also needs careful consideration, as the majority of fixatives react with protein groupings. Some fixatives precipitate proteins, e.g. alcohol, while others undergo chemical reactions with proteins, e.g. formaldehyde.

Fixatives produce the best results when used at temperatures just above freezing point. For obvious reasons, however, this is not possible in routine histology laboratories.

The size of the piece of tissue to be fixed should be as small as possible (a thickness of 0·5 cm is ideal for routine use). As the fixative penetrates rapidly, the time of fixation can be kept to a minimum. To obtain rapid fixation, the tissue should be covered by 10 to 20 times its own volume of fixative. Fixatives as a general rule tend to be acid, so for histochemical methods it is usually necessary to adjust the pH to neutrality.

FIXING SOLUTIONS

Formaldehyde

This is the most popular fixing agent in histology. It may be used on its own or in other compound fixatives. Formaldehyde, which is a gas, is normally available as a 40 per cent solution in water. When solutions of formalin are prepared, this 40 per cent solution must be taken as 100 per cent, e.g. to prepare a 10 per cent solution of formalin, 10 parts of 40 per cent formaldehyde are added to 90 parts of water.

Solutions of formalin are invariably acid, due to the formation of small amounts of formic acid in the formaldehyde. For all histochemical, and the majority of histological, techniques it is necessary to bring the pH of formalin to neutral. This can be done by employing either a buffer (sodium phosphate), or by placing calcium carbonate at the bottom of the container holding the formaldehyde solution. Fixation in acid formalin over a lengthy period produces formalin pigment, especially in blood-containing tissues (*see* page 182). If the tissue has been fixed in acid formalin over a long period of time, difficulty may be encountered in making acid dyes such as eosin stain correctly.

Formaldehyde will not fix lipids, nor will it remove them, which allows for their demonstration. The following formaldehyde solutions are amongst those used in histochemistry and histology:

(1) 10 per cent formol saline
(2) 10 per cent formalin (aqueous)
(3) 10 per cent neutral formalin
(4) 10 per cent formol calcium
(5) 10 per cent formalin in alcohol
(6) 10 per cent formol sucrose
(7) Formaldehyde vapour.

As in routine histology, formaldehyde is probably the most used fixative in histochemistry. It is an ideal fixative for tissue in which lipids are to be demonstrated, as lipids are chemically unaltered by formaldehyde fixation. Phospholipids are well preserved by formaldehyde fixation when calcium has been added to the fixative. In enzyme histochemistry, the majority of hydrolytic enzymes are well preserved with fixation in formol calcium at 4°C. The amount of enzyme activity is reduced if the fixation time is extended or if it is carried out at room temperature. Formaldehyde vapour is recommended for the fixation of freeze dried tissues and produces excellent demonstration of mucosubstances including glycogen (*see Plate 1*) and proteins. Nucleic acids are also well preserved after vapour fixation.

(N.B. The formulae for these solutions, and other compound fixatives that contain formaldehyde, will be found at the end of this chapter.)

Other aldehyde fixatives

Other aldehydes, besides formaldehyde, may be used as fixatives. They are especially useful when enzyme histochemistry is followed by electron microscopy. Sabatini, Bensch and Barrnett (1963) produced a paper dealing with nine different aldehydes. They buffered the fixatives to between pH 5·5 and 7·6. The hydrolytic enzymes worked satisfactorily after most of the fixatives, as did NADH and NADPH diaphorases. Flitney (1966), using seven different aldehydes (*see* Table 2.1), investigated the rate of fixation of these fixatives with albumen, and their effect on enzyme activity in cryostat sections. In regard to the fixation of cryostat sections, he found that aldehydes which fixed the albumen most rapidly also destroyed most enzyme activity. This could be overcome, however, by using these fast acting aldehyde fixatives for very short times, i.e. for an 8 micron cryostat section, 30 seconds to 1 minute was usually sufficient. The two aldehydes that gave good fixation with reasonable morphological preservation and with only a small amount of enzyme loss were glutaraldehyde and acrolein when used for 60 seconds. These aldehydes have not gained popularity as

TABLE 2.1

Aldehyde fixatives

Aldehyde	%	*Buffer*	*Final* pH
Acrolein	10		6·8–7·2
Glutaraldehyde	6	Phosphate buffer	7·2
Crotonaldehyde	10	Phosphate buffer	7·4
Formaldehyde	10	Phosphate buffer	7·2–7·4
Hydroxyadipaldehyde	12	Phosphate buffer	7·4
Acetaldehyde	10	Phosphate buffer	7·2–7·4
Glyoxal	4		6·8–7·2

block fixatives because of the time taken to penetrate to the centre of the tissue. The advantage to be gained by short fixation is lost.

Alcohol

This is rarely used on its own in histology because of the damage it causes by shrinkage and excessive hardening of the block. It is, however, used more often in histochemistry, especially for fixation of cryostat sections, to demonstrate enzymes. Alcohol is a good fixative as the enzymes are almost unaffected by cold alcohol (4°C) with the exception of the esterases. For the demonstration of glycogen, alcohol is occasionally used as an 80 per cent solution. This, while being an ideal fixative for glycogen, has drawbacks from a morphological point of view. When used in compound fixatives, however, alcohol will give acceptable results. It will precipitate proteins, and will remove lipids. It also makes the freezing of tissue and the subsequent sectioning difficult. The following are the more common fixatives which contain alcohol.

(1) Formol alcohol
(2) Carnoy
(3) Clarke's
(4) Gendre's fluid
(5) Acetic alcohol formalin (AAF)
(6) Wolman's fixative.

(The formulae for the above fixatives can be found at the end of this chapter.)

Osmium tetroxide

Osmic acid finds little use in routine histology and histochemistry, with the exception of the demonstration of some lipid-containing structures, although it is in constant use in electron microscopy where it is used in a 1 per cent buffered solution.

The fixation of moderate-sized pieces of tissue in osmium produces large amounts of shrinkage and uneven penetration of the tissue. It can be used to render lipids insoluble. It can also be used as a vapour fixative with freeze dried material (Tock and Pearse, 1965). This fixative is very damaging to enzymes.

Suggested fixatives for histochemical methods

Methods	*Fixatives*	*Temp* (°C)	*Block time* (h)	*Section time* (min)
Acid and alkaline phosphates	Acetone 100%	4	18	30–60
	90% Alcohol	4	24	30
	Formol calcium	4	24	30
	10% Formol saline	4	24	30
Non-specific esterase	Acetone 100%	4	18–24	30–60
E600 Resistant esterase	Formol calcium	4	24	30–60
	10% Formol saline	4	18–24	30–60
Glycogen	Gendre or Bouin	4	18–24	—
	Formol vapour after freeze drying			
Carbohydrate methods generally	10% Formol saline	22	2–24	30
	Formol alcohol	22	6–24	10–20
	90% Alcohol	22	6–24	30
	Formol vapour after freeze drying			
All types of lipids	10% Formol calcium	22	18–24	—
	10% Formol saline	22	18–24	—
	10% Neutral buffered solution	22	18–24	—
Protein Methods	Formol vapour after freeze drying	60	2	30
	10% Formol saline	22	18–24	30–60
	Carnoy	22	1	1–5
	Formol alcohol	22	6–24	5
Acridine orange technique	Carnoy	22	1	1–5
	100% Alcohol		6–24	30–60
Nucleic acid methods	Carnoy	22	1	1–5
	10% Formol saline	22	18–24	30–60
Pigment methods	10% Neutral buffered formol saline	22	18–24	30–60
Calcium	10% Neutral buffered formol saline	22	18–24	30–60

Acetone

This reagent may be used in histochemistry as a fixative of cryostat sections. The acetone is used at 0–4°C. It has frequently been used as a fixative for pieces of tissue to be processed to paraffin wax, and hydrolytic enzyme methods applied to the sections. Acetone is a fairly rapid fixative but does, in the author's experience, cause shrinkage of the tissue. It is frequently employed as the first step in the freeze substitution technique. At −70°C it will not remove much lipid material from the tissue, nor will it fix the tissue, whereas it will be substituted for the ice in the tissue. It is rarely used in any compound fixatives, certainly not in any of the standard fixatives. At 4°C, it will fix cryostat sections (5–20 microns (μ m)) in 1 hour or less and will fix small pieces of tissue overnight at 4°C.

Picric acid

This gives good fixation of tissue blocks. It is a rapid fixative that hardens the block well, without causing much shrinkage. Picric acid is used in many compound fixatives, of which Bouin's and Gendre's are the most popular. Any fixatives containing this acid are recommended for the demonstration of glycogen and histological trichrome stains. Tissue fixed in picric acid must be washed in either alcohol or water until the yellow colour of the block is removed. Lillie (1965) states that it is more rapid to process, embed and section in the normal way and to remove the yellow colour from the section before staining. Picric acid precipitates proteins and combines with some of them. In some instances, these are soluble in water, but they may be treated with alcohol first and then they become insoluble.

Mercury-containing fixatives

These fixatives are little used in histochemistry. Mercuric chloride has a rapid but uneven penetration and only thin blocks of tissue should be fixed. It produces a poor result with glycogen. If the tissue is overfixed, the blocks become hard and sections are difficult to produce. Mercuric chloride also causes a great deal of shrinkage and is therefore rarely used alone. It is usually employed in a compound fixative with formaldehyde or acetic acid. All tissue fixed in mercuric-containing fixatives will have a mercury precipitate, which must be removed by treatment with dilute iodine, followed by immersion in 3 per cent sodium thiosulphate.

FIXATIVES FOR USE IN HISTOCHEMISTRY

Acetone

Absolute acetone at 4°C

Alcohol

Alcohol 80–100 per cent, at 4°C

10 per cent Formol saline

Formaldehyde 40 per cent	100 ml
Sodium chloride	9 g
Distilled water	900 ml

10 per cent Formalin

Formaldehyde 40 per cent	10 ml
Distilled water	90 ml

10 per cent Neutral buffered formalin

Formaldehyde 40 per cent	10 ml
Distilled water	90 ml
Sodium dihydrogen phosphate (anhydrous)	350 mg
Disodium hydrogen phosphate (anhydrous)	650 mg

10 per cent Neutral formalin

Formaldehyde 40 per cent	10 ml
Distilled water	90 ml
Calcium carbonate chips to cover bottom of container	

10 per cent Formol calcium

Formaldehyde 40 per cent	10 ml
Distilled water	90 ml
Calcium chloride	1,100 mg (or until pH reaches 7·0)

Formol sucrose

Formaldehyde 40 per cent	10 ml
Sucrose	7·5 g
0·2M Phosphate buffer, pH 7·4	90 ml

Carnoy fixative

Ethyl alcohol	60 ml
Chloroform	30 ml
Glacial acetic acid	10 ml

Clarke's fixative

Absolute alcohol	75 ml
Glacial acetic acid	25 ml

Formol alcohol

Formaldehyde 40 per cent	10 ml
Absolute alcohol	80 ml
Distilled water	10 ml

Acetic alcohol formaldehyde (AAF)

Formaldehyde 40 per cent	10 ml
Glacial acetic acid	5 ml
Absolute alcohol	85 ml

Gendre's fixative

Picric acid (saturated in 95 per cent alcohol)	85 ml
Formaldehyde 40 per cent	10 ml
Glacial acetic acid	5 ml

Bouin's fixative

Picric acid (saturated aqueous)	75 ml
Formaldehyde 40 per cent	25 ml
Glacial acetic acid	5 ml

Formol sublimate

Mercuric chloride (saturated aqueous)	90 ml
Formaldehyde 40 per cent	10 ml

Flemming's fixative

1 per cent Chromic acid	60 ml
2 per cent Osmium tetroxide	16 ml
Glacial acetic acid	4 ml

Newcomer's fixative

Isopropanol	50 ml
Propionic acid	25 ml
Petroleum ether	8·3 ml
Acetone	8·3 ml
Dioxane	8·3 ml

Heidenhain's 'Susa.'

Distilled water	76 ml
Mercuric chloride	4·5 g
Sodium chloride	500 mg
Trichloracetic acid	2 g
Acetic acid	4 ml
Formaldehyde 40 per cent	20 ml

Zenker's fixative

Distilled water	95 ml
Mercuric chloride	5 g
Potassium dichromate	2.5 g
Sodium sulphate	1 g
Glacial acetic acid, added before use	5 ml

Helly's fixative

Distilled water	95 ml
Mercuric chloride	5 g
Potassium dichromate	2·5 g
Sodium sulphate	1 g
Formaldehyde 40 per cent is added before use	5 ml

6 per cent glutaraldehyde

Glutaraldehyde (25 per cent)	24 ml
0·1M Phosphate buffer, pH 7·4	76 ml

On storage, the glutaraldehyde will become acid, pH 2·5 to 3·0. The final pH of the above fixative should be checked and adjusted to 7·0 to 7·2 if necessary.

1 per cent acrolein

Acrolein	1 ml
0·1M Phosphate buffer, pH 7·4	99 ml

The final pH of this fixative should be checked and adjusted to 7·2 to 7·6 if necessary.

REFERENCES

Flitney, F. W. (1966). *Jl. R. microsc. Soc.* **85,** 353

Lillie, R. D. (1965). *Histopathological Technique and Practical Histochemistry,* New York: McGraw-Hill

Sabatini, D. D., Bensch, K. and Barrnett, R. J. (1963). *J. cell Biol.* **17,** 19

Tock, E. P. C. and Pearse, A. G. E. (1965). *Jl. R. microsc. Soc.* **84,** 519

3

Paraffin Sections

Routine paraffin sections have been produced in hospital and other laboratories for many years. In order to produce these sections in such a manner that they can be of use a number of criteria must be satisfied. The tissue in section must resemble as closely as possible its appearance in life. The most important factor is to 'fix' or preserve the tissue. This fixation also hardens the tissue, but not enough to allow thin sections to be produced from the block. To facilitate the production of these sections, the fixed tissue has to be embedded in a medium to render it firm and rigid. This is traditionally carried out by placing the tissue in paraffin wax or, for specialized procedures, in suitable resins. Few of the embedding media available are miscible with the water invariably present in the tissue and fixative. This gap is bridged by the process known as dehydration and clearing, the removal of water from the tissue blocks being attained by treatment with increasing concentrations of alcohol until no water remains. As the embedding media are not alcohol-miscible an organic solvent must be used to remove the absolute alcohol; this is the process known as 'clearing'. A number of organic solvents may be used of which chloroform, toluene and xylene are examples.

Following the removal of the alcohol, the tissues are impregnated in molten paraffin wax at 58°C. When the wax cools down to room temperature it sets as a hard block in which the tissue is contained. The support offered by the wax enables thin sections of the tissue to be cut on a microtome. These sections are ideal for treatment with the many dyes and stains available to demonstrate the histological features of the tissue.

The use of these paraffin sections in histochemistry is somewhat restricted. They can be used for the demonstration of non-enzymatic components and under carefully controlled conditions certain hydrolytic enzymes may be demonstrated but in a considerably reduced amount. The effects of routine paraffin processing on a piece of tissue are predictable. They are listed in Table 3.1.

TABLE 3.1

Effects of routine processing methods on tissue for histochemical demonstration

Fixation at room temperature Most fixatives	Loss of enzyme activity Denatured proteins (depending upon fixative and length of fixation) General diffusion of enzymes Loss of some carbohydrates Diffusion of other carbohydrates
Dehydration in alcohol (room temperature)	Loss of enzyme activity General diffusion of enzymes Loss of some lipids Shrinking, hardening
Clearing in either xylene, chloroform, toluene, etc.	Loss of enzyme activity Loss of lipids Shrinkage, hardening (depending upon clearing agent)
Wax embedding Paraffin wax, 56–60°C	Loss of enzyme activity Loss of lipids Shrinkage and hardening

It will be observed that very little enzyme activity will remain; it is possible, however, for very small amounts of hydrolytic enzymes such as alkaline phosphates to be demonstrated. The accuracy of localization is open to doubt. The alteration of standard processing methods will allow the demonstration of more enzyme activity.

While these methods seem to cause much morphological damage (e.g. shrinkage) they are well worth trying if no other means of processing the tissue are available.

The reagents that can be used to dehydrate and clear tissue for normal histological purposes are numerous. The fluids used when processing tissue for histochemistry should be as inert as possible. This causes the smallest loss of enzyme activity. If these solutions, e.g. acetone and petroleum spirit, are used at low temperatures (4°C), the retention of the enzymes is further increased. Therefore fixation, dehydration and most of the clearing stages are carried out at 4°C. For the full method see Method 1, page 19. As well as loss of enzymes with clearing agents, heat also causes a big loss in enzyme activity, especially above 40°C. It is advisable to use a paraffin wax with a melting point as low as can be conveniently handled, usually between 45°C and 54°C. The author (1966) made a comparative study of four different processing methods, and a summary of the results is given in Table 3.2.

TABLE 3.2

Results of four processing methods on five histochemical techniques

Method	*Acid phosphatase*	*Alkaline phosphatase*	*Indoxyl esterase*	*Succinate dehydrogenase*	*DPN diaphorase*
Routine paraffin	Nil	Very slight	Very slight	Nil	Nil
Specially processed paraffin (*See* method)	Slight	Moderate	Strong	Nil	Diffused moderate
Freeze dried	Slight	Strong	Moderate	Nil	Diffused moderate
Cryostat	Very strong	Very strong	Very strong	Very strong	Strong

It can be seen from the results that while no enzyme activity remained in the routine processed material, the amount in the specially processed block and the freeze dried tissue were very similar, demonstrating that the loss of enzyme activity was probably due to the paraffin wax and the heat, rather than the dehydrating solutions used.

Paraffin sections may be used for the demonstration of the following groups of substances: proteins; carbohydrates; nucleoproteins; coloured pigments, and phospholipids.

Proteins

It is possible to demonstrate most structural proteins in routine processed paraffin material, although freeze drying is the ideal method of processing. Fixation in formalin or acetic ethanol is recommended and dehydration and clearing times should be kept to a minimum.

Nucleoproteins

These may be demonstrated very successfully in routine paraffin material, Carnoy's fixative possibly being the best for this purpose.

Carbohydrates

This is a complex group of substances for which there are many different staining methods. Most of these methods will work quite satisfactorily on routine paraffin processed material, although superior results can be obtained using the freeze drying technique.

Pigments

The majority of methods used to demonstrate pigments can be carried out with routine processed paraffin material.

Lipids

These cannot be demonstrated in paraffin sections apart from phospholipids, but even with phospholipids it is preferable to use frozen sections.

Naturally occurring fluorescence

Natural fluorescence is demonstrated most efficiently in freeze dried formol vapour fixed material.

METHOD 1

Paraffin processing at 4°C

(1) Select tissue block and trim to 1·0 × 1·0 × 0·5 cm or smaller
(2) Place in precooled acetone at 4°C overnight
(3) Transfer to petroleum ether at 4°C for 1 h
(4) Transfer to petroleum ether at 4°C for 1½h
(5) Transfer to petroleum ether at 20°C for 1 h
(6) Place in 40°C paraffin wax at 42°C for 15 min
(7) Place in 40°C paraffin wax at 42°C for 15 min
(8) Embed in 40°–45°C wax

This method allows the demonstration of some of the hydrolytic enzymes, but does cause shrinkage of the block.

METHOD 2

Paraffin processing double embedding at 4°C (Gomori, 1952)

(1) Select and trim block to 1 × 0·5 cm or smaller
(2) Place blocks into precooled acetone at 4°C for 18 h
(3) Transfer to fresh acetone at 4°C for 6 h
(4) Dehydrate in acetone at 4°C for 12 h
(5) Dehydrate in acetone at 4°C for 12 h
(6) Transfer blocks to 2 per cent celloidin* at 4°C for 12 h
(7) Transfer blocks to 2 per cent celloidin at 4°C for 12 h
(8) Blot blocks to remove excess celloidin
(9) Place blocks into chloroform (1) at 20°C for 1 h
(10) Place blocks into chloroform (2) at 20°C for 2 h
(11) Embed in paraffin wax.

The method, although lengthy, does allow the demonstration of some hydrolytic enzymes. It causes less shrinkage artefact than Method 1.

REFERENCES

Bancroft, J. D. (1966). *J. med. Lab. Tech.* **23,** 105
Gomori, G. (1952). *Microscopical Histochemistry.* Chicago University Press

* In alcohol/ether 1:1.

4

Frozen Sections

The standard histological processing procedure, although capable of producing excellent sections suitable for many purposes, does have a number of drawbacks and the majority of these affect the histochemist. As far as the histochemist is concerned, routine paraffin processing alters the chemical reactions within the tissue. It will probably cause complete loss of demonstrable enzymes, the loss of other soluble substances (e.g. lipids), or the alteration and diffusion of other substances. For these reasons, and those listed below, it is necessary to be able to produce sections that have not been through this technique.

If the tissue is frozen it becomes of a consistency that will allow sections to be cut from it. The water in the tissue, on turning to ice, gives the tissue sufficient support to allow this sectioning to take place. In histochemistry there are applications where fixed tissue sections are preferred to unfixed frozen sections, for example in the demonstration of lipids and some hydrolytic enzymes; the reasons for this are discussed in the relevant chapters. The fixed tissue, with the additional water from the fixative, can also be cut frozen, and is considerably easier to handle on a freezing microtome than on a cryostat.

Frozen sections may be cut from fresh unfixed tissue and from fixed tissue (usually formalin fixed). They may be prepared using one of the following techniques.

(1) Conventional freezing microtome
(2) Standard microtomes with thermomodules attachments
(3) Cryostat.

The last technique is fully dealt with in Chapter 5. This chapter is concerned with the first two techniques.

USES OF FROZEN SECTIONS

Fresh unfixed frozen sections

These sections, which can prove very difficult to handle once they are cut, are little used today if a cryostat is available. Their main uses were and are as follows.

(1) Urgent biopsy specimens from the operating theatre
(2) Fat stains (not recommended)
(3) Histochemical methods, requiring unfixed sections, e.g. usually oxidative enzymes (dehydrogenases), glucose-6-phosphatase and others)
(4) Sections for quantitative work
(5) Immunofluorescence techniques
(6) Autoradiography.

Fixed frozen sections

These sections, which are used in many laboratories, are considerably easier to handle throughout the histochemical method than the unfixed material. Their main uses are as follows.

(1) Urgent biopsy specimens from theatre
(2) Fat stains
(3) Histochemical methods requiring fixed free-floating frozen sections, e.g. accurate localization of some hydrolytic enzymes.
(4) Fluorescent techniques
(5) Demonstration of soluble substances
(6) Autoradiography
(7) Impregnation techniques (silver methods).

The method of cutting urgent biopsy specimens is given in Method 4 at the end of this chapter.

USE OF FREEZING MICROTOME

Cutting of unfixed frozen sections

This technique involves freezing a piece of fresh tissue, 2 cm × 2 cm × 0·75 cm or smaller, onto the stage of a freezing microtome. This is accomplished by placing a drop of water on the stage and holding the tissue firmly against it with the index finger, while giving repeated blasts of carbon dioxide. The water turns to ice, thus holding the tissue firmly onto the stage. Further blasts of carbon dioxide are given until the block is completely frozen. This can be observed by the colour change of the tissue from its natural

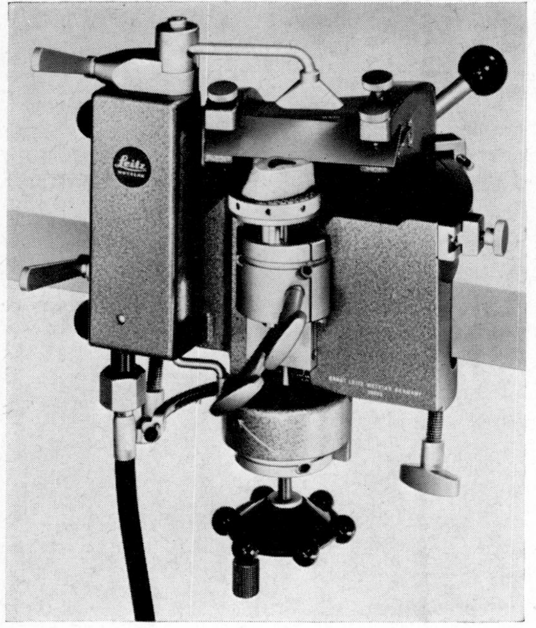

Figure 4.1 The Leitz freezing microtome, for cutting fixed or unfixed blocks. Reproduced by courtesy of Leitz Instruments Ltd.

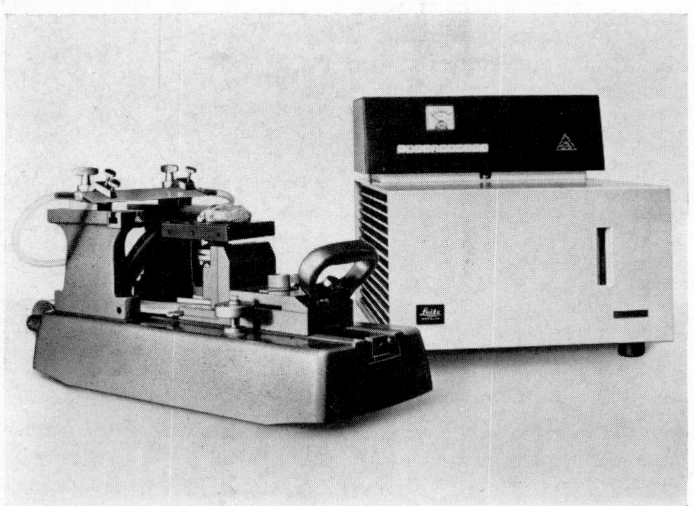

Figure 4.2 The Leitz cryomat, here being used with a base-sledge microtome. Reproduced by courtesy of Leitz Instruments Ltd.

colour to a glossy white. Once the tissue is frozen it is necessary to cool the knife. In freezing microtomes not equipped for knife-cooling with carbon dioxide gas, the knife is cooled with pieces of solid carbon dioxide. When knife and block have both been cooled, the block must be brought up to the correct cutting temperature. This is done by overcooling the tissue and then warming the surface of the block by placing a finger on it. The knife is then passed over the block. If the tissue is too cold, the sections will crumble and fragment. The block should then be warmed again, and the procedure repeated until satisfactory sections are cut. The sections should curl and remain on the knife. They are removed by stroking the finger towards the knife edge from the back of the knife, or by using a brush. The sections are placed in saline and are then ready to be mounted on slides or coverslips. Alternatively, they can be stained free-floating, as described later.

Cutting of fixed frozen sections

Fixed tissue is easier to cut on a freezing microtome than unfixed tissue but in a cryostat the situation is reversed. Formaldehyde is a good fixative for fixed frozen sections: alcohol-containing solutions should be avoided because of their low freezing point, and dichromate-containing fixatives make the tissue brittle and more difficult to cut. It is not necessary for the knife to be cooled for cutting fixed tissues, for when the sections are cut they will not form a 'slush' against the knife. The fixed tissue blocks need a warmer cutting temperature because of the increased water content of the tissue; the sections are easier to handle after cutting than are unfixed sections. Otherwise the technique is as for unfixed blocks.

Limiting factors concerning freezing microtome technique

A few of the many limiting factors of this technique are listed below.

(1) As a rule sections 10 microns or thicker only can be cut
(2) Only small thin blocks can be used
(3) Certain tissues are difficult, if not impossible, to cut
(4) Freezing artefact is likely to be present in some tissues
(5) Tissues must be fresh (if unfixed sections are required)
(6) Correct cutting temperature is difficult to maintain
(7) Lack of supporting medium causes shattering of fine structures.

Embedding tissues in gelatin

If tissues are friable, or if many small fragments are assembled to make one block, it is advisable to embed the tissue in gelatin before cutting frozen sections. One of the disadvantages of this technique is that the gelatin is frequently also stained. The technique for gelatin embedding of tissue is given at the end of this chapter in Method 3.

Fixation of blocks

The fixation of blocks of tissue for the frozen section technique depends upon the histochemical method to be carried out on the section. However, as routine fixatives, formol saline or formol calcium are recommended. It is advisable to avoid fixatives with an alcohol constituent because of the inhibitory effect of the alcohol on freezing. Fixatives causing excessive hardening of the tissue are also to be avoided.

Picking up frozen sections on slides

Many of the techniques using frozen sections call for the staining of the sections free-floating. The mounting of the section comes at the end of the process. Where possible, it is advisable to pick up the sections on slides before staining, the exception being in the demonstration of lipids by the Sudan methods.

Mounting frozen sections on slides

To pick up fixed frozen sections, coat a microscope slide with glycerin albumen and float the section onto distilled water. If the section is flat and crease-free, place the slide underneath the section and bring it upwards until it touches one edge of the section. At this point, bring the slide to the vertical position and slowly raise it out of the water. If the section is creased, allow the excess water to drain away, then replace the slide in the water until half the section is free-floating; the creases are then removed and the slide withdrawn from the water. Should the other half of the section contain creases, the slide is reversed and the exercise repeated. The sections are then drained, before being blotted and allowed to dry.

If the section is badly creased and folded when it is initially placed on the water, it can be floated onto 70 per cent alcohol for 30 seconds and then returned to the distilled water. The different surface tensions in the two solutions cause the section to spin, coming eventually to rest in a crease-free state on the top of the water.

The sections may be dried at room temperature or at 37°C.

As an alternative to using glycerin albumen to retain frozen sections on the slide, the following technique is suggested.

The section is picked up on a clean slide and blotted firmly with filter paper soaked in absolute alcohol; it is then washed in absolute alcohol. Repeat the blotting, then coat the slide in 0·5 per cent celloidin and allow to partially dry. The slide is now ready to be washed in water and to be stained. At the end of the staining technique, during the dehydration, the slide is placed in absolute alcohol/ether mixture 1:1 to remove the celloidin before being placed in xylol. This technique is unsuitable for any method demonstrating soluble substances (e.g. lipids), or impregnation methods (e.g. silver).

Staining free-floating sections

This is the method of choice when carrying out staining procedures such as oil red O, or the silver impregnation techniques. The sections, preferably fixed frozen sections, are placed into distilled water after cutting. The equipment needed for this method consists of embryo staining dishes (the same number as there are steps in the staining technique), a glass rod shaped like a hockey stick and a dissecting needle. The sections are placed in the first staining dish by manipulating the section out of the distilled water by means of the 'hockey stick'. It is possible to wrap the sections around the hockey stick without causing them any damage. A section is passed along the staining dishes in this manner until it reaches the distilled water at the end of the procedure. From the distilled water it is picked up on an albumenized slide, as described earlier, with the aid of the hockey stick or a dissecting needle.

USE OF THERMOMODULE ATTACHMENT

In recent years the technique of using thermomodules to maintain the block temperature, and in some cases the knife temperature, has been gaining popularity. The first report of this technique was by Ioffe (1956) and further papers were published by Brown and Dilly (1962) and Hardy and Rutherford (1962). All these authors stated that frozen sections could be cut with ease. Brown and Dilly listed the following five advantages that this system had over the conventional carbon dioxide technique.

(1) Convenience. The need for carbon dioxide gas is eliminated
(2) Accurate temperature control
(3) Optimal cutting temperature can be maintained indefinitely
(4) Serial sections can be cut at 5 microns
(5) Adaptability of unit for other cooling uses.

The first two papers mentioned above describe the use of the modules as a means of maintaining the block temperature. Hardy and Rutherford (1962) in a further paper, described the cooling of the knife, as well as the block, to allow for cutting of all types of

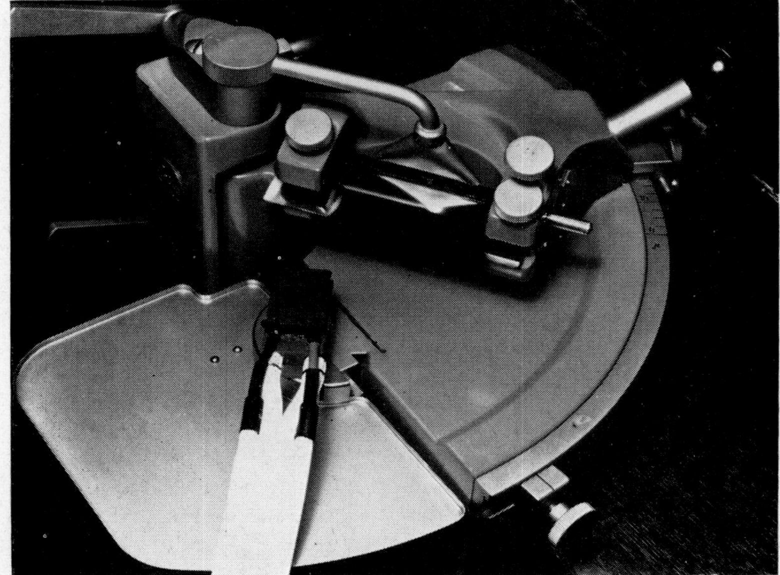

Figure 4.3 A conventional freezing microtome converted to employ thermomodules.

material. In a later paper (Rutherford, Hardy and Isherwood, 1964), the authors described the use of different microtomes with the thermoelectric equipment. For a description of how a thermomodule works readers are referred to page 58.

Using thermomodules for frozen sections

Thermoelectric modules have adaptors which allow them to be fixed onto all standard microtome stages. The modules and their electrical equipment are produced commercially.

As the thermomodules require water for the hot stage, it is necessary to place them on a bench near to a supply of running cold water. When operated under optimal conditions, the module is capable of reaching just below −30°C, and this temperature is controllable to ±1°C. To cut unfixed material, it is necessary to use the thermomodules on the knife, which can then be cooled to −20°C or below, if required.

Cutting a fixed block of tissue

A piece of fixed tissue is placed onto the microtome stage together with a drop of water. The current is turned to maximum and the block will be seen to freeze. When the block is completely frozen, the electrical supply is reduced until a satisfactory consistency of the block is obtained. It is possible to maintain the block at this temperature indefinitely.

The cutting temperature varies with the nature of the tissue, as with all frozen section techniques (the figures in Table 5.2 may be taken as a guide here). The sections are floated-out onto water or formol saline.

Cutting an unfixed block of tissue

The thermomodules are attached to the knife to cool it a few degrees below the temperature of the block. Once the knife and

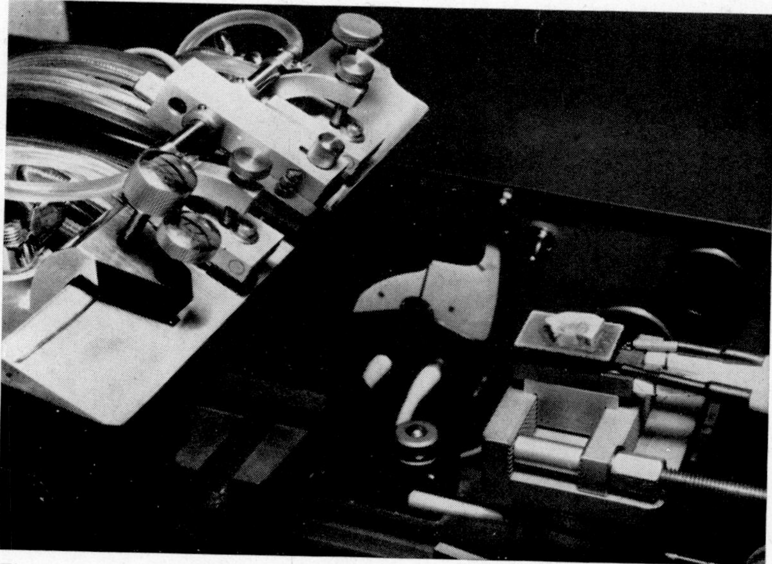

Figure 4.4 A sledge microtome with thermomodules on both knife and stage for cutting unfixed frozen sections. Reproduced by courtesy of De La Rue Frigistor Ltd.

block are at the correct temperature, it is far easier to obtain satisfactory sections of unfixed material with this method than by any other technique, apart from the cryostat. If enzyme histochemical methods are to be applied to sections produced by this technique, it is necessary to freeze the tissue by one of the procedures listed in Chapter 5 since thermomodule freezing is often not rapid enough. Otherwise the tissue is frozen by placing it on the thermomodule in the manner described above. Using this technique it is possible to obtain serial sections with a thickness of less than 10 microns.

METHOD 3

Gelatin embedding for friable tissues

(1) Fix block in 10 per cent formol saline overnight
(2) Wash out formalin by washing in running tap water for 6–8 h
(3) Place block into glycerin–gelatin mixture at 37°C for 6 h
(4) Transfer block to fresh mixture and embed in suitable mould and allow to cool
(5) Place the block of gelatin in 10 per cent formol saline overnight
(6) Trim away the excess gelatin and reimmerse in 10 per cent formol saline for 8 h or until required.

Gelatin	16 g
Glycerin	15 ml
Distilled water	70 ml
Thymol	1 crystal

METHOD 4

Cutting of frozen sections of urgent biopsy specimens

(1) On notification of an urgent biopsy, place 100 ml of 10 per cent formol saline to heat on a Bunsen burner
(2) On arrival of biopsy remove the formol saline from the boil
(3) Select block to be cut
(4) Place in hot 10 per cent formol saline for 60–90 s
(5) Wash rapidly in running tap water for 10 s
(6) Place drop of water on microtome stage
(7) Transfer tissue to the microtome stage
(8) Freeze the tissue with rapid bursts of CO_2
(9) Warm the block with finger to correct cutting temperature
(10) Cut 6–12 sections at 10–15 microns
(11) Place sections in distilled water
(12) Pick up on glass slides as indicated
(13) Blot dry with filter paper
(14) Pass rapidly over Bunsen flame
(15) Rinse in water
(16) Stain in Harris' haematoxylin for 60 s
(17) Wash off stain
(18) Differentiate in 1 per cent acid alcohol for 10 s
(19) Place in Scott's tap water (*see* page 322) for 20 s
(20) Wash in tap water for 5 s
(21) Place in 1 per cent eosin for 5 s
(22) Wash in tap water for 10 s
(23) Dehydrate through graded alcohols to:

(24) Xylene
(25) Mount in DPX.

Remarks

It is advisable to stain more than one section in case the first section floats off the slide. If difficulty is experienced in keeping the sections on the slide it would be advisable to use the technique described on page 24.

REFERENCES

BROWN, R. and Dilly, N. (1962). *J. Physiol.* **161,** No. 1 (Proceedings)
HARDY, W. S. and RUTHERFORD, T. (1962). *Nature, Lond.* **196,** 785
IOFFE, A. F. (1956). *Semiconductor Thermoelements and Thermoelectric Cooling.* London: Infroresearch Ltd.
RUTHERFORD, T., HARDY, W. S. and ISHERWOOD, P. A. (1964). *Stain Tech.* **39,** 185

5

Cryostats

The advent of the cryostat has contributed much to the rapid development of histochemistry since the early nineteen-fifties. Before the manufacture of the cryostat it was difficult, if not impossible, to consistently obtain thin sections of unfixed material with reasonable preservation and quality.

DEVELOPMENT OF CRYOSTATS

The first cryostat described in the literature was produced by Linderstrøm-Lang and Morgensen (1938) who developed their cryostat for quantitative cytochemical work. Alternate sections of equal thickness were taken for biochemical estimations and for histology. The cabinet for the cryostat was kept at approximately −20°C; this was done by means of large blocks of dry ice placed at the back of the cabinet. A fan was used to circulate the cold air from above the dry ice around the chamber. The fan was not in operation, however, while sections were being cut. A rotary microtome was used in the well insulated chamber. Another feature of this cryostat was a device which, when pressed against the knife edge, allowed flat, crease-free sections to be cut. This device was called an anti-roll plate, or guide-plate. The guide-plate assembly, though much modified from the original form, is still of great importance in the operation of the cryostat. The anti-roll plate is dealt with in detail later. Access to this early microtome was through a hinged sloping door on the front of the cabinet. In this door were two large gloved portholes through which the microtome was operated, a small stoppered port for the removal of sections, and also a window for observation. To combat one of the problems of rotary microtomes in cryostats, the microtome had a small electric heater to keep it a few degrees above freezing point. From this cryostat it was only a short step to the model produced by Coons, Leduc and Kaplan (1951).

Coons–Leduc–Kaplan cryostat

The cryostat designed by these workers was based on the earlier model, except that the cold environment was produced by refrigeration coils running round the cabinet. The latter, which was of 6 ft^3 capacity, was made of stainless steel. The operating temperature obtained with this model was between −16°C and −18°C. The cryostat was later produced commercially by the Harris Refrigeration Co. of Cambridge, Massachusetts. Later models produced by this company have operating temperatures down to −40°C. An alternative Coons-type of cryostat is produced in Germany by the Dittes Co. of Heidelberg, West Germany.

Dittes rotary cryostat

In this model a large Jung rotary microtome is used. The actuating wheel of the microtome is placed outside the cabinet, so that while the operator has his hands inside the chamber, the machine is operated by an assistant. To avoid rusting of the microtome, the Dittes cabinet is also modified to reduce the humidity. Later models are available with a foot-controlled electric motor to drive the large microtome.

Development of British cryostats

Following the arrival in Britain of the original Coons-type of cryostat and its success, there was a rapid increase in the use of cryostat-sectioned material. Coons and his colleagues had designed their instrument to provide sections for use with the fluorescent antibody technique.

The production of frozen sections for the demonstration of enzymes became a major function of the equipment, as well as the increasing use for urgent biopsy specimens.

In 1954 Pearse started to build the prototype of the Pearse–Slee cryostat. In building his cryostat, Pearse intended that seven criteria be satisfied; they were:

(1) remote control
(2) instant availability for diagnostic biopsies
(3) thermostatic control between −5°C and −20°C
(4) minimum temperature below −20°C
(5) low cost and constant running
(6) automatic delivery of sections into incubating media or fixatives, and
(7) ability to produce serial sections.

The cabinet of this cryostat was cooled by refrigeration coils running along two of the interior walls. It was capable of reaching −30°C and an accurate thermostat allowed control of temperature between −5°C and −30°C.

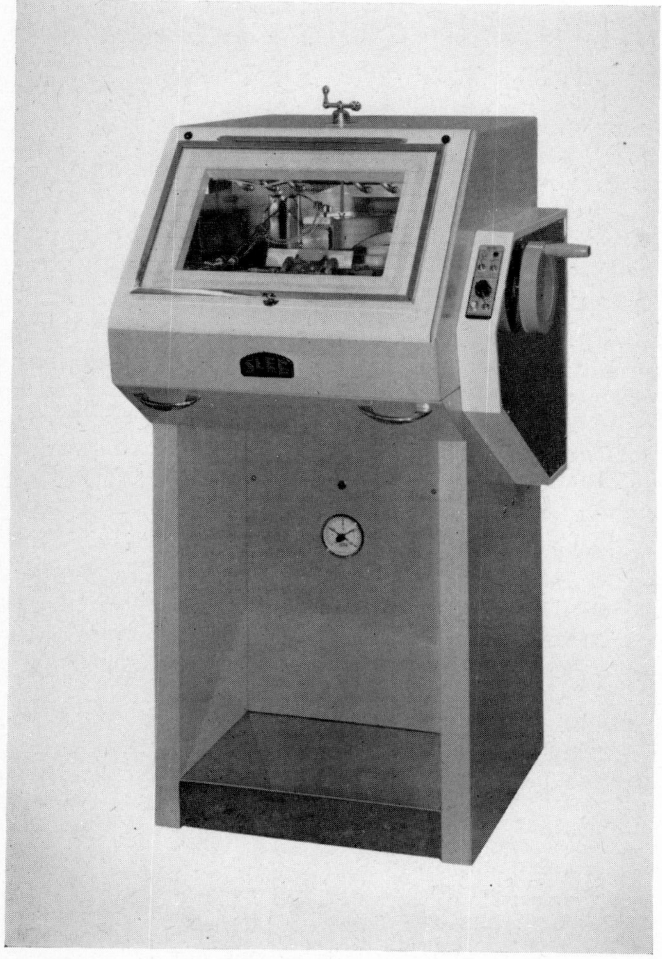

Figure 5.1 The Slee motorized cryostat containing the Slee retracting microtome. Reproduced by courtesy of Slee Medical Equipment Ltd.

The microtome in the original Pearse-Slee, and also in the first Bright cryostat, was a Cambridge rocking microtome; the controls (i.e. coarse advance, thickness setting, operating handle and anti-roll plate) were all external and could be operated through the sides or top of the chamber. The anti-roll plate was attached to the microtome and not, as in the Coons cryostat, to the knife. The front of the cryostat had a porthole for the removal of sections.

Current models

The development of the cryostat over the last twenty years has brought many improvements, as well as a diversity of choice. The

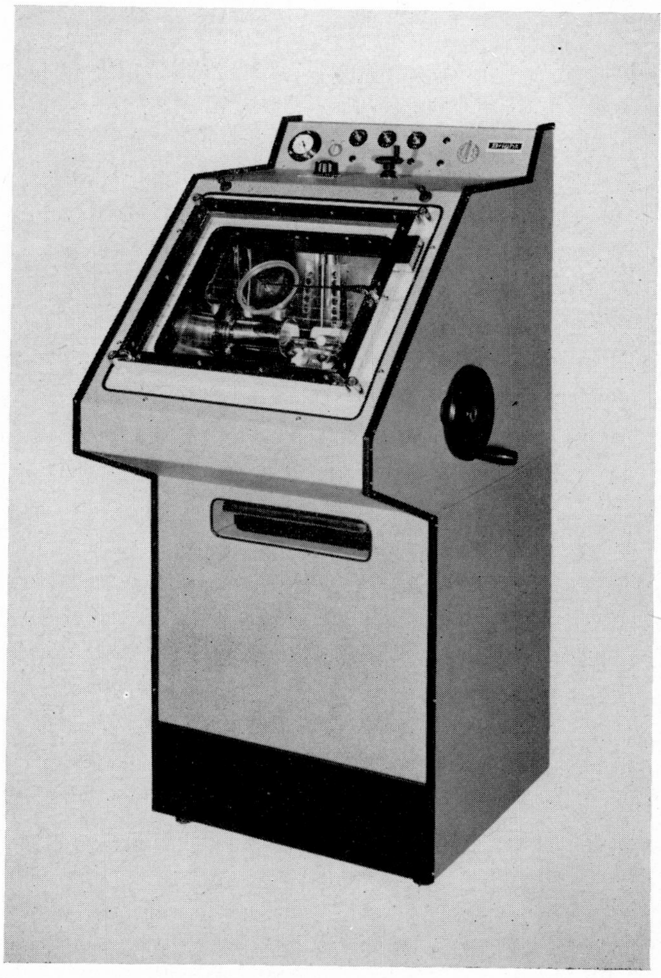

Figure 5.2 The Bright cryostat model FS/FCS. Reproduced by courtesy of Bright Refrigeration Co. Ltd.

largest single improvement has been the gradual change from the rocking microtome to the rotary. This has allowed larger and more difficult blocks to be cut, and thinner sections to be produced. Another welcome advance is the heated and hinged window which has entirely eliminated the early problems associated with the frosting of the window. The anti-roll plate, the proper adjustment of which is a major part of successful cryostat technique, has also become a more sophisticated piece of equipment with accurate micro-adjustment. Motorized cryostats have become popular in recent years; the obvious application for this type of cryostat is in the cutting of serial sections, and in some instances where the correct cutting speed is critical to success in producing the section (*see Figure 5.1*).

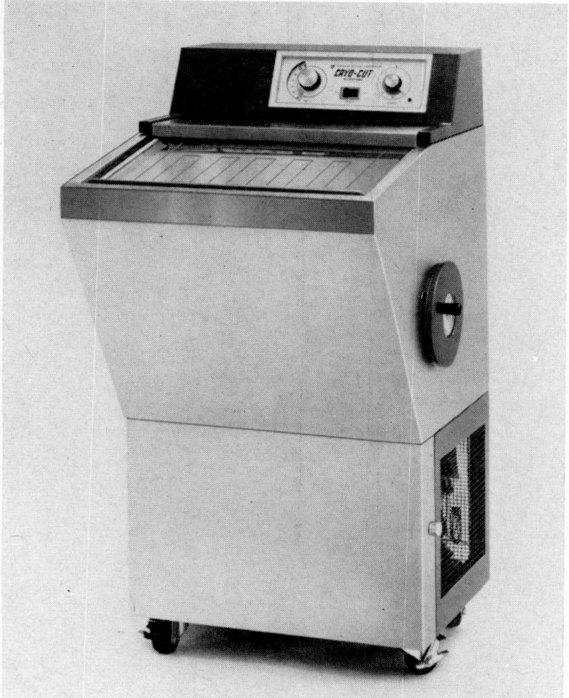

Figure 5.3 An open -top cryostat ('Cryocut') produced by the American Optical Corp. Reproduced by courtesy of American Optical Corp.

There are a number of cryostats produced commercially which are operated from above, i.e. the top is hinged and is removed when the microtome is in use. This type of cryostat (commonly manufactured in America), of which the Harris International, The Lab

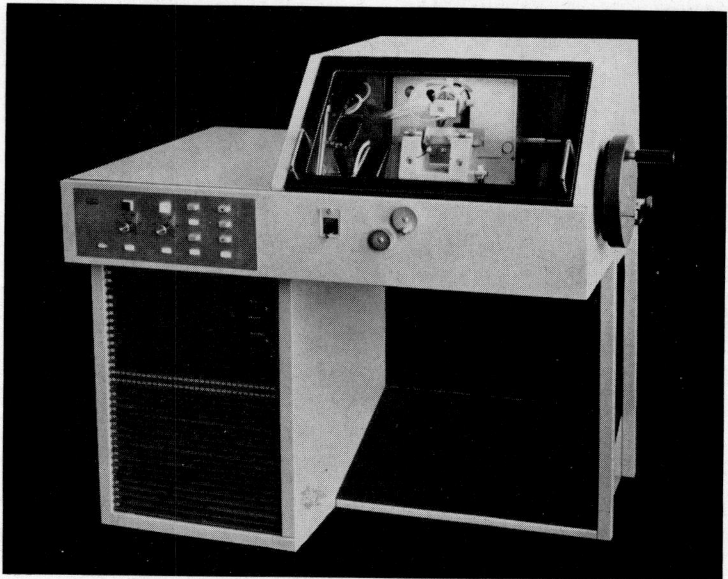

Figure 5.4 The Leitz 'Histokryotom' with automatic section removal and delivery. Reproduced by courtesy of Leitz Instruments Ltd.

Tek and the American Optical Co. cryostats (*see Figure 5.3*) are representatives, is operated under the same conditions as other models. Leitz have developed a very sophisticated cryostat known as the Histokryotom (*see Figure 5.4*). In this model the sections are automatically picked up from the knife edge onto slides contained within the cryostat. Many of the functions of this cryostat can be controlled electronically.

Thermoelectric cryostats

Thornburg and Mengers (1957) in their paper 'Analysis of Frozen Section Techniques', made the observation that if the environmental temperature was between +5°C and −5°C serial sections of 2μ m could be obtained. The advent of the use of thermomodules in frozen section techniques by Ioffe (1956), Brown and Dilly (1962), Rutherford, Hardy and Isherwood (1964), and other workers, led to the possibility of a thermoelectric cryostat being produced. The development of this machine (*see Figure 5.5*) was described by Pearse and Bancroft (1966). The results of these experiments confirmed the findings of Thornburg and Mengers that, if it is possible to vary the temperature of both the knife and block, −20°C or below is too low a figure for the environmental temperature. In the thermoelectric cryostat it is possible to vary the block, knife and chamber temperature accurately for the first time and when these temperature variables were studied, the following facts emerged.

(1) Each tissue has its own optimal block (cutting) temperature

(2) Each tissue has its own optimal knife temperature

(3) The chamber temperature is sufficiently cold if maintained at −5°C.

Tables 5.1 and 5.2, reproduced from the Pearse and Bancroft paper, give the temperature optima for cutting of rat tissue, both unfixed and fixed.

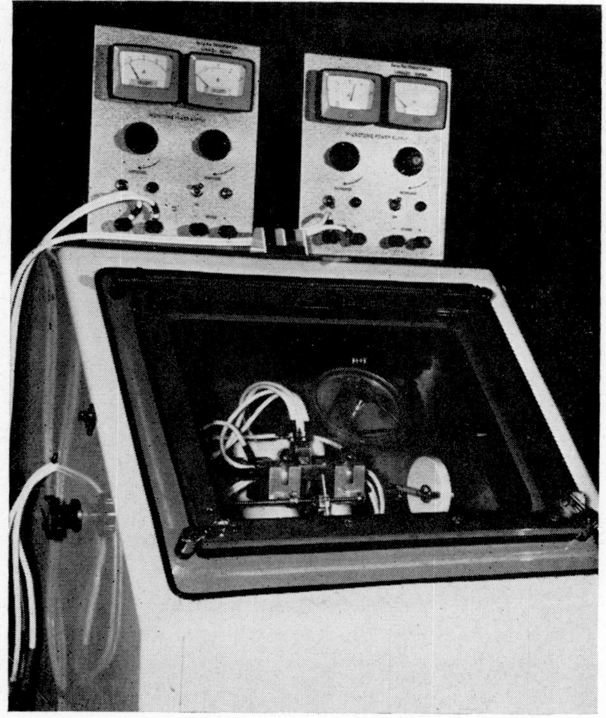

Figure 5.5 The prototype thermoelectric cryostat.

Unfixed and fixed tissues need different handling; the treatments are discussed separately.

CRYOSTAT TECHNIQUE

The production of thin, artefact-free sections in the cryostat is dependent upon a number of factors. These are:

(1) satisfactory preparation of tissue
(2) cryostat temperature (involving both tissue block and knife)
(3) microtome
(4) adjustment of anti-roll plate.

All these factors must be correct before successful sections can be consistently produced.

TABLE 5.1

Temperature optima for the frigistorized cryostat (unfixed rat tissue)

Tissue	*Knife temperature* (°C)	*Block temperature* (°C)	*Environmental temperature* (°C)
Liver	−18	−10	−5
Kidney	−15	−8	−5
Skin	−35	−10	−5
Keloid	−35	−12	−5
Patella	−40	−18	−5
Brain	−18	−15	−5
Thyroid	−20	−10	−5

TABLE 5.2

Temperature optima for the frigistorized cryostat (fixed rat tissue)

Tissue	*Knife temperature* (°C)	*Block temperature* (°C)	*Environmental temperature* (°C)
Liver	−15	−8	−5
Kidney	−10	−8	−5
Skin	−35	−5	−5
Keloid	−35	−5	−5
Patella	−40	−20	−5
Brain	−15	−8	−5
Thyroid	−25	−12	−5

PREPARATION OF MATERIAL

Tissues to be cut in a cryostat can be either fresh frozen, i.e. unfixed, or fixed (usually with formol calcium) followed by suitable freezing.

Preparation of fresh tissue (unfixed)

To produce cryostat sections of good quality two criteria must be satisfied. The tissue must be fresh; sections produced from autopsy material are inferior to those cut from fresh surgical material. Equally important is the initial freezing of the tissue; the rate of freezing is critical. The faster the quenching, the better the tissue will be preserved. Slow freezing of tissue will produce ice crystal artefact in some tissues. The water in the tissue acts as the embedding medium, giving the tissue hardness when frozen. For this reason tissue frozen by one of the techniques using very low temperatures should be allowed to warm up to a suitable cutting temperature before trimming.

Tissue may be frozen in the following ways.

(a) Solid carbon dioxide ('cardice')
(b) Cardice mixtures, e.g. cardice/acetone
(c) Carbon dioxide gas (from a pressure cylinder)
(d) Liquefied gases
(e) Cold contact
(f) Aerosol sprays.

It is necessary to freeze the tissue as rapidly as possible to avoid ice crystal formation. The rate and level of production of ice usually vary with the water content of the tissue to be frozen.

Solid carbon dioxide (cardice)

This is one of the slowest satisfactory means of freezing. The tissue is placed onto a block holder with a drop of water and two pieces of cardice are held against the sides of the metal block holder. Freezing occurs by conduction and a white line can be observed passing through the tissue until it is all frozen. This method, despite its slowness, is popular in routine histology laboratories when the cryostat is only used for urgent biopsies from the operating theatre. Cardice is supplied in 28-lb blocks*. The lower the temperature of storage, the longer the cardice will last, but with storage at 4°C two blocks will give a constant supply for one week.

Cardice mixtures

This technique is similar to the previous one, except that the cardice is crushed into a fine powder. It is then placed in a Thermos flask and an organic solvent is added until a slush is obtained. This will remain all day in a vacuum flask, allowing many blocks to be frozen. The freezing technique is to lower the metal block holder into the slush until only a $\frac{1}{4}$ in is clear and then place a drop of water and the tissue on the block holder. Care must be taken with this method, especially if histochemical techniques are going to be applied to the sections, so that the block does not become contaminated with the solvent.

Carbon dioxide gas

The freezing of tissue by carbon dioxide gas is carried out by using a piece of equipment like the Slee bench freezer (*Figure 5.8*) which is designed to take the block holders on a small platform under which the gas is fed from a cylinder. The block holders must have holes on each side for the gas to pass through. The freezer has a Perspex

* Available from Distillers Co. Limited.

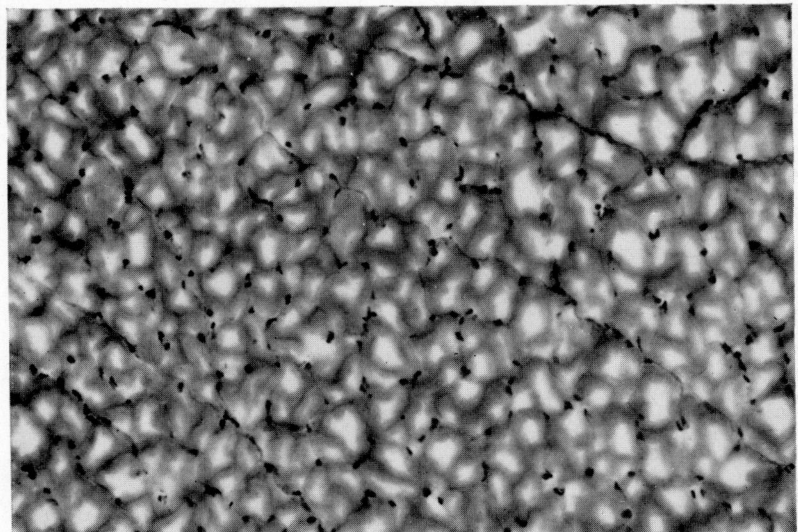

Figure 5.6 Freezing artefact caused by freezing muscle with solid carbon dioxide. Note the non-staining central area of each fibre. Compare with Figure 5.7. (Van Gieson × 220).
(Reduced to two-thirds in reproduction)

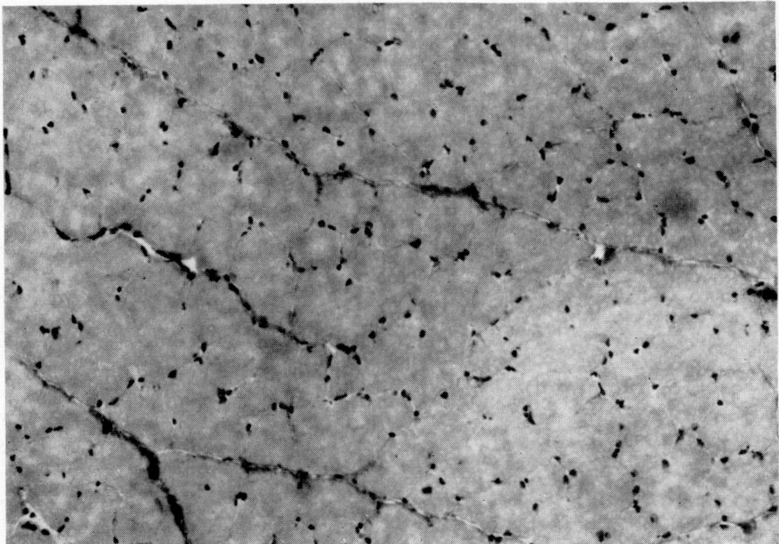

Figure 5.7 Muscle frozen with liquid nitrogen. Note absence of freezing artefact. (Van Gieson × 220).
(Reduced to two-thirds in reproduction)

lid from which the gas is returned to aid the rapid freezing of the block. It is possible to adapt a conventional freezing microtome for the same purpose, although freezing is slower.

Liquefied gases

This method is the most rapid of those available to the majority of laboratories practising histochemistry. The most readily available gases are liquid air or liquid nitrogen, and a Thermos flask filled with either will usually last for a full day. Liquid nitrogen is the safer of the two. If tissue needs to be frozen daily it is probably worthwhile to have a supply of liquid nitrogen delivered to the laboratory. A suitable container (*Figure 5.9*) is available to hold 25 litres; taking into account the loss of nitrogen during storage and filling one Thermos flask a day, this amount would last for almost two weeks. The cost of liquid nitrogen itself is small.

The freezing of tissue in liquid nitrogen is rapid enough for most purposes. The material can be frozen either directly onto the block holder, or by placing the tissue onto a piece of aluminium foil and plunging both into the liquid nitrogen. If the second technique is used, the frozen tissue can be stored in polythene bags in the deep freeze until required. A difficulty of freezing tissue with liquefied gases is the cracking of the block. The larger the piece of tissue, the more likely is cracking to occur, although fibrous types of tissue tend to crack less than softer ones like liver. With large blocks and soft tissue (liver etc.) a little practice is necessary before this cracking can be avoided.

Cold contact

The technique suggested by Cunningham *et al.* (1962), involving the pre-chilling of glass tubes to $-70°C$ and below, is a useful method. The tubes are kept corked at this temperature and when the tissue is ready for freezing the cork is removed and the tissue placed against the inside of the tube. Freezing is rapid and the method is suitable for almost all tissues, muscle being the exception. An advantage of using this technique is that a ready means of storage is available for material which is not required for immediate cutting. Within this group falls the technique utilizing metal cooled by the refrigeration coils of the cryostat. In some instances these do not give low enough temperatures to produce rapid and adequate initial freezing of some tissues.

Aerosol sprays

Recently some commercial firms have marketed aerosol freezing sprays containing gases liquefied under pressure e.g. dichlorodifluoromethane. Tissue from urgent biopsy specimens can be

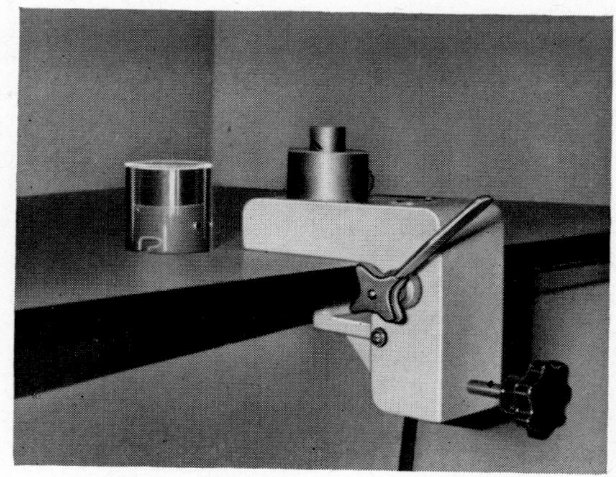

Figure 5.8 Bench freezer manufactured by the Slee company for attachment to carbon dioxide cylinders for easy freezing of tissue blocks.

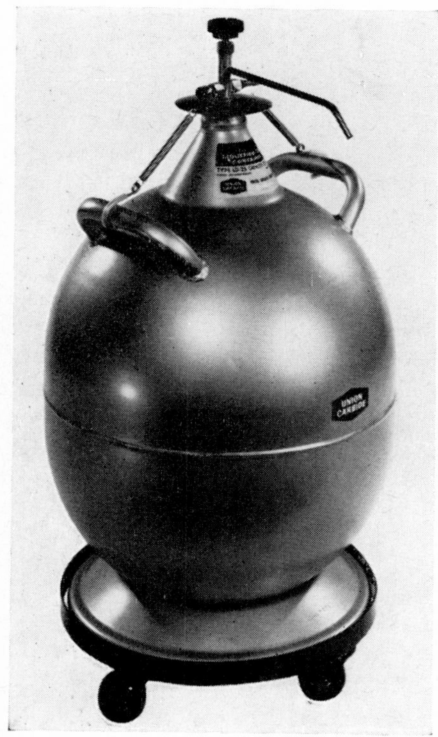

Figure 5.9 A container, suitable for holding 25 litres of liquid nitrogen, which can be replenished weekly. Reproduced by courtesy of Union Carbide Ltd.

satisfactorily frozen on the block holder by this technique, although the freezing is neither rapid nor even enough for most histochemical methods. The big advantage of these sprays is their simplicity and easy availability, with minimal storage problems.

Freezing of muscle

Muscle is the most difficult of routine biopsy tissues to freeze without serious artefact, and to obtain satisfactory results three conditions must be fulfilled. First, the piece of muscle selected must be small (not exceeding 5 mm $\times$ 4 mm). Secondly it must be left for 10–25 minutes in a moist atmosphere to avoid subsequent contraction artefact and, finally, it must be frozen by the most rapid means, usually liquefied gases. *Figures 5.6* and *5.7* show the difference when two different freezing techniques are used. Other tissues are satisfactorily frozen by any of the above techniques and if a choice has to be made between them, the final decision must take into account availability of the freezing reagent.

Preparation of fixed tissue

For the demonstration of hydrolytic enzymes and other substances affected by diffusion, prefixation in 10 per cent formol calcium at 4°C is advised. This will ensure more precise localization of the enzyme than by freezing the tissue unfixed. Tissue to be treated in this way is fixed for 18 hours in cold formol calcium, followed by a similar time in gum sucrose (*see* Method 5). It is important that after fixation and subsequent treatment the tissue is blotted as dry as possible before freezing. The excess water in the tissue will make the block very hard when it is frozen. Contrary to the need for rapid freezing of unfixed tissue, fixed blocks should be frozen relatively slowly to avoid tissue damage when this excess of water is frozen; hence liquid nitrogen is not recommended.

The sectioning of fixed tissue is considerably more difficult than that of unfixed material. This is due to the extra hardness of the tissue block. Block temperatures of below −20°C will cause damage to the microtome knife. The temperature of the cryostat should be raised to between −5°C and −10°C depending upon the tissue; this is usually sufficient for suitable sections to be cut. In cases of difficulty further cooling of the knife with cardice will probably help. Sections cut from tissue treated in this way have a tendency to float off the slide or coverslip; to overcome this, the slides or coverslips should be treated with a 2 per cent gelatin–formaldehyde solution (*see* Method 99).

CRYOSTAT TEMPERATURE

This is of vital importance for the consistent production of thin, artefact-free sections. The majority of the standard cryostats have thermostats to regulate the chamber temperature between −5°C and −30°C. It is also possible to cool the knife and block further with cardice to temperatures approaching −70°C. The use of cardice, however, does not allow for accurate control of the knife or tissue temperature, although arbitrary cooling of the knife with cardice may occasionally enable a satisfactory section to be produced under sub-optimal cryostat conditions. Accurate control of cryostat conditions can only be obtained by using the thermoelectric cryostat equipped so that the block and knife temperature can be varied accurately and independently within a few moments.

The development of the thermoelectric cryostat showed that each tissue has its own optimal cutting temperature; kidney and liver will cut best in a conventional cryostat at −15°C to −18°C, while muscle will cut more easily at −23°C to −25°C. Formalin-fixed material will cut satisfactorily at −8°C to −12°C, depending upon the tissue. All the above figures are the chamber and knife temperatures. It is important that the tissue should not be too cold during cutting. If the tissue is below —30°C it will be brittle and the resistance to cutting such that the block may fracture into many pieces and the knife will be badly damaged. After a block has been frozen it is advisable to leave it in the cryostat for 10 minutes to reach chamber temperature, so when urgent biopsies are being cut it is better to use carbon dioxide for the initial freezing to minimize this waiting period. If the unfixed block is too warm the sections will stick to the top of the knife in a wet mass. If the anti-roll plate is too warm, the sections will stick to that also. Most tissues, however, will cut successfully at −15°C to −22°C.

ANTI-ROLL PLATE

The anti-roll plate (or guide-plate, as it is sometimes called) was originally a piece of glass, usually a microscope slide, with two strips of Sellotape running down the vertical edges of the plate. The two strips of Sellotape cut from a standard roll are approximately 70 microns thick. The plate is sprayed with polytetrafluoroethylene (P.T.F.E.) to reduce the friction between the plate and the section as it is being cut. The anti-roll plate is carried in a holder which is usually attached to the microtome. In the newer models of the Bright cryostat the anti-roll plate is a shaped piece of perspex (*see Figure 5.10*) with spacer screws instead of Sellotape. It is possible and necessary to be able to adjust the angle, height and alignment of the plate to the knife. To produce satisfactory, crease-free, flat sections it is vital that the operator of the cryostat fully understands the use of the anti-roll plate and is capable of adjusting it correctly. All types of anti-roll plate are now micro-adjustable (*see Figure 5.11*). The tendency of sections of all tissues, when they are being cut in the cryostat, is to curl upwards. The anti-roll plate must be in a position

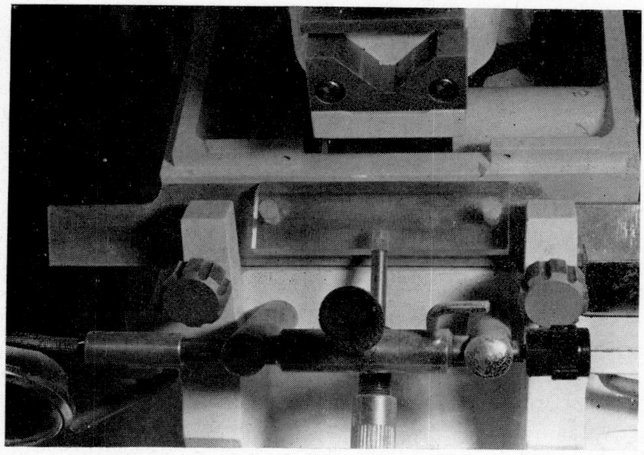

Figure 5.10 The Bright perspex anti-roll plate. The height is adjusted by the bottom nut; the two perspex screws in the anti-roll plate act as 'spacers'.

to guide the section downwards and to leave it resting on the knife face. The two strips of Sellotape rest against the knife when the anti-roll plate is in position, the thickness of the Sellotape (or spacer screws) allowing a sufficient gap for the section to pass down. For

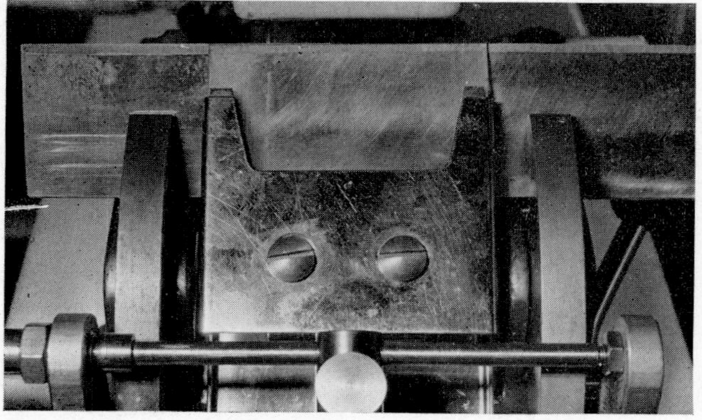

Figure 5.11 The anti-roll plate in the Pearse-Slee cryostat. Accurate height adjustment is by the two screws in the anti-roll plate holder.

the production of good sections, the following five points should be observed with the anti-roll plate.

(1) Anti-roll plate cold (cabinet temperature)
(2) Anti-roll plate firmly held in holder
(3) Sellotape cut flush with top of anti-roll plate (if Sellotape used)
(4) Top edge of anti-roll plate not damaged
(5) Good coating of PTFE on anti-roll plate (if glass plate used).

Setting the anti-roll plate in the correct position can cause a new operator considerable trouble, but with practice it is possible to fit a new anti-roll plate in the correct position within 30 seconds or so. No set position can be claimed for the anti-roll plate as the angle and height will vary according to the angle at which the knife is set in the microtome and the method of sharpening the knife. General conditions for setting the anti-roll plate are that the top of the plate appears fractionally above the knife and the angle of the anti-roll plate to the knife is 20°. This angle applies to a new knife. After adjusting the anti-roll plate, it is important to allow the plate to cool down to the cabinet temperature before attempting to cut sections.

MICROTOMES

The early British cryostats employed the Cambridge rocking microtome. This microtome was ideal from a mechanical point of view at sub-zero temperatures, as no use is made of sliding parts. It also needed only minor alteration to fit the anti-roll plate. The disadvantages of this microtome, however, are the limitation of the size of block that can be cut, and the problems of cutting hard pieces of tissue. This led to the choice of rotary microtomes for these cryostats. In the U.K. these are rotary rocking microtomes, either the Cambridge or the Slee, both of which incorporate many of the mechanical advantages of the Cambridge rocker, but at the same time are capable of cutting larger and tougher blocks more easily. The Slee rotary microtome has a retracting stroke which makes it ideal for serial sectioning of frozen tissue. Of the cryostats produced in America the majority are top-opening, compared with the British front-opening models. The American cryostats usually employ a more sophisticated type of rotary microtome, which from a mechanical point of view is less suited to operating at low temperatures but is more rigid and provides better support for difficult tissues. The two major British manufacturers both produce cryostats that house the Leitz base sledge; these models are used for neurohistology, neurohistochemistry, bone sections and whole body (rat) autoradiography. Due to the weight of the microtome, they need to be motor-driven. This allows for an infinitely variable cutting speed which enables many types of tissue to be cut. The application of motor-drive to the cryostat is also applicable to the rotary microtomes and this type of cryostat is a decided advantage when cutting serial sections from a block; this refinement is probably not necessary in a routine surgical laboratory.

Microtome knives

Any knife designed for the microtome in the cryostat will cut satisfactory sections when new. The difficulties occur when the knife needs resharpening.

The fact that the anti-roll plate has to be adjusted against the knife edge raises problems in regard to sharpening the knife. If the knife is frequently honed by hand, the facet on the knife does not allow the anti-roll plate to be correctly adjusted. This difficulty can be delayed by using a knife back, but the problem remains. The use of automatic knife sharpeners is better, but these also produce a facet. In the author's experience, the best results are obtained by having the knives reground. The knife, when in need of sharpening, is removed from the cryostat, dried and sent away to be reground. The cost is not high and when the knife is returned it is ready to be placed into the cryostat without any further attention. If the knife is stropped it has a fine edge, which is soon removed by the hard frozen blocks. Unless very thin sections are required it is advisable not to treat the knife in any way after regrinding.

METHOD 5

Preparation of tissue for prefixed cryostat sectioning

(1) Remove tissue as rapidly as possible from the body
(2) Cut into pieces 1 cm × 1 cm × 0·5 cm
(3) Place into 10 per cent formol calcium at 4°C overnight. (*See* page 13)
(4) Wash in running tap water for 5 min
(5) Place in gum sucrose solution for 24 h (*see* page 240)
(6) Blot as dry as possible
(7) Freeze tissue and mount on block holder.

Note. A more detailed method for enzyme work is Method 99.

METHOD 6

Rapid staining of cryostat sections (haematoxylin-eosin)

(1) Fix sections in formol–acetic–alcohol for 40 s
(2) Rinse rapidly in tap water
(3) Stain in Harris haematoxylin at 37°C for 30 s
(4) Rinse rapidly in tap water

(5) Differentiate in 1 per cent acid alcohol
(6) Rinse in Scott's tap water (*see* page 322)
(7) Rinse rapidly in tap water
(8) Stain in 1 per cent eosin for 10 s
(9) Rinse rapidly in tap water
(10) Dehydrate through graded alcohols to xylene and mount.

METHOD 7

Preparation of lung tissue for satisfactory cryostat sectioning (Tyler and Pearse, 1965)

(1) With animal tissue inject 4 per cent gelatin into the lung
(2) Remove lungs from animal and place in running cold water (to congeal gelatin) for 5–10 min
(3) Slice lung to required size
(4) Freeze lung by one of the techniques in Chapter 1.

If only a small piece of lung is available, i.e. biopsy specimen, infiltrate the lung with as much gelatin as possible before freezing.

Note. Tyler and Pearse recorded no difference between injected and uninjected lungs with the enzyme methods. Using uninjected lung however, only small fragments of section could be obtained.

REFERENCES

Brown, R. and Dilly, N. (1962). *J. Physiol.* **161,** No. 1 (proceedings)
Coons, A. H. Leduc, E. H. and Kaplan, M. N. (1951). *J. exp. Med.* **93,** 173
Cunningham, G. J., Bitensky, L., Chayen, J. and Silcox, A. A. (1962). *Ann. Histochim.* **6,** 433
Ioffe, A. F. (1956). In *Semiconductor Thermoelements and Thermoelectric Cooling*, London: Infroresearch Ltd.
Linderstrøm-Lang, K. and Morgenson, K. R. (1938). *C.R. Lab. Carlsberg, Serie Chim.* **23,** 37
Pearse, A. G. E. and Bancroft, J. D. (1966). *Jl. R. microsc. Soc.* **85,** 385
Rutherford, T., Hardy, W. S. and Isherwood, P. A. (1964). *Stain Tech.* **39,** 185
Thornburg, W. and Mengers, P. E. (1957) *J. Histochem. Cytochem.* **5,** 47
Tyler, W. S. and Pearse, A. G. E. (1965). *Thorax* **20,** 149

6

Freeze Drying and Freeze Substitution

In simple terms freeze drying is the rapid freezing of tissue, followed by the removal of water under vacuum whilst the tissue remains frozen. Freeze substitution is a variant of the freeze drying technique in which the water in the frozen tissue is replaced by an organic solvent at sub zero temperatures. Freeze substitution is not carried out under vacuum.

The technique of freeze drying is probably the most misunderstood of the histochemical processing methods. It is a common error for freeze drying to be regarded as a method of fixation; this is not so. The fixation of freeze dried material can be accomplished by two means: (1) vapour fixation of the block before impregnation with wax; and (2) fixation of the embedded sections before staining. A comparison is sometimes made between freeze dried sections and unfixed frozen (cryostat) sections. The important difference in freeze dried material, apart from the embedding in paraffin wax, is that the disruptive effects of thawing of the frozen sections is avoided, all the unbound water having been removed while the tissue is below freezing point. The importance of this fact is frequently overlooked in the appraisal of these two techniques.

Reasons for freeze drying

The standard methods of tissue preparation involving fixation, dehydration, clearing and embedding in paraffin wax have a number of drawbacks for the histochemist. These procedures affect tissue by causing loss of some soluble substances, by the alteration of chemically reactive groups and by the displacement of cell constituents caused by the penetration of the various fluids. Some of the advantages obtained with freeze drying are, however, lost when the freeze dried tissue is embedded. This applies particularly to enzymes, especially the oxidative types. For the critical demonstration of carbohydrates, proteins and some hydrolytic enzymes freeze drying is ideal.

FREEZE DRYING TECHNIQUE

This involves the tissue being frozen rapidly to preserve its chemical composition and cell structure much as it was in life. The unbound water is removed from the tissue by means that cause little or no change to its chemical composition. Once the tissue is dry it is embedded and sectioned. The technique of freeze drying can be divided into four parts.

(1) Freezing the tissue (quenching)
(2) Drying the tissue (dehydration)
(3) Fixation
(4) Embedding and sectioning.

Quenching

It is necessary to quench the tissue rapidly, for the more rapid the quenching, the smaller the ice crystals formed and, the smaller the ice crystals, the more the tissue will retain its original appearance. Many workers have tried to avoid this ice-crystal artefact by soaking the tissue in different reagents before freezing, glycerin and gelatin being the most popular, but without much success. To obtain a fast rate of cooling, a quenching liquid with a high rate of thermal conductivity is required. This fact has been stressed by many workers, including Simpson (1941). The requirements are for a solution of high thermal conductivity and with as low a temperature as possible. If a solution with low thermal conductivity is used, a layer of vaporized gas is formed around the block, slowing down the transference of heat from the tissue to the freezing medium. In recent years many different solutions have been tried, Gersh (1932) used liquid air at −195°C. Although this will freeze the tissue at this temperature, it has, unfortunately, a low thermal conductivity. Other agents tried include ethyl alcohol cooled by liquid air, isopentane cooled by liquid nitrogen and pentane cooled to −125°C. Bell (1952) recommended the use of dichlorodifluoromethane (Arcton 12), the coolant used in domestic refrigerators. The gas is condensed into a beaker, and the beaker containing the liquid Arcton is then placed carefully into a flask of liquid nitrogen. When the Arcton freezes the beaker is removed from the flask, and as the Arcton starts to thaw (at −158°C) the tissues for freeze drying are immersed in the liquid. A recent advance is to use

Arcton 22 (Freon 22), recommended by Rebhun (1965) and Pearse (1968) as the fastest quenching agent. It is used in the manner described for Arcton 12. Other workers prefer different liquids. Moberger, Lindström and Anderson (1954) used pure propane cooled with liquid nitrogen.

One problem with quenching is that certain tissues will crack, due to differential expansion of the tissue during freezing. Liver is especially vulnerable and care must be taken when quenching large pieces. It is advisable to quench the tissues by placing them on a strip of aluminium foil and immersing them in the liquid.

Eränkö (1954) pointed out that a much faster rate of cooling could be achieved by placing the tissue between two strips of copper previously cooled by immersion in liquid nitrogen. However, the majority of blocks for freeze drying are irregularly shaped so this method cannot often be used.

Dehydration or drying

This phase of the freeze drying technique consumes virtually all the time involved. If a slice of fresh kidney weighs 100 mg there will be 75–80 mg of water which must be removed during the drying phase. A satisfactory means of removing this large amount of water has to be employed without damage to the tissue.

Drying of the tissue will occur when heat is supplied to the ice crystals in it, thus causing water molecules to vaporize from their free surfaces. According to Stephenson (1953), after the molecules sublime they pass either into the vacuum chamber through the dry shell of the tissue, or they return to the interface between the dry shell and the frozen wet tissue. Although both processes may take place simultaneously, it is considered that the majority of the water molecules pass into the vacuum chamber to be absorbed by the vapour traps.

The drying phase is carried out in a vacuum at a higher temperature than that of the initial quenching. If the temperature of the tissue is maintained at −40°C in a vacuum of 10·3 torr, or better, then under these conditions, relative heat is being supplied to the tissue and the pressure of the environment around the tissue is lower than the vapour pressure of the ice, so that the latter sublimes, while the tissue remains solid and the growth of ice crystals is delayed. According to Pearse (1960), the temperature of the tissue during the drying phase is critical. He suggested that −30°C to −40°C is the best temperature range since ice vaporizes ten times more slowly at −60°C than at −40°C. If a reasonably short drying time is required, it is important not to have the tissue too cold, although care must be taken to ensure that the temperature during drying does not rise above $-30°C$. When the ice sublimes from the tissue it leaves a dry outer shell. Through this dry shell of tissue the remaining ice has to pass during sublimation and must not damage the extremely delicate tissue of the already dried outer shell. The relative heat necessary to complete the drying of the tissue must pass through this dry shell. Unfortunately, the dry outer shell is a poor conductor of heat but nevertheless relative heat must be continually supplied to the wet core of the tissue. The amount of heat supplied must be carefully controlled since too much heat will cause damage to the dry shell of the tissue and too little heat will not allow efficient drying of the remaining wet core. When the water molecules have left the dry shell of the tissue and have entered the vacuum chamber, they are removed by a vapour trap. These traps are usually one or more of two main types.

(1) A chemical trap (e.g. phosphorus pentoxide)
(2) A cold trap (which may be a liquid gas, e.g. nitrogen or air *or* a mixture of solid carbon dioxide with alcohol or acetone).

A common chemical trap employs phosphorous pentoxide which is a desiccant and when placed into the vacuum chamber will absorb water molecules reaching it. The container is usually placed between the tissue and the vacuum pump line.

The second type of trap is usually called a 'cold finger'. It consists of a piece of Quickfit glassware shaped like a finger. The 'nail' end of the finger is usually placed about 5 cm from the tissue. The cold finger is filled with liquid nitrogen or other refrigerating fluid and placed into the drying chamber some 5 cm away from the tissue. The water molecules passing from the tissue attach themselves to the cold finger. There are many opinions about the correct distance of cold fingers from the tissue during the drying phase. Most of this literature is complicated, involving unconfirmed complex mathematical theory, which is beyond the scope of this book.

Many attempts have been made to reduce the drying time of the pieces of tissue. These attempts have been frustrated mainly for two reasons. First, the drier the tissue becomes the more difficult it is to remove the remaining water molecules through the dry shell, which provides a strong resistance to them. Secondly the amount of heat that can be supplied to the piece of tissue during the drying phase is strictly limited, because the temperature of the tissue must not be raised above $-30°C$. If it is, damage will occur to the dry shell of the tissue. Workers in the past have carefully dried blocks for 12–48 hours maintaining the heat to the tissue at $-40°C$ to $-50°C$, and then for the last hour they have raised the temperature from $-40°C$ to $-10°C$. It is in this hour that damage due to ice crystal formation may occur, because there is still a considerable amount of water remaining. It is imperative, then, that the drying of the tissue be carried out at the same temperature throughout, preferably between −35°C and −55°C. The temperature should not be allowed to rise above −30°C with the vacuum pump operating unless the operator is in no doubt that the tissue is completely dry. When the tissue block is dry, it is possible to remove the block from the freeze dryer without causing any apparent damage to it. If the tissue is completely dry it can be left at room temperature and in the normal laboratory atmosphere without any outward change. A piece of tissue that is only partially dry, however, will start to rehydrate as soon as it is removed from the freeze dryer and left in the laboratory atmosphere; this water probably spreads outwards from the undried core.

Fixation

For the majority of histochemical techniques freeze dried tissue requires subsequent fixation. The method of choice is to fix by *vapour fixation* of the freeze dried block, although sections may be

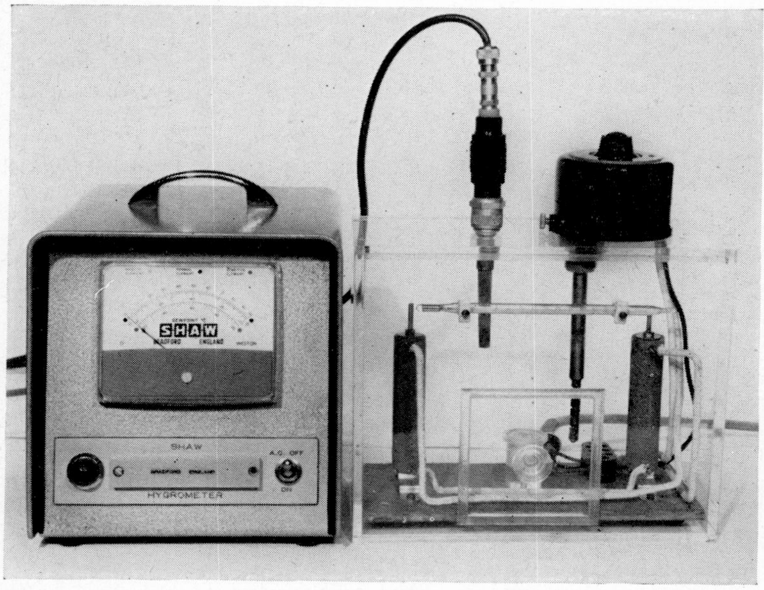

Figure 6.1 Apparatus used to fix blocks of freeze dried tissue. The temperature of the container is thermostatically controlled; the moisture content is read by using the hygrometer.

fixed after suitable embedding and cutting. Fixative vapours may be introduced into the drying chamber of the freeze dryer, but this is not recommended. The best results are obtained by vapour-fixing the block in a special piece of equipment in which it is possible to vary the temperature and moisture content of the surrounding atmosphere (*see Figure 6.1*). Control of the moisture content is particularly important for the demonstration of catecholamines in the tissue.

A number of substances are suitable for use as vapour fixatives, notably formaldehyde, glutaraldehyde and osmium tetroxide. The easiest to use, and the most successful, is formaldehyde vapour which gives excellent preservation of the tissue and good localization of most substances, particularly carbohydrates and proteins. Formaldehyde vapour is produced by heating paraformaldehyde powder at 60°C (*see* Method 12, page 65).

An alternative method of fixation is to fix the sections cut from the unfixed embedded block, using any of the standard aqueous fixatives. The accuracy of localization of the substances to be demonstrated is usually much inferior to that obtained with vapour fixation.

Embedding

When the tissue has been dried, and possibly vapour-fixed, it is ready for the embedding stage of the process. Many different embedding media can be used, the most popular being paraffin wax, but the choice depends on the structures and substances to be demonstrated. Lipids and enzymes are usually better demonstrated after embedding in polyester wax or even Carbowax despite some problems associated with infiltration of Carbowax into dry tissue. In many freeze dryers the embedding process takes place within the freeze dryer without the vacuum being broken. The paraffin wax must be placed in the dryer before the tissue and degassed under vacuum (*see* Method 11). When freeze drying is complete, the temperature is raised from −40°C to one or two degrees above the melting point of the paraffin wax. The tissue is then impregnated with the wax whilst still under vacuum. This technique, while admirable in many respects, has the disadvantage, in the author's experience, of occasionally causing damage to the tissue.

As long as the tissue is dry, the best policy is to remove it from the dryer after it has reached room temperature and then either place it immediately in degassed paraffin wax in a normal histological vacuum embedding bath or expose to vapour fixation, followed by paraffin wax embedding. The tissue is then embedded in fresh wax and is ready for cutting.

Cutting of paraffin-embedded freeze dried blocks

This presents only minor difficulties to an experienced histology technician. The blocks, fixed or unfixed, tend to be more brittle than routine processed paraffin blocks, and should be embedded in paraffin wax with a high content of plastic polymer. Cooling of both block and knife is usually sufficient to overcome the problem caused by the brittle nature of the block. From properly impregnated paraffin blocks of freeze dried material it is possible to cut serial sections of 3 microns with little difficulty. It appears more difficult to cut unusually thick sections than thin ones, due probably to the brittleness of the block.

Floating out of sections of unfixed freeze dried blocks

This presents much more of a problem than the cutting of the sections. Because of their hygroscopic nature unfixed sections cannot be floated out on to a waterbath in the normal way. Sections cut from blocks of vapour-fixed material can be left on warm water for a limited time before being picked up on slides. The most common floating out solutions for unfixed sections are:

(1) 70 per cent alcohol at 40–50°C
(2) 10 per cent formol saline at 45°C
(3) 10 per cent formol calcium at 45°C
(4) 18 per cent sodium sulphate at 45°C
(5) warm mercury at 40°C (toxic)
(6) dry mounting on a warm slide.

Each of these techniques has its own disadvantages. The first three allow perfectly flat sections to be picked up on slides, but the sections are subject to fixation and, in the case of 70 per cent alcohol, to loss of some lipid substances. The floating out of sections on warm mercury (warm mercury is toxic and care must be taken) involves no fixation or loss of any substances; the method is more difficult than most floating out procedures and some practice is required before repeatable success is obtained. An important factor is to keep the mercury as clean as possible. This means frequent filtering if many sections or blocks are to be cut. The method of floating out on mercury was first used by Harris, Sloane and King (1950).

The last method, favoured by many workers, is to coat microscope slides with glycerin albumen and to place them on a hotplate at 45°C. The section is cut, placed on the dry warm slide, and then flattened by finger pressure. Whilst this method causes least damage to the section, crease-free sections are rarely obtained. Furthermore, it is more difficult to keep the sections from floating off the slide during the subsequent staining technique. Careful consideration must be given when deciding which floating out method to use, and it may be necessary to use more than one method while cutting the same block, in order to obtain the best possible results from the stains or reactions to be carried out.

Embedding in media other than paraffin wax

Embedding in water-soluble waxes, the most common of which is Carbowax, has been used with freeze dried blocks. The main advantage is that no heat and no organic solvents are required for removal of the wax. The wax can be removed from the slide with water. The use of this method in routine histology laboratories has been restricted because of the difficulties of floating out the sections. Water cannot be used, and removing the creases is also a problem. With freeze dried blocks the same difficulties occur and, in the author's experience, difficulty is also encountered in getting the Carbowax to penetrate into completely dry tissues. If the block of tissue is slightly wet the Carbowax will penetrate.

As an alternative to embedding in paraffin wax, it is possible to double-embed blocks (*see* Method 13). This technique (Burstone, 1956), takes considerably longer, but if the substance to be demonstrated will resist the procedures involved, it is possible to obtain sections of a higher standard than can be obtained by any other method. The method is given in full at the end of this chapter (Method 13). It involves processing through alcohols and celloidin at deep-freeze temperatures before finally embedding in paraffin wax. An advantage is that sections can be floated out onto warm water in the usual manner. Burstone (1956) used this method to demonstrate hydrolytic enzymes in freeze dried material. The subject is more fully discussed in Chapter 15.

An acrylic resin such as methacrylate, used much as the electron microscopists use it, is sometimes preferred as an embedding medium when thin or very thin sections are required. Polymerization of methacrylate or other resins is achieved by heating at 50°C for eighteen hours or at 60°C overnight, and for this reason, the method is only used for specialized techniques.

Applications of freeze dried material

Freeze dried material has many applications. Pearse (1960) placed them under the following four main headings.

(1) Examination of unfixed material in inert media by physical methods

(2) Examination of unfixed material by microincineration or by treatment with buffer extractions, etc.

(3) Examination of suitably fixed or unfixed material by histochemical and conventional histological methods

(4) Examination by autoradiographic techniques.

Unfixed material in inert media

Unfixed freeze dried sections can be examined by phase contrast microscopy, polarized light, dark-field illumination and fluorescent microscopy.

Extraction with buffer solutions and microincineration

The proteins of freeze dried sections are said to be almost completely undenatured and therefore it is possible to test their solubility in different buffer solutions. Following the extraction, the section is fixed and a suitable reaction for the protein may be carried out alongside a control section to help establish the quantity extracted.

Microincineration is a technique carried out to determine the presence of inorganic elements in the tissue sections. It is important that fixation and processing of the tissue must not alter its mineral content. Freeze dried sections are therefore ideal for this purpose; the method is discussed in Chapter 19.

Fixed and unfixed sections and staining techniques

The choice of a fixative with freeze dried sections is dictated by the components to be demonstrated or the particular histological staining method to be applied. All the routine histological stains can be used on freeze dried sections, although the staining times must be reduced, possibly by one third for the majority of methods. It is also possible to demonstrate enzymes, but the use of the heat, paraffin wax and a combination of the two, reduce the degree of enzyme activity and its localization is open to question. For mucin and other mucopolysaccharides this is probably the best means of demonstration. A comprehensive study was carried out by Tock and Pearse (1965) and readers are referred to this for details.

Examination by autoradiographic techniques

Freeze dried sections are worth consideration when water soluble isotopes are to be used and their usefulness should be compared with that of frozen sections.

HISTORY AND TYPES OF FREEZE DRYERS

There have been many different types of freeze dryers developed over the years. The drying times of the tissues have varied from a few hours to many days and the slices of tissue dried in some cases were very small indeed. Mann in 1902 described that Leewenhoek, one of the founders of microscopical science, prepared samples of muscle by a method of freeze drying as early as 1720. However, the method was not really exploited until the end of the 19th century when liquefied gases became available. Altman in 1890 described a method which involved drying small fragments of tissue *in vacuo* over concentrated sulphuric acid. After several days it was possible to remove the tissue and embed it in paraffin wax. Altman stated that this method eliminated histological shrinkage. The second major advance in freeze drying technique was made by Gersh (1932). His equipment, with its various modifications by many people, including Stowell (1951), Jensen (1954) and Burstone (1956), is basically the equipment that is still used in laboratories today. Gersh used a Dewar flask containing liquid ammonia, which was hermetically sealed to the drying chamber. The temperature inside

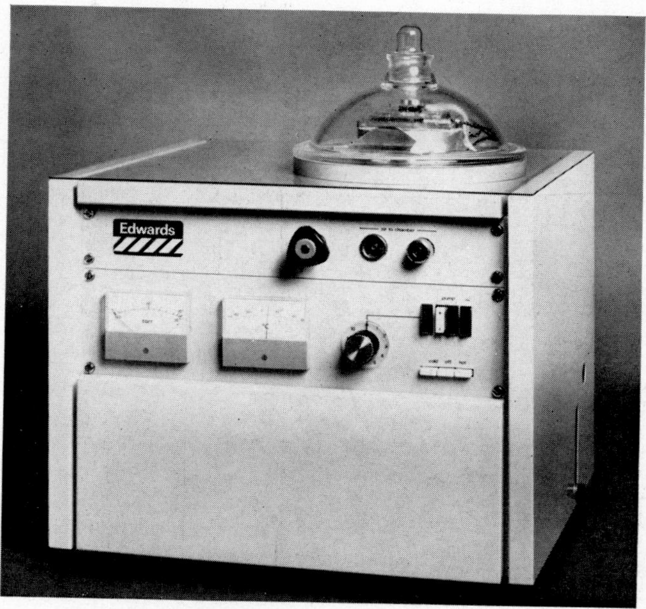

Figure 6.2 The Speedivac–Pearse thermoelectric freeze-dryer. Reproduced by courtesy of Edwards High Vacuum Ltd.

the chamber was −22°C. To obtain the vacuum, two pumps were used, a rotary pump and a mercury vapour diffusion pump. He used a phophorus pentoxide vapour trap. He also incorporated a compartment for the vacuum-embedding of the tissue.

Two years later Goodspeed and Uber (1934), instead of using liquid gases as a means of cooling the tissue, placed the drying tube in a mechanically refrigerated chamber at −29°C. A single mechanical pump was employed and phosphorus pentoxide was used in the vapour trap. Goodspeed and Uber removed the tissue from their dryer before wax-embedding. A method of freeze drying based on the use of a dry gas moving over the frozen tissues to remove the water evaporating from them was reported by Treffenburg (1953), Jansen (1954) and Kramer and Hill (1956). Some provision for drying the air and maintaining the low temperature of the air and specimens was required during dehydration. Kramer and Hill used a mixture of carbon dioxide snow and cellulose in a vacuum flask to cool the chamber and to supply a stream of dry gas. The drying time claimed for this type of freeze dryer is 10–24 h for small pieces of tissue.

The next significant advance in the field of freeze drying was made by Pearse (1963) who designed a freeze dryer to operate with thermoelectric modules. This freeze dryer (*Figure 6.2*) was subsequently produced commercially by Edwards High Vacuum Ltd. The tissue is kept at the required temperature throughout the drying phase by the use of thermomodules. At this point, before describing thermoelectric freeze drying, a brief explanation of how a thermomodule works may be necessary.

HOW A THERMOMODULE WORKS

The thermomodules produce cold by means of a phenomenon known as the *Peltier effect*. When a direct current is passed across the junction of two dissimilar metals, heat is emitted or absorbed according to the direction of the current. Recent advances in the technology of semiconducting materials have led to the production of thermoelements with considerable refrigerating capacity. The modules consist of an array of bismuth telluride couples, connected in series by copper strips which serve both as electrical conductors and for heat transmission. When a current of direct electricity is passed through the module, heat is absorbed on one side, and evolved on the other. Anodized aluminium plates are bonded to the faces of the module.

With the hot face of the module at 27°C, the cold face of the module is capable of attaining −30°C. The cooling produced by the module is dependent upon the amount of the operating current, thereby providing a simple technique for precise temperature control. If the polarity of the electricity supply is reversed, a heating effect can be produced instead of a cooling one.

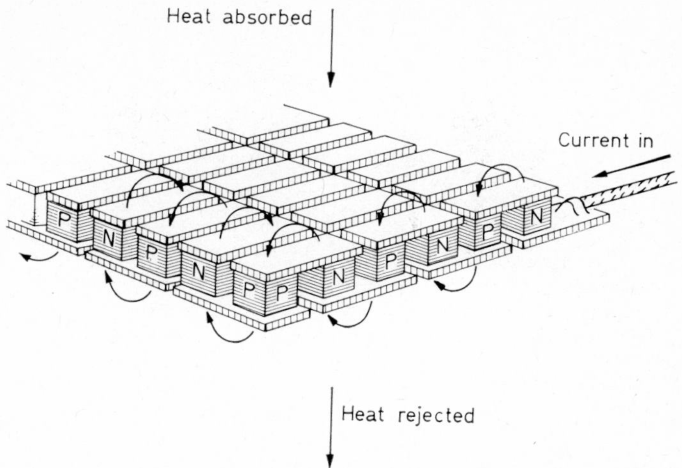

Figure 6.3 The above demonstrates how the cold surface is obtained. Reproduced by courtesy of De La Rue Frigistor Ltd.

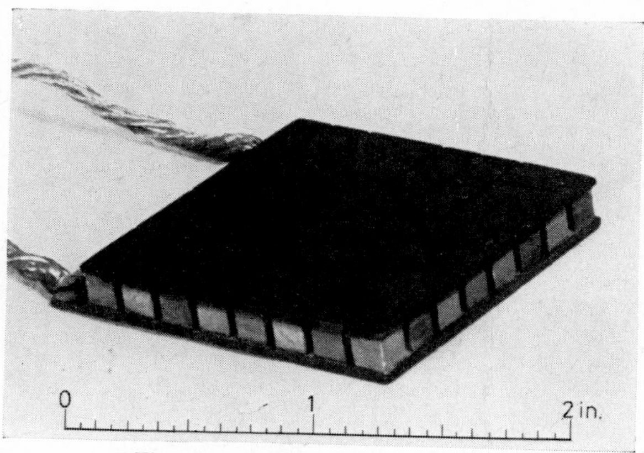

Figure 6.4 A thermoelectric module.

THERMOELECTRIC FREEZE DRYING

To obtain a satisfactory working range of temperatures, +60°C or more (to melt the embedding wax, if required) to below −60°C, it is necessary to use more than one module. These thermomodules are arranged in a cascade effect (*Figure 6.5*), the base set of modules having more than the top in the ratio of 4:1. This is to allow the

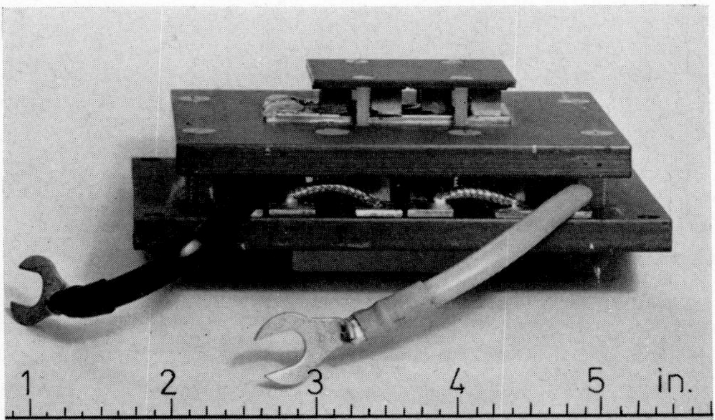

Figure 6.5 The cascade effect of modules to produce a colder top surface.

heat produced by the warm face of the top set of modules to be satisfactorily removed by the cold face of the bottom set, allowing the top surface of the top module to drop below −60°C if necessary.

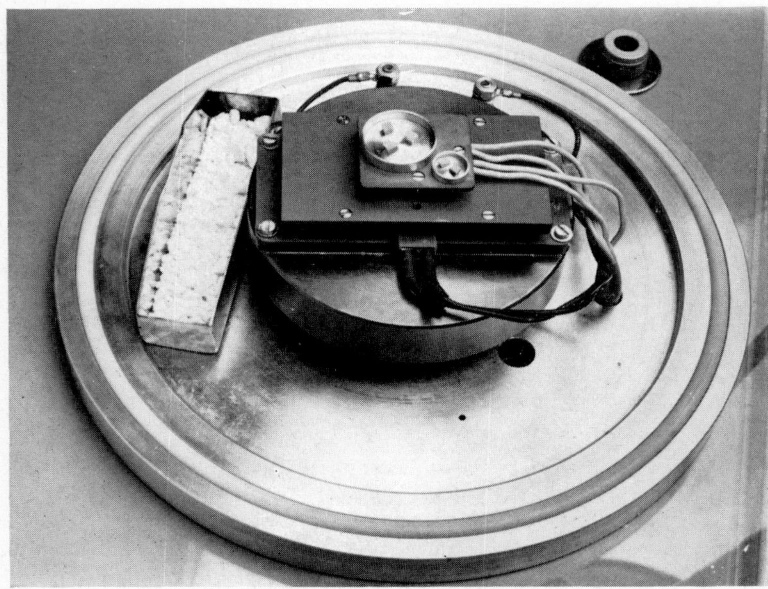

Figure 6.6 The thermoelectric modules as used in the freeze dryer. Note the container of phosphorus pentoxide to absorb the water molecules leaving the tissue. Reproduced by courtesy of Edwards High Vacuum Ltd.

The heat from the base set of modules is removed by cold running water.

This use of thermomodules obviates the necessity for employing liquefied gases or deep freeze cabinets during the drying phase. It also allows more accurate control of the drying temperature by the simple means of controlling the current supply to the modules. It can be seen from *Figure 6.2* that the vacuum pump and electrical

TABLE 6.1

Drying times using thermoelectric freeze dryer

Thickness of tissue (mm)	*Drying temperature* (°C)	*Drying times* (h)
1	−30	$1\frac{1}{2}$–2
1	−40	2–$2\frac{1}{2}$
1	−50	3–4
1	−60	6–$6\frac{1}{2}$
2	−30	3–$3\frac{1}{2}$
2	−40	4–$4\frac{1}{2}$
2	−50	5–6
2	−60	8–10
3	−30	4–5
3	−40	5–$5\frac{1}{2}$
3	−50	7–8
3	−60	Dry overnight
4	−30	5–6
4	−40	$6\frac{1}{2}$–7
4	−50	Dry overnight
4	−60	Dry overnight

The above drying times were determined by using liver, kidney and spleen. Many factors influence the drying time of tissues. The above table is included as a general guide.

system are set into the base of the cabinet, while the modules are mounted on the top and are covered by a desiccator lid. The area covered by this desiccator lid is the drying chamber. The controls are mounted on the front panel of the cabinet with two gauge dials giving the module temperature and the vapour pressure. The controls allow the operator to isolate the drying chamber from the vacuum pump and to regulate the temperature of the thermomodules from +60°C to −60°C. The vapour trap usually used in the freeze dryer is phosphorus pentoxide, contained in two boats placed near the vacuum line. Although the temperature of the module is held at −40°C during freeze drying, there is a temperature gradient above the tissue and at the desiccator lid it reaches approximately

+15°C. The temperature difference between −40°C to +15°C facilitates the drying of the tissue to such an extent that in four hours a 4 mm slice of tissue at −40°C will be dry. The majority of other types of freeze dryers need 12 hours or more to complete drying. The block may simply be placed on the module, or it may be firmly attached by ice. Drying occurs faster when the tissue rests on the surface of the module.

In summary, freeze driers may be of the following types.

(1) Vacuum chambers cooled by liquid or solid refrigerators
(2) Vacuum chambers cooled by mechanical refrigerators
(3) Refrigerated drying tube through which dry gas passes
(4) Thermoelectric.

The first three types are now largely of historical interest in Britain. The thermoelectric type with its accurate temperature control and its efficient drying ability is now the most widely used type of freeze dryer. For a detailed comparison of the theoretical aspects of the different freeze dryers readers are referred to Pearse (1968), Chapter 3.

FREEZE SUBSTITUTION

The technique of freeze substitution was originally described by Simpson (1941) as an alternative technique to freeze drying. The tissue is frozen as rapidly as possible, and the ice replaced or 'substituted' by leaving the tissue in dehydrating solutions (usually an organic solvent) at sub zero temperatures. The technique can be divided into three stages.

(1) Quenching or freezing
(2) Substitution
(3) Embedding.

Quenching

The tissue for freeze substitution should be absolutely fresh and frozen as rapidly as possible. To obtain good results, the quenching must be as fast as possible, for, as with freeze drying, damage by ice crystal formation will ruin the end result. The blocks to be substituted should be small and frozen in a bath super-cooled to 190° by liquid nitrogen. The technique described in Method 8 for freeze drying is ideal for this technique.

Substitution

The ice in the tissue can be substituted in two types of solutions either (a) a pure dehydrating solution or (b) a dehydrating solution containing a fixative. Consideration must be given in the latter case to the effect of the fixative at the substituting temperature. The use of a fixative such as picric acid, mercuric chloride or 1 per cent osmium tetroxide in the dehydrating solution is normally used for morphological studies and not for critical histochemical work. Substitution has been carried out in a wide range of temperatures from −20°C down to −130°C. The majority of the work has been carried out at around −70°. The temperature at which the substitution is performed is important for a number of reasons; the lower the temperature the less the growth of ice crystals, and the lower the temperature the slower the penetration of the substituting fluid.

A number of solutions may be used to substitute the ice in the tissue, the two most common being ethanol or acetone.

The penetration of the dehydrating solution will normally take up to about six days at −70°C. Agitation during substitution should be employed as often as possible.

Embedding

When the tissue is thought to be fully dehydrated it is transferred to a refrigerator at 4°C. When the substituting fluid has reached this temperature the tissue is immersed in chloroform at 4°C overnight and then in chloroform at room temperature before embedding in either paraffin wax or polyester wax.

SECTION FREEZE-SUBSTITUTION

As more sophisticated techniques are developed with the cryostat, section freeze-substitution has become a simpler and less time-consuming procedure than block substitution (Chang and Hori, 1961; and Chang, 1965). The tissue is frozen as for freeze drying, sectioned at as low a temperature as possible, and the sections are transferred direct to cold acetone at −70°C overnight. From the acetone they are picked up on slides and allowed to dry. For the demonstration of oxidative enzymes the sections should be coated with celloidin.

The advantage of freeze-substituted cryostat sections over normal cryostat sections is that the water is removed without the sections thawing and thus avoiding the diffusion which usually occurs during thawing; it must be remembered that diffusion will occur during the incubating phase of the histochemical technique. Whether the results obtained by section freeze-substitution are superior to the standard prefixed cryostat sections is a matter for debate.

METHOD 8

Quenching—equipment required

Dewar flask full of liquid nitrogen or liquid air
Cylinder of Arcton 22 or Freon 22 (I.C.I. Ltd.)
50 ml Pyrex beaker
Copper discs or aluminium foil
Pair forceps
Scalpel

(1) Obtain fresh tissue and slice into pieces no thicker than 5 mm
(2) Into a 50 ml Pyrex beaker run 20 ml Arcton 22
(3) Place beaker into a Dewar flask containing liquid nitrogen
(4) Take care not to let the beaker slip below the surface of the nitrogen
(5) Wait for the Arcton 22 to freeze (5 min or less)
(6) Remove beaker of frozen Arcton 22 and stand on bench
(7) Place tissue on copper disc or strip of aluminium
(8) As Arcton 22 begins to thaw plunge the tissue on the strip or disc into Arcton for 40 s
(9) Remove tissue from the beaker of Arcton 22 and transfer to the freeze dryer

METHOD 9

Quenching

(1) Liquid nitrogen in Dewar flask
(2) Place two copper discs into flask for 2 min
(3) Remove discs from coolant
(4) Place tissue between the discs for 30 s
(5) Remove tissue and place in freeze dryer

METHOD 10

Operating the thermoelectric freeze dryer (with wax-embedding outside freeze dryer)

(1) Switch on vacuum pump
(2) Turn on tap water
(3) Switch on current to thermomodules set to maximum
(4) Fill containers with phosphorus pentoxide
(5) Check that temperature is below −40°C
(6) Break vacuum by isolating pump and removing desiccator lid
(7) Place containers of phosphorus pentoxide in chamber

(8) Place tissue previously quenched by Method 8 or 9 on the module surface
(9) Evacuate chamber by opening isolation valve
(10) Set module temperature (usually −40°C to −60°C)
(11) Check (a) temperature is correct; (b) vacuum reading correct
(12) Leave to dry (*see* Table 6.1 for approximate time)
(13) When dry, isolate chamber and switch off vacuum pump
(14) Switch off current to modules
(15) Turn off running water
(16) Let tissue reach room temperature
(17) Remove tissue from drying chamber
(18) Place in molten degassed paraffin wax **or**
(19) Fix in vapour as in Method 12
(20) Embed

METHOD 11

Alternative method of freeze drying to Method 10

(1) Switch on vacuum pump
(2) Set modules to heat and switch current on
(3) Place molten paraffin wax in brass boat, and place on module surface
(4) Evacuate chamber
(5) Check temperature is two or three degrees above melting point of the wax
(6) After degassing the wax, reverse current and cool the modules till the wax is solid
(7) Isolate chamber and remove boat from module surface
(8) Remove wax from centre of boat, to enable tissue to be in contact with metal surface and put in tissue
(9) Replace boat in freeze dryer
(10) Evacuate chamber
(11) Continue from Step (3) Method 10 until Step (13)
(12) When tissue is dry reverse current and start to heat the boat
(13) Watch for paraffin wax to melt then control temperature to 3°C above the melting point of wax while infiltrating the tissue
(14) Wait for 10 min
(15) Isolate pump
(16) Remove tissue and embed in fresh degassed paraffin wax

METHOD 12

Formol vapour fixation of freeze dried blocks

(1) Quench as in Method 8 or 9

(2) Freeze dry as in Method 10 until Step (17)
(3) Place tissue in airtight vessel containing a quantity of paraformaldehyde and with variable temperature and humidity control between +20°C and +70°C
(4) Leave for 1–3 h usually at +60°C
(5) Remove tissue and switch off heat
(6) Place tissue in molten paraffin wax in embedding bath, for 30 min or longer depending upon size of tissue
(7) Embed in fresh wax

METHOD 13

Double embedding of freeze dried blocks

(1) Quench as in Method 8 or 9
(2) Freeze dry as in Method 10 till Step (13)
(3) Place tissue in alcohol/ether 1:1 at —70°C for 3 h
(4) Place tissue in 2 per cent celloidin (in alcohol/ether, 1:1) at —70°C for 16 h
(5) Excess celloidin removed by blotting
(6) Place tissue in chloroform at −70°C for 1 h
(7) Place tissue in fresh chloroform at −70°C for 1 h
(8) Place tissue in chloroform and allow to reach room temperature
(9) Place tissue in paraffin wax for 1–2 h
(10) Embed

METHOD 14

Block freeze-substitution

Reagents required

(1) Liquid nitrogen or liquid air
(2) Arcton 22 or Freon 22
(3) Acetone
(4) Chloroform
(5) Paraffin wax

Technique

(1) Obtain small fresh slices of tissue
(2) Quench by placing in Arcton 22 precooled by liquid nitrogen
(3) Place frozen tissue in precooled acetone −70°C for 2–5 days
(4) Transfer tissue to chloroform at −70°C for 2–3 h
(5) Allow chloroform to reach room temperature slowly
(6) Fresh chloroform at room temperature for 1 h
(7) Transfer sections to paraffin wax
(8) Fresh paraffin—then embed

METHOD 15

Section freeze-substitution (Chang and Hori, 1961)

Equipment required

(1) Cryostat
(2) Liquid nitrogen or liquid air
(3) Arcton 22 or Freon 22
(4) 0·5 per cent Celloidin, solution in alcohol/ether 1:1
(5) Acetone

Technique

(1) Obtain fresh slices of tissue
(2) Quench by placing in Arcton precooled with liquid nitrogen
(3) Transfer block to cryostat and cut sections at as low a temperature as possible
(4) Drop the sections in precooled acetone
(5) Transfer acetone to −70°C for 18–24 h
(6) Mount sections on coverglasses (coat with Celloidin if necessary).

REFERENCES

ALTMAN, R. (1890). *Die Elementarorganismen und ihre Beziehungen zur Zellen*, Liepzig
BELL, L. G. E. (1952). *Nature, Lond.* **170,** 717
BURSTONE, M. S. (1956). *J. Natn. Cancer Inst.* **17,** 49
CHANG, J. P. and HORI, S. A. (1961). *J. Histochem. Cytochem.* **9,** 292
ERÄNKÖ, O. (1954). *Acta anat.* **22,** 231
GERSH, I. (1932). *Anat. Rec.* **53,** 309
GOODSPEED, T. H. and UBER, F. M. (1934). *Proc. nant. Acad. Sci., U.S.A.* **20,** 495
HARRIS, J. E., SLOANE, J. F. and KING, D. T. (1950). *Nature, Lond.* **166,** 25
JANSEN, M. T. (1954). *Expl Cell. Res.* **7,** 318
JENSEN, W. A. (1954). *Expl Cell. Res.* **7,** 572
KRAMER, H. and HILL, R. S. (1956). *Q. Jl microsc. Sci.* **97,** 144
MANN, G. (1902). *Physiological Histology*, Oxford: Clarendon Press
MOBERGER, C., LINDSTRÖM, B. and ANDERSON, L. (1954). *Expl Cell. Res.* **6,** 228
PEARSE, A. G. E. (1960. *Histochemistry, Theoretical and Applied.* London: Churchill
— (1963). *J. scient. Instrum.* **40,** 176
— (1968). *Histochemistry, Theoretical and Applied*, 3rd Edn. vol. 1, London: Churchill
REBHUN, L. I. (1965). *Fedn. Proc.* **24,** S15, 217
SIMPSON. W. L. (1941). *Anat. Rec.* **80,** 173 and 329
STEPHENSON, J. L. (1953). *Bull. math. Biophys.* **15,** 411
STOWELL, R. E. (1951). *Stain Technol.* **26,** 105
TOCK, E. P. C. and PEARSE, A. G. E. (1965). *Jl R microsc. Soc.* **84,** 519
TREFFENBURG, L. (1953). *Ark. Zool.* **4,** 295

7

Carbohydrates

The term carbohydrate was originally used to describe compounds containing only carbon, hydrogen and oxygen. Subsequently other substances that are functionally and structurally similar have been included. It is not possible to demonstrate many of the individual carbohydrates at the present time because of their solubility. Various groups of these carbohydrates can be shown by the techniques described in this chapter.

The nomenclature of carbohydrates is very confused for technologists and histopathologists and is becoming more so as the result of recent attempts to integrate a more accurate biochemical classification into the loose working classification used by histologists. Traditionally, histological technologists and pathologists have used the terms 'mucins' and 'acid mucopolysaccharides' to describe some of the groups of carbohydrates. Histochemical methods produce little actual chemical information in regard to content of the carbohydrate in comparison to a biochemical test. The term mucosubstance was recommended by Spicer, Leppi and Stoward (1965) as a suitable name for carbohydrate-rich, but biochemically undefined, substances seen in tissues. A histochemical classification of mucosubstances cannot be compared to a biochemical classification because of the lack of specific information forthcoming from the histochemical reaction. At the same time some of the mucosubstances seen histochemically have not been characterized biochemically. Jeanloz (1960) recommended that the prefix 'muco' should be omitted from descriptions of carbohydrates, and Pearse (1968) produced a biochemical classification of common mucosubstances omitting the use of the prefix 'muco', as well as producing a histochemical classification. It would be too confusing in this chapter to relate the mucosubstances demonstrated histochemically to their counterparts in a biochemical classification. The classification shown in Table 7.1 goes some way as an introduction in relating the two. It is based upon the writings of Meyer (1953; 1966); Spicer, Leppi and Stoward (1965); Pearse (1968); and Cook (1972; 1974). The term mucosubstance will be used throughout this chapter and can be defined as substances which contain hexosamine sugars in combination with differing amounts of proteins, and, in some instances, lipids. Some of these carbohydrates are known as neutral mucosubstances. They usually have free hexose groups available and are hence demonstrated by the Periodic Acid–Schiff reaction, ('periodate reactive'). Other carbohydrates contain acid radicals and are known as acid mucosubstances. The type of acid and its position on the reactive molecule will determine some of the histochemical reactions.

In their paper Spicer, Leppi and Stoward (1965) recommended that tissue mucosubstances should be classified by (1) site; (2) their reactivity to histochemical methods; and (3) lability to enzyme digestion. An example of this nomenclature would be 'connective tissue mucosubstance, Alcian Blue positive and resistant to testicular hyaluronidase'.

The biochemical terms homoglycan, heteroglycan, glycosaminoglycan and glycosaminoglucuronoglycan, are being increasingly used by pathologists and histochemists. These terms, unless used

TABLE 7.1

Carbohydrates

(1) Polysaccharides—glycogen (periodate reactive)
(2) Neutral mucosubstances (periodate reactive)
(3) Acid mucosubstances
  Sulphated
  (i) Connective tissue mucopolysaccharides (periodate unreactive)
    (a) keratan sulphate, heparin and dermatan sulphate (stable to testicular hyaluronidase)
    (b) chondroitin sulphates (labile to testicular hyaluronidase)
  (ii) Epithelial sulphomucins (stable to testicular hyaluronidase)
    (a) sulphate esters on vic-glycols
    (b) sulphate esters not on vic-glycols
    (c) a group exist as periodate reactive (*see* text)

  Non-sulphated
  (i) Connective tissue (periodate unreactive)
    (a) hexuronic acid-rich–hyaluronic acid (labile to testicular hyaluronidase)
    (b) sialic acid-rich
  (ii) Epithelial sialomucins (periodate reactivity variable)
    (a) sialic acid-rich (labile to sialidase)
    (b) sialic acid-rich (stable to sialidase)
(4) Mucoproteins
(5) Mucolipids

accurately and in their proper context, only lead to further confusion in an already confusing nomenclature. Readers are referred to chapter 10 of Pearse (1968) for an explanation of this terminology.

Polysaccharides

Glycogen

This is the only member of the polysaccharide group which can normally be demonstrated histochemically in tissue sections. Glycogen, which is polymerized glucose, is a neutral polysaccharide; it is a storage carbohydrate and accumulates in the hepatocytes in the liver. It is also demonstrable in skeletal and cardiac muscle, as well as in many organs of the newborn. Glycogen will rapidly break down to glucose after death, so it is imperative to obtain rapid and adequate fixation. A great deal has been written about the fixation of glycogen, especially in regard to its possible solubility in water. Conflicting opinions are still expressed about the choice of fixative, whether to use alcoholic fixatives, picric acid fixatives or any standard solution. Lillie (1947) showed that little or no loss of glycogen was observed after formol saline fixation, followed by a lengthy wash in running tap water. Personally I prefer to use Gendre's fixative at 4°C on thin slices of tissue. Mercury-containing fixatives should be avoided. During room temperature fixation,

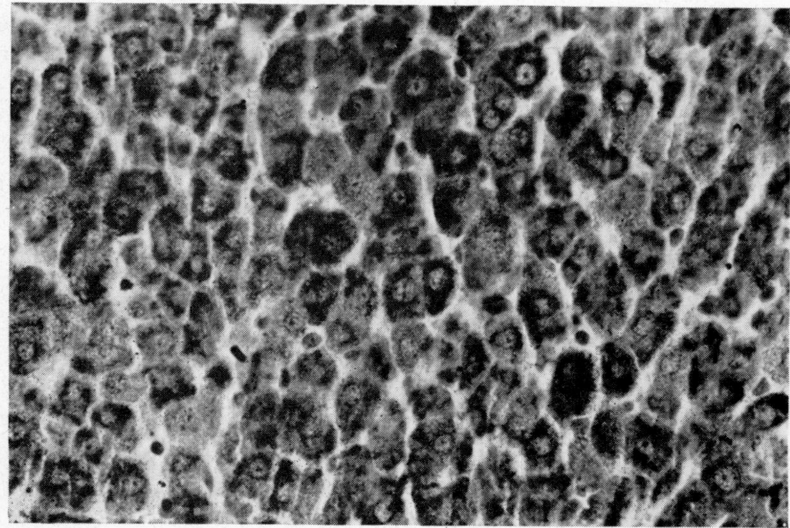

Figure 7.1 Rat liver freeze dried formalin-vapour fixed. Note the absence of 'streaming effect' and that the glycogen is located around the nucleus. (× *370*)

glycogen becomes insoluble and the classical streaming artefact is produced; this may be avoided by using Gendre's fixative at 4°C or by freeze drying (*see Figure 7.1*).

Leske and Mayersbach (1969) and Lake (1970) reported that unfixed cryostat sections are superior to conventional paraffin processing for the demonstration of glycogen. Celloidinization is necessary to avoid loss of unfixed glycogen during staining.

Glycogen can be routinely demonstrated by Best's Carmine, Schiff methods, silver techniques or by iodine. The silver and iodine methods are the least specific and are little used today. The Best's Carmine method can prove capricious and a known positive control should always be used; accurate differentiation is also an important aspect of the technique. The PAS methods are probably the most specific available for glycogen, although other reactive carbohydrate substances will be positive. For this reason enzyme digestion techniques and positive controls should be employed.

Diastase digestion of glycogen

This technique allows for the specific demonstration of glycogen when using the Periodic Acid–Schiff and Best's Carmine methods. Diastase will digest glycogen from a section whilst other PAS-positive, carbohydrate material, resistant to diastase digestion, will remain. Amylase (diastase) is used as a 0·5–1 per cent solution in phosphate buffer pH 6 or distilled water; this solution needs to be freshly prepared. A watch should be kept on the stock diastase as this seems to deteriorate within six months or so. Saliva, which contains amylase, will usually work well. Sections for digestion are either placed in 0·5–1 per cent diastase at 37°C for 40 minutes or up to one hour at room temperature. Saliva is used for the same times. Diastase can be used before or after staining with Best's Carmine but only before staining with the PAS reaction.

Celloidinization of sections

There is considerable dispute in the literature about the necessity for using celloidin. At one time it was considered that celloidinization prevented loss of glycogen from the section, when in contact with water. A number of workers now consider that little or no loss of glycogen occurs after fixation during staining; however celloidinization does prevent diastase from digesting glycogen in control sections. Unfixed cryostat sections to be used for the demonstration of glycogen will need to be coated with 0·25 per cent celloidin.

Neutral mucosubstances

These contain sugars and normally have free hexose groups available, but do not contain any free acid radicles or sulphate esters. These mucosubstances are found in the stomach, intestines and prostate. They show a positive PAS reaction (periodate reactive), and a variable result with Southgate's Mucicarmine (Cook, 1968).

Acid mucosubstances

This is the largest of the groups of mucosubstances and can, in the first instance, be divided into sulphated and non-sulphated (carboxylated) mucosubstances.

Sulphated

These mucosubstances can also be conveniently divided into two sub-groups, the connective-tissue sulphated mucosubstances, and the epithelial sulphate mucosubstances (epithelial sulphomucins). The connective-tissue sulphated mucosubstances contain either sulphated glucuronic acids, such as the chondroitin sulphates and heparan sulphate, or keratan sulphate. The chondroitin sulphate-containing acid mucosubstances are labile to testicular hyaluronidase but the other connective-tissue sulphated mucosubstances are resistant to digestion by this enzyme. The connective-tissue sulphated mucosubstances are found in skin, cartilage, heart valves and aorta; they are also known as the strongly acidic and strongly sulphated mucosubstances. They are usually periodate unreactive, stain with Alcian Blue at pH 0·5 and are metachromatic with Azure 'A' at pH 0·5.

The epithelial sulphated mucosubstances (epithelial sulphomucins) also contain sulphate esters, but in different combination to those discussed above. They are found in the submandibular salivary glands, and in duodenal and colonic goblet cells. They are also known as weakly sulphated mucosubstances, and their staining reactions differ from those of the strongly sulphated mucosubstances in that the optimal pH level with Toluidine Blue is raised from 0·5 to 2·0 and with Alcian Blue from 0·5 to 1·5. They are resistant to testicular hyaluronidase and may be periodate reactive with the exception of an epithelial mucosubstance produced by bronchial serous glands (Lamb and Reid, 1970), which is Periodic acid–Schiff positive.

Non-sulphated (carboxylated)

This group of mucosubstances may also be conveniently separated into sub-groups, by their site, content, and by their response to enzyme digestion techniques. The classification by site is based on whether the substance is found in the epithelium or connective tissue, and the classification by content is based on whether the acid radical present is sialic acid or a hexuronic acid.

Connective-tissue non-sulphated mucosubstances are rich in hexuronic acid and possibly sialic acid. The hexuronic acid-rich

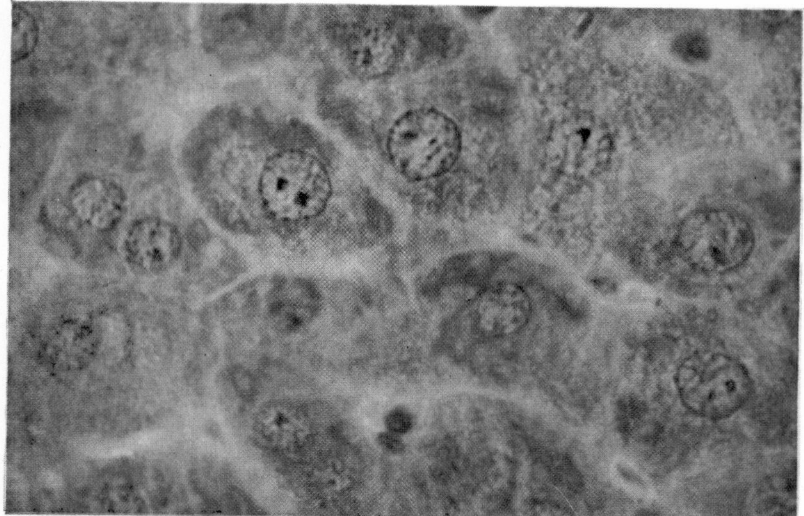

Plate 1 Glycogen demonstrated by the PAS reaction on freeze dried liver. Note the absence of diffusion artefact ('streaming artefact'). (Magnification × *985)*

(Reduced to nine-tenths in reproduction)

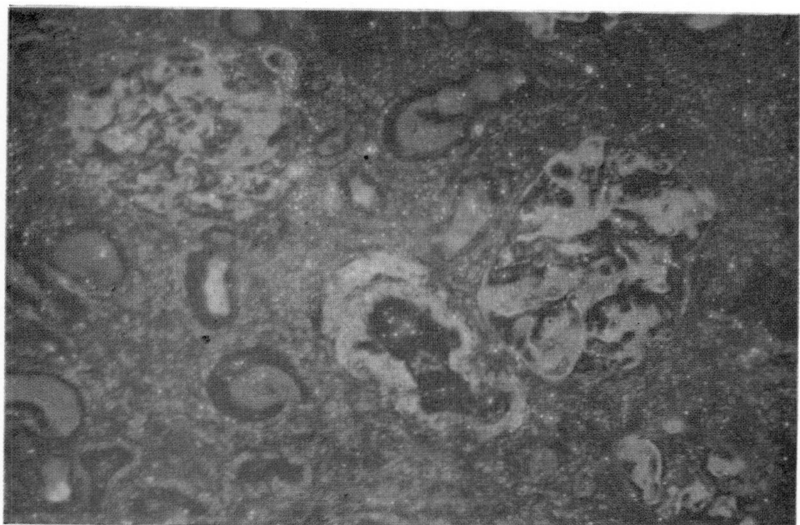

Plate 2 Amyloid demonstrated by the fluorescent Congo Red technique. The amyloid fluoresces strongly red even when the Congo Red staining of the section is so faint as to be not visible by normal light microscopy. (Method 49, Magnification × *100)*

(Reduced to nine-tenths in reproduction)

Sigma London Chemical Company Ltd. have kindly contributed towards the cost of these colour plates.

mucosubstances contain large amounts of hyaluronic acid. The reactive components are the carboxyl groups. These substances react with Alcian Blue at pH 2·5 and with metachromatic dyes at pH 6. They are periodate unreactive, and are labile to testicular hyaluronidase. The existence of a sialic acid-rich connective-tissue mucosubstance is still in doubt; it may be a minor component of cartilage.

Epithelial non-sulphated mucosubstances contain as their acid radical, sialic acid, and are often called epithelial sialomucins. The sialic acid is in combination with the reactive carboxyl groups. They show identical reactions with metachromatic dyes and Alcian Blue to the hexuronic acid-rich mucosubstances discussed above, but they are usually periodate reactive (PAS-positive). In addition they are not affected by testicular hyaluronidase. Most of these epithelial sialomucins are labile to sialidase, but Lev and Spicer (1964) described a sialomucin which was resistant to sialidase digestion. Cook (1968) described these mucosubstances in human gastric pyloric glands.

Mucoproteins

Mucoproteins are complex substances in which the polysaccharide is chemically combined with a protein. The carbohydrate content of mucoproteins (hexosamine) exceeds 4 per cent of the total weight, compared with glycoproteins which have less than 4 per cent. There is no specific method for mucoproteins. They are positive by the PAS method but are negative with the Toluidine Blue technique. It may be necessary to apply a protein method to see if a positive result is obtained at the same site as the PAS-positive material. If this is the case, it may indicate a mucoprotein. The method used to demonstrate mucoproteins is the PAS method (*see* Method 19).

They are found in the beta cells of the pituitary, in basement membranes and other sites.

Mucolipids

These are similar to glycolipids and are a mixture of polysaccharide and fatty acid complexes. They are found in tissues as cerebrosides and gangliosides (*see* Chapter 10); they usually give a positive PAS reaction and in frozen sections can be stained by lipid methods.

Preparation of tissue

Sections for the demonstration of carbohydrates can be prepared by the majority of the standard techniques. Freeze drying, followed by vapour fixation, gives the best results (Tock and Pearse, 1965) (*see Figure 7.2 a, b*). Frozen sections are not ideal because of the deleterious effects of freezing and thawing on localization. Paraffin sections normally give acceptable results after either formol saline or formol mercury fixation.

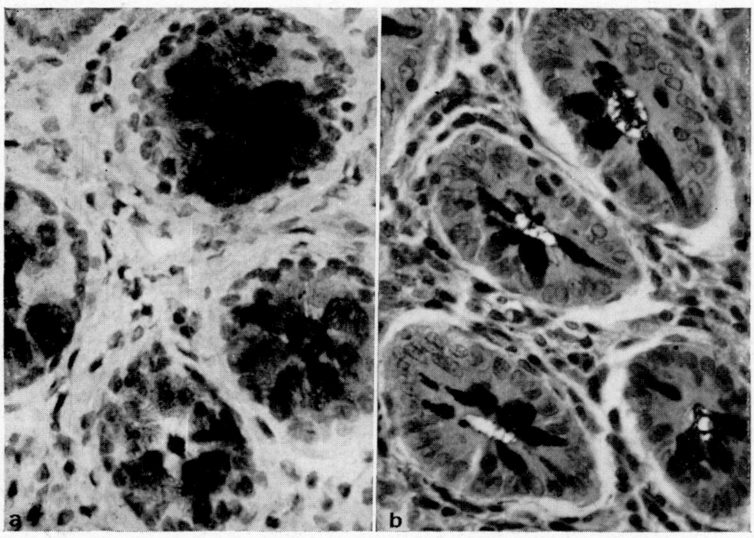

Figure 7.2a Rat colon, post-fixed cryostat section stained by PAS reaction (×600). *b Identical tissue prepared by freeze drying then stained by PAS reaction. Note the much improved localization of stained mucosubstances with this technique.* (×600)
(Reduced to two-thirds in reproduction)

There are a considerable number of methods available to demonstrate mucosubstances. Many of these techniques are relatively new and whilst being more complicated the new methods produce more accurate information. The methods listed below and to be found at the end of the chapter are a mixture of the traditional and new methods along with suitable control methods.

Mucicarmine	—Mucosubstances (variable results)	Method 18
Periodic Acid–Schiff	—Neutral mucosubstances; glycogen	Method 19
Bauer–Feulgen	—Neutral mucosubstances; glycogen	Method 16
Best's Carmine	—Glycogen	Method 17
Alcian Blue (pH 2·5)	—Acid mucosubstances	Method 22
Alcian Blue (CEC)	—Sulphated and carboxylated mucosubstances	Method 23

Dialysed Iron	—Acid mucosubstances	Method 26
Azure 'A'	—Acid mucosubstances	Method 27
Toluidine Blue	—Acid mucosubstances	Method 28
Low Iron Diamine	—Acid mucosubstances	Method 29
Alcian Blue–PAS	—Neutral mucosubstances and acid mucosubstances	Method 24
Aldehyde Fuchsin–Alcian Blue	—Sulphated and carboxylated mucosubstances	Method 25
High Diamine	—Sulphated and carboxylated mucosubstances	Method 30
'Mild' Methylation	—Sulphated mucosubstances	Method 32
Methylation and Saponification	—Carboxylated mucosubstances	Method 33
Sialidase Digestion	—Sialic acid containing carboxylated mucosubstances	Method 35
Hyaluronidase Digestion	—Hyaluronic and Choridroitin sulphate-containing mucosubstances;	Method 34
Aldehyde Blocking	—1,-2 glycol groups	Method 31

Bauer–Feulgen

Bauer (1933) suggested this method for the demonstration of glycogen. Oxidation of the glycogen is carried out with 4 per cent chromic acid, followed by staining with Schiff's reagent. Lillie (1951) pointed out that carbohydrates other than those of 1,-2 glycol groups will be over-oxidized and hence will not affect the staining. The advantage of this method is that it gives superior results on cryostat or frozen sections to the Best's Carmine method.

Best's Carmine

This method was introduced by Best (1906). It has been modified slightly over the years, but basically, the method remains the same. The mechanism of staining is unknown. It is, however, reasonably selective in staining glycogen. Mucin is also stained, but is pale in comparison to the glycogen. If difficulty is encountered, a control section incubated with diastase can be used. The method occasionally fails to work and a section known to contain glycogen should always be used as a control. The solubility of glycogen in water, according to some workers, necessitates the use of celloidin during the staining procedure; in practice, however, this is not necessary. The staining method, while ideal for the demonstration of glycogen in paraffin sections and freeze dried material, is not as satisfactory for frozen sections and to demonstrate glycogen in this type of section, it is advisable to use the Bauer—Feulgen method discussed above.

Mucicarmine method (Mayer, 1896; modified by Southgate, 1927)

This technique is an old-established method for acid-mucosubstances. It is empirical and it appears to have relatively high specificity for acid mucosubstances, although the reaction that takes place is not known. Southgate added aluminium hydroxide to the staining solution; this produced more contrast between the mucin and the background as well as making the method more reliable.

PAS reaction

This technique is the one on which much of the carbohydrate histochemistry depends, and is a method in routine use in many laboratories.

The reaction is based upon the fact that periodic acid will oxidize 1,2-glycol groups to produce aldehydes which are coloured by Schiff's reagent. The PAS reaction can be used to demonstrate a wide variety of substances, and because of this, it is necessary to use blocking techniques and controls to produce specific results whenever possible.

Oxidation

Periodic acid is the standard oxidizing agent, although it is possible to use others. The use of chromic acid in the Bauer–Feulgen technique has already been described; potassium permanganate (Casella, 1942) and lead tetra-acetate (Crippa, 1951) may be used when demonstrating mucin. Periodic acid attacks 1,2-glycols and 1,2-amino-alcohols, breaking the carbon chain and oxidizing the adjacent groups of aldehydes. An advantage of using periodic acid

TABLE 7.2
Oxidizing Agents

Oxidizing agents	*Strength*	*Solvent*	*For demonstrating*	*Reference*	*Method*
Periodic acid	0·5%	Distilled water	Carbohydrates	McManus, 1946	—
Periodic acid	1·0%	Distilled water	Carbohydrates	Mowry, 1952	19
Potassium permanganate	5%	Distilled water	Mucin	Casella, 1942	—
Lead tetra-acetate		Acetic acid	Mucin	Crippa, 1951	—
Chromic acid	4%	Distilled water	Glycogen	Bauer, 1933	16
Periodic acid	0·8%	90% Alcohol	Carbohydrates	Hotchkiss, 1948	—
Performic acid	Soln.	See p. 160	Lipids	Pearse, 1951	62
Peracetic acid	Soln.		Lipids	Lillie, 1952	—

as the oxidizing agent is that it will rarely over-oxidize the material beyond aldehydes. Oxidation is carried out for five minutes with a 0·5 per cent aqueous solution. This solution is reasonably stable, and may be used repeatedly for at least one month.

Schiff's reagent

This reagent, developed for chemical work, was introduced by Schiff in 1866. There are many modifications of the original formula and all the accepted ones give a good result. It is produced by the reaction of basic fuchsin with sulphurous acid to produce a colourless solution, fuchsin–sulphurous acid (Casselman, 1962), or, as it is more commonly known, Schiff's reagent. Sulphurous acid breaks the quinoid structure of basic fuchsin. In this state, the solution is clear, but if it is then applied to a section containing an aldehyde, the quinoid structure is restored and a coloured product is formed at the site of the aldehydes.

The preparation of Schiff's reagents can cause difficulty. Not all batches of basic fuchsin are the same and some will fail to work for unknown reasons. The instructions should be followed carefully for the type of Schiff's reagent being prepared. Most techniques call for the addition of acid to the hot distilled water-dye solution. In the author's experience, if the dye solution is too warm, a precipitate is formed, which increases on storage. Schiff's reagent should be discarded after use, as contamination can occur if it is returned to the container. It should be stored at 4°C in a dark bottle (Lhotka and Davenport, 1949), and freshly prepared each month (Pearse, 1960). With these three conditions, few problems should be encountered with the method.

Casselman (1962) stated that maximum colour intensity is reached after 10 minutes staining time, while other workers leave for 20 minutes or longer. After treatment with Schiff's reagent, many techniques indicate sulphite rinses before washing in water. [Pearse (1960) considered that for use with the PAS reaction in routine histology and histochemistry, this is not necessary.] In practice, very little difference can be detected. Two variations of Schiff's reagent are recommended: (1) de Tomasi (1936), *see* Method 20; and (2) Barger and DeLamater (1948), *see* Method 20.

Alcian Blue

This dye, whilst not being absolutely specific, is considered the most specific dye available for acid mucosubstances. As a technique in histochemistry it was introduced by Steedman (1950). It is a copper phthalocyanin dye giving a brilliant green-blue colour. It is thought that Alcian Blue stains by salt linkage to the acidic groups in acid mucosubstances. If the staining time is kept short, only acid mucosubstances will be coloured. If the pH of the Alcian Blue is altered it is possible to distinguish between some of the different acid mucosubstances. At pH 2·5 most of the acid mucosubstances are stained. By lowering the pH to 1·0 both the weakly and strongly sulphated acid mucosubstances will be demonstrated, whilst at pH 0·2 only the strongly sulphated mucosubstances will take up the stain. As Cook (1974) points out, frequently no clear cut separation of the different acid mucins can be obtained. An alternative

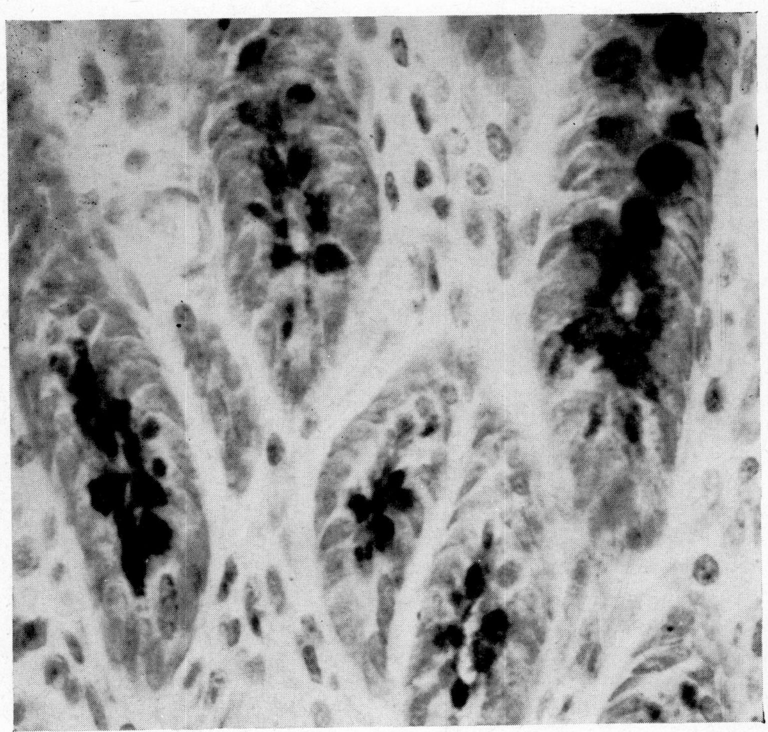

Figure 7.3 Rat colon freeze dried formalin-vapour fixed. Alcian Blue for acid mucosubstances. (×640)
(Reduced to nine-tenths in reproduction)

technique is to use the critical electrolyte concentration (CEC) method introduced by Scott and Dorling (1965). The technique is based on the assumption that electrolytes, e.g. magnesium chloride, when incorporated into the Alcian Blue staining solution will compete with Alcian Blue molecules for the reactive constituents of the acid mucosubstances. Below 0·06 mol/l magnesium chloride, both carboxylated and sulphated mucosubstances will stain; above 0·3 mol/l, only the sulphated mucosubstances will take up the Alcian Blue. The CEC technique has recently been criticised by Goldstein and Horobin (1974) on theoretical grounds. The Alcian Blue method can be combined with the PAS reaction (to distinguish between acid and neutral mucosubstances). It may also be used with aldehyde fuchsin to separate the sulphated and carboxylated mucosubstances.

Colloidal iron method

The technique to demonstrate acid mucopolysaccharides by using colloidal iron was first described by Hale (1946). This method is not specific, but gives reproducible results which are acceptable when used in conjunction with other methods.

The method depends upon the affinity of acidic-tissue components for colloidal iron at low pH levels. The acidic tissue combines with the iron, which is then demonstrated by the Prussian Blue reaction. It is necessary to stain a control slide by the Prussian Blue method alone, because of the possibility of iron already present in the section. The pH of the colloidal iron solution is important. Mowry (1958) stated that if the colloidal iron solution is below pH 1·3, the technique is more selective. Many workers have produced modifications of the original method to increase its specificity. The technique given (Method 26) is that published by Mowry (1958), after Müller (1955–56). The Colloidal Iron method is frequently used as a combination technique, e.g. with the PAS method, or using a neutral red counterstain.

Metachromatic staining

The majority of acid mucosubstances are capable of exhibiting metachromasia under the correct conditions. A number of dyes, of which Azure 'A', thionin and Toluidine Blue are the most popular, can be used. These dyes, when used in dilute solutions, will react with acid mucosubstances to produce a colour different from that of the dye itself, whilst the remaining tissue components stain the colour of the dye. The dyes given above are blue but stain acid mucosubstances red. This red staining is termed 'metachromatic' and the blue staining 'orthochromatic'. The metachromatic staining produced with these dyes is to some extent alcohol-labile, and for this reason sections should be mounted in glycerin jelly. Some workers feel that true metachromasia is only seen after dehydration through graded alcohols, whilst others recommend dehydrating through tertiary butyl alcohol. The less intense metachromatic staining is certainly removed by alcohol treatment. I feel that the sections should be examined in distilled water before mounting as well as after mounting. If the metachromatic dyes are applied to acid mucosubstances at different pH levels, it is also possible to identify separate acid mucosubstances, as the acidic strongly-sulphated mucins are positive at pH 2·0, but negative at pH 6·0. The method given on page 93 produces a reasonably alcohol-resistant metachromasia, while Toluidine Blue (Method 28) is a general technique.

Diamine methods

These were first introduced into histochemistry by Spicer (1961, 1965); N.N'dimethyl-phenyl-enediamine-dihydrochloride can be used to demonstrate a number of different mucins. The methods involve the oxidation of a mixture of the meta and para forms of the above salt by ferric chloride to form a black substance which is selectively bound to certain mucosubstances. When the diamine salt is used in low concentrations (low diamine method), most sialomucins and sulphated mucosubstances stain. At a higher concentration of the diamine salts (high diamine method) only the sulphated mucosubstances are demonstrated. Both methods are followed by staining with Alcian Blue at pH 2·5 to show non-sulphated acid mucosubstances.

Table 7.3

Acid Mucosubstances

Acid mucosubstance	*Content*	*Sites*	*Staining results*					
			Alcian Blue pH 0·5	*Alcian Blue* pH 2·5	*Azure* 'A' pH 2·0	*Azure* 'A' pH 6·0	*PAS*	*Digestion techniques*
Sulphated								
Connective tissue	Strongly acidic	Skin cartilage	Blue	Weak+ or neg	Red	NEG	NEG	'Active' methylation
Epithelial	Weakly acidic	Colonic goblet cells	Weak +	Blue	Red	Weak	Weak	'Active' methylation
Epithelial	Strongly acidic	Bronchial serious glands	Blue	Weak+ or neg	Red	NEG	Red	'Active' methylation
Non-Sulphated (carboxylated)								
Connective tissue	Hexuronic acid-rich	Synovium, umbilical cord	NEG	Blue	NEG	Red	NEG	Hyaluronidase
Epithelial	Sialomucins	Salivary, bronchial glands	NEG	Blue	NEG	Red	Red	Sialidase
Epithelial	Enzyme resistant sulphate-containing	Duodenal goblet cells	NEG	Blue	NEG	Red	Red	Sulphuric acid hydrolysis

BLOCKING AND ENZYME METHODS

These techniques are employed in histochemical techniques for mucosubstances to improve the specificity of the method or to realize more information. These control techniques are divided into two groups:

(i) *Blocking*—This is a method in which a 'blocking' agent will combine with a tissue element chemically to prevent a colour reaction taking place with a dye solution. In this situation the presence of a reacting radical can be shown by its failure to stain in one section, whilst staining in a parallel section without the blocking agent. These blocking techniques can be either 'irreversible' or 'reversible'. The first type of reaction will permanently destroy the reactive groups within the section. The second will temporarily block the reactive groups by formation of chemical derivatives; this type of effect can be reversed by using suitable chemical solutions. An example of blocking techniques is the aldehyde blocking in the Periodic Acid–Schiff reaction.

(ii) *Enzyme digestion methods*—These techniques are used where it is known that an enzyme will digest specific acid mucosubstances. Two sections are stained, one after the enzyme treatment and one with no treatment. This should show the specific substance by its disappearance from the treated section. Neither the blocking nor the digestion techniques are infallible; with the enzyme methods failure is often due to the use of impure enzymes and for this reason suitable positive and negative controls should be used.

Use of controls

The necessity of using controls with blocking and enzyme methods is perhaps obvious, but it is a point that is frequently overlooked. Cook (1972) discussed the matter of suitable controls in detail; he advocated the use of positive and negative controls along with the test section. Negative controls are required in the case of non-specific reactivity. To prevent this, along with the test section, a duplicate test section and a second positive control should be employed. These two sections will pass through all the reagents except the actual blocking agent or enzyme, including any buffers and solvents used. Positive controls are sections of tissue known to contain the mucosubstance that is to be demonstrated. They are treated in a similar manner to the test section. In all, Cook recommends that as well as the 'test section' the three controls discussed above should be used.

BLOCKING TECHNIQUES

Blocking of aldehydes

This can be carried out by using a number of different methods. Treatment with acetic anhydride will block 1:2 glycol groups by acetylation. This technique is reversible by treatment with potassium hydroxide (saponification). Method 31 (Lillie, 1965; McManus and Cason, 1950) uses three sections. A negative result with the test section with this method indicates that 1:2 glycol groups were originally responsible for the colouration of Schiff's reagent.

Methylation

This technique can be used to block one or more of the reactive groups of acid mucosubstances. The method uses a methanol–hydrochloric acid solution. Spicer (1960) divided the method into 'mild' when used at 37°C for 4 hours, and 'active' when employed at 60°C for 4 hours. Using mild methylation, only carboxyl groups are blocked, by forming methyl esters. In using 'active' methylation at 60°C, all carboxyl and sulphate esters are blocked; the carboxyl groups are methylated whilst the sulphate groups are hydrolyzed. This situation shows both reversible blocking, for the treatment with a strong alkali will restore the staining characteristics of the carboxyl groups, but the sulphate groups being hydrolyzed are irreversibly blocked. The methylation methods given as methods 32 and 33 are those from Spicer (1960).

Saponification

This is the restoration of the reactive carboxyl groups after methylation. 1 per cent potassium hydroxide in 70 per cent alcohol is usually used. The method is of doubtful value since it is known that false positive staining and false negativity are frequent after saponification (Cook, 1974).

Sulphation

This is the technique of introducing sulphate esters into mucosubstances to enable a subsequent reaction with metachromatic dyes. Lewis and Grillo (1959) described a method for sulphating glycogen.

ENZYME DIGESTION METHODS

Three enzymes are commonly used in the elucidation of acid mucosubstances. The first, diastase, has been considered in the discussion of glycogen. The other enzymes are hyaluronidase and sialidase.

Hyaluronidase

This enzyme will digest hyaluronic acid and the chondroitin sulphates A and C. For routine purposes testicular hyaluronidase is used for the digestion techniques. It is normally used as a 0·1 per cent solution in phosphate buffer.

Sialidase

Sialidase (neuraminidase) is used to digest the majority of sialic acid-containing mucosubstances. Tissue sections are incubated for 18 hours in the enzyme solution. Calcium chloride is included as an activator for the enzyme. Following treatment the sections are stained by Alcian Blue (pH 2·5). As indicated earlier some sialomucins are resistant to this enzyme digestion; however sulphuric acid hydrolysis will block both forms of sialic acids.

METHOD 16

Glycogen: Bauer–Feulgen Method (Bauer, 1933)

Reagents required

(1) Chromium trioxide
(2) Schiff's reagent
(3) Sodium metabisulphite
(4) Hydrochloric acid
(5) Distilled water

Staining solutions

(1) *Oxidizing solution (4 per cent chromic acid)*

Chromium trioxide	4 g
Distilled water	100 ml

(2) *Schiff's reagent (see* page 87)

(3) *Sulphurous acid rinse*

10 per cent sodium metabisulphite	5·0 ml
Hydrochloric acid	5·0 ml (*see* page 325)
Distilled water	90 ml

Sections

This method is recommended for the demonstration of glycogen in frozen sections (cryostat, etc.).

Staining method

(1) Bring all sections to water	
(2) Place in solution (1) (chromic acid)	30 min
(3) Wash well in tap water	10 min
(4) Place sections in Schiff's reagent (solution 2)	15 min
(5) Transfer to solution (3) (sulphurous acid rinse)	2 min
(6) Transfer to fresh solution (3) (sulphurous acid rinse)	2 min

(7) Transfer to fresh solution (3) (sulphurous acid rinse) 2 min
(8) Wash in tap water 5 min
(9) Counterstain in haematoxylin 2–5 min
(10) Wash in tap water 5 min
(11) Dehydrate through graded alcohols to xylene
(12) Mount in DPX

Results

Glycogen: red
Nuclei: blue

Remarks

This technique gives the best result for demonstrating glycogen in frozen sections. Other carbohydrate substances are over-oxidized and are not stained.

METHOD 17

Glycogen: Best's Carmine method (Best, 1905)

Reagents required

(1) Carmine
(2) Potassium carbonate
(3) Potassium chloride
(4) Ammonia (·880)
(5) Methyl alcohol
(6) Absolute alcohol
(7) Distilled water

Preparation of solutions

(1) *Best's carmine stock solution*

Carmine	2 g
Potassium carbonate	1 g
Potassium chloride	5 g
Distilled water	60 ml

Boil the solution gently for 5 min, allow to cool, then filter. To the filtrate add 20 ml of ammonia (·880).

(2) *Best's carmine staining solution*

Stock solution	12 ml
Ammonia (·880)	18 ml
Methyl alcohol	18 ml

(3) *Best's differentiator*

Absolute alcohol	8 ml
Methyl alcohol	4 ml
Distilled water	10 ml

Sections

Paraffin sections
Freeze dried sections (recommended)
Frozen sections

Staining method

(1)	Bring sections from xylene to 70 per cent alcohol	
(2)	Place sections in 1 per cent celloidin*	5 min
(3)	Transfer sections to tap water	
(4)	Stain in alum haematoxylin	10–15 min
(5)	Wash briefly in tap water	
(6)	Stain in solution (2) (Best's carmine staining solution)	30 min
(7)	No water, rinse sections in 2 changes of solution (3)	20 s
(8)	Wash sections in 90 per cent alcohol	briefly
(9)	Place in absolute alcohol	
(10)	Transfer to xylene	
(11)	Mount in DPX	

Results

Glycogen: red
Nuclei: blue.

* Optional.

METHOD 18

Mucosubstances: Mucicarmine (Mayer, 1896; modified by Southgate, 1927)

Reagents required

(1) Carmine
(2) Aluminium hydroxide
(3) Aluminium chloride (anhydrous)
(4) Absolute alcohol
(5) Distilled water

Staining solution

Carmine	1 g
Aluminium hydroxide	1 g
Distilled water	50 ml
Absolute alcohol	50 ml
Shake, then add	
Aluminium chloride	500 mg

The solution is boiled for 3 min. It is advisable to use a 250 ml flask. After boiling, the solution is allowed to cool to room temperature and is made up to the original volume with 50 per cent alcohol and filtered. This solution is stable for about 12 months. For use, dilute 1:4 with distilled water. Store at 4°C.

Sections

All types

Staining method

(1) Bring sections to tap water	
(2) Stain nuclei with haematoxylin	10 min
(3) Wash in tap water	5 min
(4) Differentiate in 1 per cent acid alcohol	
(5) Wash in running tap water	5 min
(6) Stain in staining solution	30 min
(7) Wash in tap water	2 min
(8) Dehydrate through graded alcohols to	
(9) Xylene, and mount in DPX	

Results

Mucosubstances: red
Nuclei: blue.

METHOD 19

Carbohydrates: PAS reaction

Reagents required

(1) Periodic acid
(2) Basic fuchsin
(3) Hydrochloric acid
(4) Sodium metabisulphite
(5) Activated charcoal
(6) Distilled water

Solution 1—Periodic acid 1 per cent

Periodic acid	1 g
Distilled water	100 ml

Solution 2—Schiff's reagent (de Tomasi) (see page 87).

Sections

All types

Staining method

(1) Bring all sections to water	
(2) Place sections in (periodic acid) solution (1)	5–8 min

(3) Wash in tap water 3 min
(4) Wash in distilled water 1 min
(5) Treat with Schiff's reagent (solution 2) 15 min
(6) Wash in tap water 10 min
(7) Counterstain in haematoxylin
(8) Wash in tap water 5 min
(9) Differentiate if necessary in 1 per cent acid alcohol
(10) Wash in tap water 5 min
(11) Dehydrate through graded alcohols to xylene and
(12) Mount in DPX

Results

PAS-positive material: magenta
Nuclei: blue.

METHOD 20

Preparation of Schiff's reagents

(1) *de Tomasi* (1936)

Dissolve 1 g of basic fuchsin in 200 ml of distilled water and boil. Shake the solution for 5 min and allow to cool. When the temperature is down to 50°C, filter and to the filtrate add 20 ml N-hydrochloric acid. Cool to 25°C and add 1 g of sodium metabisulphite. Store the solution in the dark, overnight. To this solution, add 2 g of activated charcoal and shake for 1 min. Filter and store the filtrate in a dark bottle at 4°C.

Note. Always allow the aliquot of solution to reach room temperature before use and discard it after use to avoid contamination of stock solution.

(2) *Barger and DeLamater* (1948)

Dissolve 1 g of basic fuchsin in 400 ml of boiling distilled water, cool to 50°C and filter. To the filtrate add 1 ml of thionyl chloride. Stand in the dark overnight. Add 2 g of activated charcoal, shake well and filter. Store the filtrate at 4°C in a dark bottle.

Note. Allow the aliquot of Schiff's solution to reach room temperature before use and discard it after use.

METHOD 21

Diastase digestion for glycogen (Lillie, 1949)

Reagents required

(1) Malt diastase

(2) 0·02 M Phosphate buffer, pH 6·0
(3) Sodium chloride

Preparation of solution

Malt diastase	500 mg
0·02 M Phosphate buffer, pH 6·0	50 ml
Sodium chloride	400 mg

Staining method

(1) Bring all sections down to water
(2) Treat sections with diastase solution for 1 h at 22°C or 40 min at 37°C
(3) Rinse in water
(4) Employ histochemical method

Remarks

(1) This digestion should be carried out before celloidinization of the sections
(2) Human saliva may also be used, instead of malt diastase, for the digestion of glycogen.

METHOD 22

Acid mucosubstances: Alcian Blue (Steedman, 1950) modified

Reagents required

(1) Alcian Blue
(2) 3 per cent acetic acid
(3) 10 per cent sulphuric acid
(4) Mayer's carmalum

Staining solutions

Alcian Blue pH 2·5

Alcian Blue	1 g
3 per cent acetic acid	100 ml

Alcian Blue pH 0·2

Alcian Blue	1 g
10 per cent sulphuric acid	100 ml

Sections

All types, freeze dried recommended

Staining method

(1) Bring all sections to water
(2) Stain in Alcian Blue solution of choice 5 min

(3) Wash briefly in distilled water
(4) Counterstain in Mayer's carmalum — 2 min
(5) Wash in tap water
(6) Dehydrate through graded alcohols to xylene
(7) Mount in DPX

Results

Alcian Blue pH 0·2: strongly sulphated acid mucosubstances blue
Alcian Blue pH 2·5: most acid mucosubstances blue

Remarks

(1) Alcian Blue stains should be filtered before use
(2) Counterstaining should always be light
(3) For critical staining see Method 23.

METHOD 23

Acid mucosubstances: Alcian Blue (CEC Method) Scott and Dorling (1965)

Reagents required

(1) Alcian Blue
(2) Acetate buffer pH 5·8
(3) Magnesium chloride

Stock Alcian Blue stain

Alcian Blue	50 mg
Acetate buffer pH 5·8	100 ml

This stock solution is used with the necessary amount of magnesium chloride. To obtain the following molarities the stated figure of magnesium chloride should be added to 100 ml of the stock Alcian Blue solution.

0·6 M = 1·2 g, 0·3 M = 6·1 g, 0·5 M = 10·15 g, 0·7 M = 14·2 g, 0·9 M = 18·3 g.

Sections

All types

Staining method

(1) Bring all sections to water
(2) Stain in Alcian Blue solution for at least 4 hours, overnight preferably
(3) Rinse in distilled water
(4) Dehydrate through graded alcohols to xylene
(5) Mount in DPX

Results

Positive with 0·06 M carboxyl and sulphated mucosubstances
Positive with 0·3 M weakly and strongly sulphated mucosubstances
Positive with 0·5 M strongly sulphated mucosubstances
Positive with 0·7 M highly sulphated connective tissue mucins
Positive with 0·9 M keratan sulphate only

Remarks

(1) Background staining can occur with the low molarity solutions
(2) For comments of specificity of method *see* page 78
(3) Counterstain is optional.

METHOD 24

Alcian Blue—PAS method (Mowry, 1956)

Reagents required

(1) Alcian Blue solution
(2) 1 per cent periodic acid
(3) Schiff's reagent

Staining solutions

(1) Alcian Blue pH 2·5. *See* solution on page 88
(2) Schiff's reagent. *See* page 87.

Staining method

(1)	Bring all sections to water	
(2)	Stain in Alcian Blue solution	5 min
(3)	Wash in distilled water	
(4)	Oxidize in 1 per cent periodic acid	5 min
(5)	Wash well in distilled water	
(6)	Place in Schiff's reagent	8 min
(7)	Wash well in running tap water	10 min
(8)	Counterstain lightly in Mayer's haematoxylin if required	
(9)	Differentiate in 1 per cent acid alcohol, blue, etc.	
(10)	Dehydrate through graded alcohols to xylene	
(11)	Mount in DPX	

Results

Acid mucosubstances: blue
Neutral mucosubstances: red
Mixtures: purple

Remarks

(1) A good method to separate acid and neutral mucosubstances

(2) As Cook (1974) states, the method if negative can be taken to mean that a given substance is unlikely to be a mucosubstance.

METHOD 25

Sulphated and carboxylated mucosubstances: Aldehyde Fuchsin–Alcian Blue (Spicer and Meyer, 1960)

Reagents required

(1) Basic fuchsin
(2) Conc. HCl
(3) Paraldehyde
(4) Alcian Blue
(5) Acetic acid

Staining solutions

(1) *Aldehyde fuchsin stain*

Basic fuchsin	1 g
60 per cent alcohol	100 ml
Hydrochloric acid (conc.)	1 ml
Paraldehyde	2 ml

Dissolve the dye in the alcohol, then add the acid and paraldehyde. Leave until stain is deep purple, 3–4 days.

(2) *Alcian Blue*

Alcian Blue	1 g
3 per cent acetic acid	100 ml

Staining method

(1) Bring all sections to water
(2) Stain in aldehyde fuchsin stain — 20 min
(3) Rinse well in 70 per cent alcohol
(4) Wash in tap water
(5) Stain in Alcian Blue solution — 5 min
(6) Wash in tap water
(7) Dehydrate through graded alcohols to xylene
(8) Mount in DPX

Results

Strongly sulphated mucosubstances: deep purple
Weakly sulphated mucosubstances: purple
Carboxyl mucosubstances: blue

Remarks

(1) Aldehyde fuchsin is not specific for sulphated mucosubstances

(2) The aldehyde fuchsin is a capricious stain that deteriorates and should be replaced every 2 months. Store at 4°C.

METHOD 26

Acid mucosubstances: Dialysed Iron method (Hale, 1946; modified by Müller, 1955; and Mowry, 1958)

Reagents required

(1) Ferric chloride
(2) Acetic acid
(3) Hydrochloric acid
(4) Potassium ferrocyanide
(5) Distilled water

Preparation of solutions

(1) *Stock colloidal iron solution*

29 per cent ferric chloride	2·2 ml
Distilled water	125 ml

Pour the ferric chloride into boiling distilled water and stir well. The solution will turn dark red; at this point it is removed from the heat and allowed to cool. It is important that the solution is boiling when the ferric chloride is added.

(2) *Staining solution of collodial iron*

Glacial acetic acid	5 ml
Distilled water	15 ml
Stock colloidal iron solution	20 ml

(3) *Acid ferrocyanide mixture*

Potassium ferrocyanide	2 g
Hydrochloric acid (conc.)	2 ml
Distilled water	98 ml

The potassium ferrocyanide is dissolved in the distilled water and the hydrochloric acid is added to this solution.

Sections

All types

Staining methods

(1) Bring all sections to water
(2) Rinse in 12 per cent acetic acid
(3) Stain in solution (2), collodial iron solution — 1 h
(4) Rinse in 12 per cent acetic acid, 4 changes, 3 min each
(5) Treat section with acid ferrocyanide, solution (3) — 20 min
(6) Wash in distilled water

(7) Wash in tap water 5 min
(8) Counterstain in Mayer's Carmalum 10 min
(9) Wash in tap water
(10) Dehydrate through graded alcohols
(11) To xylene and mount in DPX

Results

Acid mucosubstances: bright blue
Nuclei: red

Remarks

Some workers prefer to use the Feulgen reaction as a counterstain.

METHOD 27

Acid mucosubstances: Azure 'A' (Hughesdon, 1949)

Reagents required

(1) 0·2 per cent Azure A (aqueous)
(2) 5 per cent oxalic acid (aqueous)
(3) 1 per cent potassium permanganate (aqueous)
(4) 0·2 per cent uranyl nitrate (aqueous)

Sections

All types

Staining method

(1) Bring all sections to water
(2) Treat with 1 per cent potassium permanganate 5 min
(3) Wash in tap water
(4) Bleach in 5 per cent oxalic acid
(5) Wash well in running tap water
(6) Stain in 0·2 per cent Azure A 5 min
(7) Rinse briefly in water
(8) Differentiate in 0·2 per cent uranyl nitrate 10–20 s
(9) Wash briefly in water, blot dry
(10) Dehydrate through graded alcohols to xylene
(11) Mount in DPX

Results

Acid mucosubstances: purple-red
Nuclei, backgrounds: blue

Remarks

The staining obtained with this method is reasonably alcohol-fast.

METHOD 28

Acid mucosubstances: Toluidine Blue method (Kramer and Windrum, 1955)

Reagents required

(1) Toluidine Blue
(2) Absolute alcohol
(3) Distilled water

Staining solution

Toluidine Blue	100 mg
Absolute alcohol	30 ml
Distilled water	70 ml

Sections

Frozen sections (formalin-fixed)
Cryostat post-fixed
Cryostat pre-fixed
Paraffin sections
Freeze dried

Staining method

(1) Bring all sections to water
(2) Stain in Toluidine Blue solution 15 min
(3) Wash one section in distilled water and mount in glycerin jelly
(4) Rinse another section in 95 per cent alcohol
(5) Rinse in absolute alcohol
(6) Clear in xylene and mount in DPX

Results

Acid mucosubstances: pink (metachromatic)
Nuclei: blue

Remarks

A comparison is made between the two slides, *see* text.
Azure A can be used instead of Toluidine Blue and is preferred by some workers.

METHOD 29

Low Iron Diamine method for acid mucosubstances (Spicer 1965; Leppi and Spicer, 1967)

Reagents required

N,N-dimethyl-m-phenylenediamine dihydrochloride

N,N-dimethyl-p-phenylenediamine dihydrochloride
40 per cent ferric chloride
3 per cent acetic acid
Alcian Blue

Preparation of staining solutions

(1) *Diamine solution*

N,N-dimethyl-m-phenylenediamine dihydrochloride	30 mg
N,N-dimethyl-p-phenylenediamine dihydrochloride	5 mg

Dissolve the salts in 50 ml of distilled water and add 0·5 ml of 40 per cent ferric chloride. It must be freshly prepared or the method will fail.

(2) *Alcian Blue pH 2·5* (*see* page 88)

Sections

All types

Staining method

(1) Bring sections to water	
(2) Stain in diamine solution	18 h
(3) Rinse rapidly in distilled water	
(4) Stain in Alcian Blue solution	5 min
(5) Briefly rinse in tap water	
(6) Dehydrate through graded alcohols	
(7) Mount in DPX	

Results

Sulphated and non-sulphated mucosubstances: black
Some acidic non-sulphated mucosubstances: blue

Remarks

Neutral mucosubstances may be demonstrated by this method and by the high diamine method, if an additional section is oxidized in 1 per cent periodic acid followed by a wash in tap water before staining in the diamine solution. Neutral mucosubstances in the oxidized section will stain purple-grey.

METHOD 30

High Iron Diamine method for sulphated mucosubstances (Spicer, 1965; Leppi and Spicer, 1967)

Reagents required

(1) N,N-dimethyl-m-phenylenediamine dihydrochloride

(2) N,N-dimethyl-p-phenylenediamine dihydrochloride
(3) 40 per cent ferric chloride
(4) Alcian Blue
(5) Acetic acid

Preparation of solutions

(1) *Diamine solution*

N,N-dimethyl-m-phenylenediamine dihydrochloride	120 mg
N,N-dimethyl-p-phenylenediamine dihydrochloride	20 mg

Dissolve the salts in 50 ml of distilled water then add 40 per cent ferric chloride 1·4 ml. Check pH of solution which should be 1·5. The solution must be freshly prepared.

(2) *Alcian Blue solution pH 2·5* (*see* page 88)

Sections

All types

Staining method

(1) Bring all sections to water
(2) Stain in diamine solution for 18 h
(3) Wash in water
(4) Stain in Alcian Blue solution for 5 min
(5) Wash in water
(6) Dehydrate through graded alcohols to xylene
(7) Mount in DPX

Results

Sulphated mucosubstances: black
Non-sulphated mucosubstances: blue

METHOD 31

Blocking of Aldehyde Groups by Acetylation (Lillie, 1965, McManus and Cason, 1950)

Reagents required

(1) Acetic anhydride
(2) Dry pyridine
(3) Potassium hydroxide
(4) Periodic acid
(5) Schiff's reagent

Preparation of solutions

(1) *Acetic anhydride solution*

Acetic anhydride	16 ml

Dry pyridine	24 ml

(2) *Potassium hydroxide solution*

Potassium hydroxide	1 g
Absolute alcohol	70 ml
Distilled water	30 ml

(3) *1 per cent periodic acid*

(4) *Schiff's reagent* (*see* page 87)

Sections

All types

Suitable control sections

Previous known positive control

Method

(1) Bring three sections to water, label 1, 2 and 3
(2) Place sections numbered 1 and 2 in acetic anhydride solution 1–24 h. Leave section 3 in distilled water
(3) Rinse sections 1 and 2 in distilled water
(4) Treat section labelled 2 in KOH solution for 30 min
(5) Rinse section 2 in distilled water
(6) Apply Schiff's routine to all sections (*see* Method 19)

Results

A positive result with sections numbered 1 and 3 with a negative result with no. 2 indicates the reaction was due to 1:2 glycol groups.

METHOD 32

'Mild'/Methylation for Blocking of Carboxylated Mucins (Spicer, 1960)

Reagents required

(1) Hydrochloric acid
(2) Methanol
(3) Alcian Blue
(4) Acetic acid

Preparation of staining solutions

(1) *Methylation solution*

Methanol	50 ml
Hydrochloric acid (conc.)	0·4 ml

(2) *Alcian Blue pH 2·5* (*see* page 88)

Sections

All types

Suitable control sections

2 previous known positive controls sections and 2 test sections

Method

(1) Bring two positive and two control sections to water
(2) Treat one positive and one control section with methylation solution at 37°C for 4 h. Leave other two sections in distilled water at 37°C for 4 h
(3) Wash all sections in tap water
(4) Stain in Alcian Blue solution 5 min
(5) Wash in tap water
(6) Dehydrate through graded alcohols to xylene and
(7) Mount in DPX

Results

Non-sulphated carboxylated mucosubstances: unstained
Sulphated mucosubstances: blue

Remarks

Untreated positive control should be stained.

METHOD 33

Methylation and Saponification—Alcian Blue for carboxy lated mucosubstances (Spicer and Lillie, 1959)

Reagents required

(1) Methanol
(2) Hydrochloric acid
(3) Potassium hydroxide
(4) Alcian Blue
(5) Acetic acid

Preparation of solutions

(1) *Methylating solution* (*see* previous method, page 97)
(2) *Saponification solution*

Potassium hydroxide	1 g
Absolute alcohol	70 ml
Distilled water	30 ml

(3) *Alcian Blue solution pH 2·5* (*see* page 88)

Sections

All types

Suitable control sections

3 test sections and 3 control sections required

Method

(1) Clearly number both test and control slides 1, 2 and 3
(2) Bring all sections to 70 per cent alcohol and celloidinize
(3) Down to water
(4) Place the test and control sections numbered 1 and 2 in methylating solution at 60°C for 5 h. The sections labelled 3 are placed in distilled water at 60°C for 5 h
(5) Wash all the sections in tap water 5 min
(6) Treat sections labelled 1 with saponification solution for 30 min. Leave sections numbered 2 and 3 in 70 per cent alcohol for 30 min
(7) Wash sections in water 5 min
(8) Place in 70 per cent alcohol
(9) Remove celloidin in alcohol and ether 50:50
(10) Rinse in 70 per cent alcohol
(11) Wash in water
(12) Stain all sections in Alcian Blue solution 5 min
(13) Rinse in tap water
(14) Use suitable background counterstain
(15) Wash in water
(16) Dehydrate through graded alcohols to xylene
(17) Mount in DPX

Results

Sections numbered 1 = carboxylated mucosubstances: blue
Sections numbered 2 = sulphated and carboxylated mucosubstances: blocked, no blue staining
Sections numbered 3 = all acid mucosubstances: blue

Remarks

(1) On some occasions this method works well, on others it appears capricious
(2) During saponification sections will tend to float off the sides.

METHOD 34

Hyaluronidase digestion: Alcian Blue

Reagents required

(1) Testicular hyaluronidase
(2) Phosphate buffer pH 6·7
(3) Alcian Blue solution

Preparation of solutions

(1) *Hyaluronidase solution*
Testicular hyaluronidase (600 units/mg) 10 mg

Phosphate buffer pH 6·7 10 ml (*see* page 327)

(2) *Alcian Blue solution either pH 2·5 or pH 0·5* (*see Remarks*)

Sections

All types

Suitable control sections

Known positive containing hyaluronic acid or chondroitin sulphates

Staining method

(1) Bring two test and two control sections to distilled water

(2) Treat one test and one control section with hyaluronidase solution at 37°C for 3 h. The other two sections are placed in buffer solution only, at 37°C for 3 h

(3) Wash all sections in water

(4) Stain in Alcian Blue solution 5 min

(5) Wash in water

(6) Counterstain in Mayer's Carmalum 5 min

(7) Wash in water

(8) Dehydrate through graded alcohols to xylene

(9) Mount in DPX

Results

Hyaluronic acid and chondroitin sulphates: negative
Other acid mucosubstances: blue
Nuclei: red

Remarks

(1) Loss of staining in the test section after digestion compared with the section incubated in buffer only indicates the presence of one or more of the hyaluronidase labile mucosubstances.

(2) If Alcian Blue at pH 0·5 is employed, any highly sulphated mucosubstances will be shown.

METHOD 35

Sialidase digestion: Alcian Blue (Spicer *et al.*, 1962)

Reagents required

(1) Sialidase
(2) Acetate buffer pH 5·5
(3) Calcium chloride
(4) Alcian Blue solution

Preparation of solutions

(1) *Sialidase*

Neuraminidase available ready prepared from Koch-Light Ltd.	1 ml
Acetate buffer, pH 5·5	4 ml
Calcium chloride	50 mg

(2) *Alcian Blue solution pH 2·5* (See page 88)

Sections

All types

Suitable control sections

Known positive containing sialic acid

Staining method

(1) Bring 2 test and 2 control sections to water

(2) Treat 1 test and 1 control section with sialidase solution at 37°C for 18 h. Incubate the other 2 sections with buffer solution only at 37°C for 18 h

(3) Wash well in tap water

(4) Stain in Alcian Blue pH 2·5 for 5 min

(5) Wash in water

(6) Counterstain in Mayer's Carmalum

(7) Wash in water

(8) Dehydrate through graded alcohols to xylene and

(9) Mount in DPX

Results

Sialidase labile sialomucins: unstained
Other acid mucosubstances: blue
Nuclei: red

REFERENCES

Barger, J. D. and De Lameter, E. D. (1948). *Science* **108,** 121
Bauer, H. (1933). *Z. Mikrosk. anat. Forsch.* **33,** 143
Best, F. (1906). *Z. Wiess Mikrosk.* **23,** 319
Casella, C. (1942). *Anat. Anz.* **93,** 289
Casselman, W. G. B. (1962). *Histochemical Technique,* London: Methuen
Cook, H. C. (1968). *J. med. Lab. Technol.* **25,** 13
— (1972). *Human Tissue Mucins (Laboratory Aid Series),* London: Butterworths
— (1974). *Manual of Histological Demonstration Techniques,* London: Butterworths
Crippa, A. (1951). *Boll. Soc. ital. Sper.* **27,** 599
Goldstein, D. J. and Horobin, R. W. (1974). *Histochem. J.* **6,** 157
Hale, C. W. (1946). *Nature, Lond.* **157,** 802
Hughesdon, P. E. (1949). *Jl. R. microsc. Soc.* **69,** 1
Jeanloz, R. W. (1960). *Arthritis Rheum.* **3,** 223

KRAMER, H. and WINDRUM, G. M. (1955). *J. Histochem. Cytochem.* **3,** 227
LAKE, B. (1970). *Histochemical J.* **2,** 441
LAMB, D. and REID. L. (1970). *J. Path.* **100,** 127
LEPPI, J. J. and SPICER, S. S. (1967). *Anat. Rec.* **159,** 179
LESKE, R. and MAYERSBACH, H. (1969). *J. Histochem. Cytochem.* **17,** 527
LEV, R. and SPICER, S. S. (1964). *J. Histochem. Cytochem.* **12,** 309
LEWIS, P. R. and GRILLO, T. A. I. (1959). *Histochemie* **1,** 391
LHOTKA, J. F. and DAVENPORT, H. A. (1949). *Stain Technol.* **24,** 237
LILLIE, R. D. (1947). *Bull. int. Ass. med. Mus.* **27,** 33
— (1949). *Anat. Rec.* **103,** 611
— (1951). *Stain Technol.* **26,** 123
— (1965). *Histopathologic Technique and Practical Histochemistry,* New York: McGraw-Hill
McMANUS, J. F. A. and CASON, J. E. (1950). *J. exp. Med.* **91,** 651
MAYER, P. (1896). *Über Schlumfärbung mit Zool Stel Neapel* **12,** 303
MEYER, K. (1953). In '*Some Conjugated Proteins*', Symposium Rutgers University, New York
— (1966). Introduction Mucopolysaccharides. *Fedn. Proc.* **25,** 1032
MOWRY, R. W. (1956). *J. Histochem. Cytochem.* **4,** 407
— R. W. (1958). *Lab. Invest.* **7,** 566
MÜLLER, G. (1955). *Acta. Histochem.* **2,** 68
PEARSE, A. G. E. (1960). *Histochemistry Theoretical and Applied.* London: Churchill Livingstone
— (1968). *Histochemistry Theoretical and Applied* Vol. 1, London: Churchill Livingstone
SCOTT, J. E. and DORLING, J. (1965). *Histochemie* **5,** 221
SOUTHGATE, H. W. (1927). *J. Path. Bact.* **30,** 729
SPICER, S. S. (1960). *J. Histochem. Cytochem.* **8,** 18
— (1961). *Amer. J. clin. Path.* **36,** 393
— (1965). *J. Histochem. Cytochem.* **13,** 211
— LEPPI, T. J. and STOWARD, P. J. (1965). *J. Histochem. Cytochem.* **13,** 599
— and LILLIE, R. D. (1959). *J. Histochem. Cytochem.* **7,** 123
— and MEYER, E. (1960). *Amer. J. clin. Path.* **33,** 453
— NEUBECKER, R. D., WARREN, L. and HENSON, J. G. (1962). *J. natn. Cancer Inst.* **29,** 963
STEEDMAN, H. F. (1950). *Q. Jl. microsc. Sci.* **91,** 477
TOCK, E. P. C. and PEARSE, A. G. E. (1965). *Jl. R. microsc. Soc.* **84,** 519
DE TOMASI, J. A. (1936). *Stain Technol.* **11,** 137

8

Proteins and Amino Acids

Proteins are the third of the components that go to make up cell cytoplasm, the other two being lipids and carbohydrates. Similar problems of identification apply to the proteins as to the other two, mainly because of the intermingling of all three components. Proteins are to be found in all cells and tissues. The actual demonstration of protein material is not difficult, but the identification of any particular protein is.

Proteins may be very simply classified as shown in Table 8.1.

TABLE 8.1

Simple proteins	*Conjugated proteins*
Albumins	Lipoproteins
Globulins	Mucoproteins
Fibrous proteins	Glycoproteins
Histones and others	Nucleoproteins

The simple proteins are the naturally occurring proteins that upon hydrolysis will yield amino acids only. These can be divided into fibrous proteins (e.g. collagen, keratin and fibrin), and globular proteins (e.g. albumin, globulin). The first group are mainly insoluble in water, but the second are freely soluble. Because of their insolubility, it is much easier to demonstrate the fibrous proteins than the globular ones.

The conjugated proteins consist of simple proteins combined with a non-protein material, for example, lipids in lipoproteins and nucleic acids in nucleoproteins.

Demonstration of fibrous proteins

The commonly occurring fibrous proteins such as collagen, reticulin, elastin, fibrin/fibrinoid and keratin are easily demonstrated using routine histopathological staining methods. All, with the exceptions of reticulin, are easily seen in haematoxylin and eosin stained sections, and are usually strongly eosinophilic.

Collagen can be demonstrated by the red acid fuchsin in the Van Gieson stain, and by certain components of the various trichrome stains. The finer fibres of reticulin are demonstrated by silver reduction methods, and elastic fibres can be stained by resorcin or orcein. Fibrin/fibrinoid, derived from circulating plasma proteins, is stained dark-blue by Mallory's PTAH method and bright red by the MSB technique developed by Lendrum *et al.* Because fibrin/fibrinoid has a high tryptophan content it can also be demonstrated in tissues by the DMAB-nitrite method of Adams (*see* page 120). Keratin has a particularly high content of the sulphur-containing amino acid, cystine, and the keratin which forms hair is particularly richly endowed with this amino acid. Mature keratin will therefore be demonstrable by the DDD or Mercury Orange methods which depend on the presence of disulphide linkages.

Methods for proteins and amino acids

The methods discussed below do not demonstrate the protein molecule as a whole, but are dependent on the presence of certain types of reactive groups or special types of linkages within the protein molecule. These groups or linkages reside within certain of the amino acids making up the protein, and so these methods enable some conclusion to be drawn about the amino acids present in the tissue section. Unfortunately this whole segment of amino-acid histochemistry is confused because of the uncertainty about the specificity of the methods used.

Histochemical reactions are available for some, but not all, of the reactive groups of the protein molecule. The groups and linkages for which histochemical methods exist are enumerated below.

(1) Protein-bound amino groups (e.g. lysine) Methods 36, 37, 38

(2) Disulphide and sulphydryl linkages (e.g. in cystine and cysteine) Methods 39, 40, 41, 42

(3) Guanidyl groups (e.g. in arginine) Method 43

(4) Indole groups (e.g. tryptophan and tryptamine) Method 44

(5) Phenyl groups (e.g. tyrosine) Methods 45, 46

Protein-bound amino groups

Amino groups of lysine, ornithine and terminal peptides cannot be demonstrated individually, but the group as a whole may be demonstrated. The simplest and most reliable methods are the Ninhydrin–Schiff method of Yasuma and Ichikawa (1953), the DNFB (dinitrofluorobenzene) method of Sanger (1945, 1950), modified by both Danielli and Burstone, and the hydroxynaphthaldehyde method of Weiss, Tsou and Seligman (1954). The DNFB method performed in the manner given in Method 37 demonstrates sulphydryl groups and the hydroxyphenyl groups of tyrosine, as well as the protein-bound amino groups. Nevertheless this does not detract from its value as a general protein stain; various blocking techniques enable the method to be used more specifically if desired.

Disulphide and sulphydryl linkages

These sulphur-containing groups are found in the amino acids cystine, cysteine and methionine. Reduction of the disulphide linkage (-S-S) will give the sulphydryl group (-S-H). Lillie, (1965) stated that great caution must be exercised when distinguishing between the two groups. The best methods available for the demonstration of the sulphydryl and disulphide groups are the dihydroxydinaphthyldisulphide method of Barrnett and Seligman (1952) (the DDD method) and the Mercury Orange method of Bennett and Watts (1958). The demonstration of disulphide groups with the former method depends upon the reduction of these groups to sulphydryl. (*See* Method 40.) Alternatively, the performic acid–alcian blue method of Adams and Sloper (1955, 1956) may be used for disulphide groups, but it is less sensitive than the others.

Guanidyl groups

The only amino acid containing the guanidyl group which is demonstrable histochemically in human tissue is arginine. The histochemical method is based on the well known Sakaguchi reaction, in which a red colour develops when arginine reacts with α-naphthol and hypochlorite in an alkaline solution. The original biochemical reaction was modified by Baker (1947) for histochemical use; the orange-red colour which develops is transient, so the preparation must be examined immediately. To obtain satisfactory results the tissue must contain a high concentration of arginine; testis is particularly rich in arginine.

Indole groups

The indole-containing amino acids which can be demonstrated histochemically are tryptophan and tryptamine. Of the many methods available the most reliable is the DMAB-nitrite method of Adams (1957). (*See Figure 8.1*). The best results are obtained using freeze dried sections which have been fixed in formalin vapour; sites of high concentration of typtophan show an intense blue colour.

Phenyl groups

The only amino acid which contains the hydroxyphenyl group and which can be demonstrated histochemically is tyrosine. Because tyrosine is such a very frequent component of almost all tissue proteins, the methods for tyrosine can be regarded as demonstrating protein in general. The histochemical methods available are the Millon reaction modified by Baker (1956), and the diazonium coupling method of Glenner and Lillie (1959).

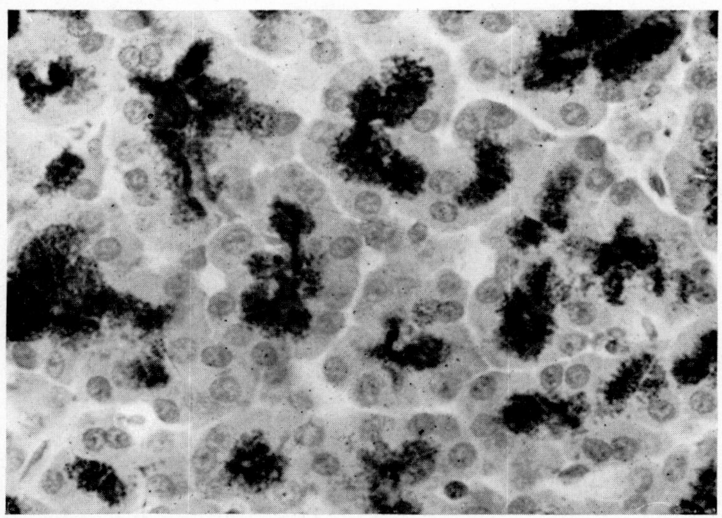

Figure 8.1 Rat pancreas. DMAB method for tryptophan. Tissue prepared by freeze drying and formalin vapour fixation. Counterstained by Mayer's carmalum (× 350).
(Reduced to seven-tenths in reproduction)

STAINING METHODS

Ninhydrin–Schiff for amino groups

Ninhydrin at neutral pH will react with α-amino groups. Yasuma and Ichikawa (1953) published the first histochemical technique that involved the use of ninhydrin. The α-amino group reacts with ninhydrin and yields an aldehyde. This is then demonstrated by Schiff's reagent. The precise nature of the reaction is not known although the results appear to be specific. Ninhydrin is normally used as an 0·5 per cent solution in absolute alcohol and at 37°C. Fixation is best carried out in neutral formol saline.

DNFB method for amino, sulphydryl and hydroxy-phenyl groups

Dinitrofluorobenzene (DNFB) has frequently been used as a reagent for protein end groups. It reacts with free amino groups in proteins, the amino groups of lysine and hydroxylysine, the hydroxyphenyl groups of tyrosine and the sulphydryl groups of cysteine. The end product of the DNFB–amino group reaction is coloured yellow, whereas the product of the DNFB–tyrosine reaction is colourless. This colourless product can be made visible by diazotization and subsequent coupling with a phenol or aromatic amine. The most suitable coupling agent is 'H-acid' (8-amino-1-naphthol-3:6-disulphonic acid) which gives an insoluble reddish-purple deposit as a final reaction product. Burstone considered that the DNFB–H-acid combination could be satisfactorily used to demonstrate primary amino groups (e.g. lysine) and hydroxy groups (e.g. tyrosine). More specific separation of staining due to amino, sulphydryl and aromatic hydroxyl groups can be obtained by using specific blocking agents before performing the DNFB reaction. This problem is dealt with by Pearse (1968).

Hydroxynaphthaldehyde methods for amino groups

Weiss, Tsou and Seligman (1954) suggested the use of 3-hydroxy-2-naphthaldehyde for the demonstration of protein-bound amino groups at pH 8·5. The primary reaction product is post-coupled with a diazonium salt at pH 7·4 to form a blue colour. Formalin fixation may partially suppress the reaction, although a positive result may still be obtained after routine formalin fixation provided that there are a large number of reactive amino groups.

The dihydroxyldinaphthyldisulphide method for S-S and S-H groups

This method, known as the DDD reaction, was published by Barrnett and Seligman (1953–1954). The method with modifications can be used to demonstrate: (1) sulphydryl groups and disulphide linkages; (2) sulphydryl groups only; and (3) disulphide linkages. The methods are basically the same. For the first method, thioglycollic acid splits the disulphide linkages and forms sulphydryl groups. These, together with any pre-existing sulphydryl groups, are then demonstrated. Both types of sulphydryl groups react with the DDD reagent and the primary reaction product, which is colourless, is then coupled with the diazonium salt fast blue B. The colour of the final reaction product is blue.

The method is considered by many authors to be very specific, but unfortunately, the intensity of the positive blue colour is not very strong. If the reaction is required for the demonstration of pre-existing sulphydryl groups only, the thioglycollic acid stage is omitted, and the disulphide linkages are not then demonstrated since the bond is not broken. To demonstrate disulphide linkages only, it is necessary to use N-ethyl maleimide to block the existing sulphydryl groups. The disulphide linkages are then reduced to sulphydryl groups and demonstrated by the method. Barrnett and Seligman (1954) stated that a weak reducing agent must be used, otherwise the N-ethyl maleimide blocking of the sulphydryl may be reversed. They recommended 10 per cent potassium cyanide for this purpose.

The Mercury Orange method for S-H Groups

This was published by Bennett and Watts (1958). The reagent used is now called Mercury Orange. It was originally called Red Sulphydryl Reagent (R.S.R.) but this name has now passed out of use. The method is said to be specific for sulphydryl groups (Bennett and Watts, 1958; Barka and Anderson, 1963). The sulphydryl groups react with Mercury Orange to form a mercaptide, which is coloured and visible with the light microscope. The colour however, is not intense.

Performic Acid–Alcian Blue method for S-S groups

This technique was introduced by Adams and Sloper (1955), (1956), for the demonstration of cysteine in paraffin sections. The technique can also be applied to cryostat and freeze dried material, the latter giving the best results of the three. The authors used Pearse's performic acid (freshly made daily), to oxidize the cysteine to cysteine sulphuric acid. This was subsequently stained using the basic dye, Alcian Blue. It is important that the pH of the Alcian Blue solution should not be less than 0·2 otherwise the localization is unsatisfactory. Adams (1965) stated that for disulphide groups (-S-S) and sulphydryl groups (-SH), the specificity and selectivity of the method are good.

Sakaguchi method for arginine

It is difficult to obtain consistent results using this technique. The intensity of the final colour is sometimes weak and is unstable, so sections must be examined immediately. Various modifications have appeared since the original paper. In his paper, Sakaguchi described the reaction of α-naphthol with arginine in the presence of strong alkali, to give a red colour. Baker's (1947) modification of this method is probably the best. Other naphthols have been tried and in some cases a more stable colour reaction can be obtained;

among these may be mentioned 8-hydroxyquinoline (Warren and McManus, 1951) and 2:4-dichloro-α-naphthol. It is important that the sections used for this method are not too thin; satisfactory results are obtained using sections of about 15 microns. They show the weak colour reaction better and are more able to withstand the technique which is very destructive to sections.

The DMAB-nitrite method for tryptophan

Histochemical techniques for the demonstration of tryptophan have been given by Glenner (1957), Adams (1957) and Glenner and Lillie (1957). The methods described by these authors employ *p*-dimethylaminobenzaldehyde (DMAB). The difference between the Glenner and Adams techniques is in the composition of the oxidizing solutions. The Glenner and Lillie method is a post-coupling technique. The method of Adams is recommended because it is easy to carry out and the results are usually reproducible. In the Adams method, the tryptophan reacts with *p*-dimethylaminobenzaldehyde to produce a compound known as β-carboline. Oxidation of this product by nitrite solution produces a blue pigment.

The Millon reaction for tyrosine

This reaction, known to biochemists for many years, has been modified for histochemical purposes. The two best and most popular methods are those of Bensley and Gersh (1933) and of Baker (1956). The method, which is specific for tyrosine, has one disadvantage in that it gives a weak colour reaction. The recommended method, and the one considered here, is a modification of Baker's (1956).

It was shown by Meyer (1864) that if mercuric chloride is applied to tyrosine in the presence of potassium nitrite in an acid solution, a red colour is produced. The various modifications of the method have centred around the choice of the mercuric salt to be used. Baker (1956) found that Folin's reagent gave him the strongest reaction (Folin and Ciocalteu, 1927; and Folin and Marenzi, 1929). In this reagent, mercuric sulphate is used with sulphuric acid. Baker (1956) also experimented with fixation, and found that formaldehyde-fixed tissue gave stronger coloration than tissues treated with other routine fixatives. To produce a satisfactory colour reaction it is necessary to heat the mercuric sulphate solution. Generally speaking, the higher the temperature, the more intense the colour. Baker heated celloidin sections to above 90°C. Other types of sections are heated to 70°C, when a reddish pink colour may be obtained at the sites of tyrosine. Alternative methods for the demonstration of tyrosine are the diazotization coupling method of Glenner and Lillie (1959) and the DNFB method of Danielli (1950).

Diazotization-coupling method for tyrosine

This method, developed by Glenner and Lillie in 1959, was based on earlier work by Lillie (1957) who claimed that prolonged nitrosation of tyrosine led to the formation of diazonium nitrates. These diazonium nitrates could subsequently be coupled with amines in alkaline solution to give coloured products. The histochemical method uses 'S-acid' (8 amino 1-naphthol-5-sulphonic acid) as the coupling amine and the incubations are carried out in the dark.

TABLE 8.2

Protein Staining Methods

Method	*Application*	*References*
Millon Reaction	Tyrosine (Phenyl group)	Millon, 1849 Bensley and Gersh, 1933 Baker, 1956
Sakaguchi	Arginine (Guanidyl group)	Sakaguchi, 1925 Baker, 1947
Mercury Orange	Sulphydryl groups	Bennett and Watts, 1958
DDD Reaction	Sulphydryl groups Disulphide linkages	Barrnett and Seligman, 1952/1953; 1954
Diazotization with H-Acid	Tyrosine (Phenyl group)	Glenner and Lillie, 1959
DMAB Method	Trytophan (Indole groups)	Adams, 1957 Glenner, 1957 Glenner and Lillie, 1957
Performic Acid–Alcian Blue	Disulphide groups	Adams and Sloper, 1955; 1956
DFNB Method	Sulphydryl groups Amino groups Tyrosine	Sanger, 1945 Sanger, 1945 Danielli, (1950) Burstone (1955)
Ninhydrin–Schiff	Amino groups	Yasuma and Itchikawa, 1952
Hydroxynaphthaldehyde	Amino groups	Weiss, Tsou and Seligman (1954)

This list is not complete, many other methods exist, but it indicates the more common techniques.

FIXATIVES

For most purposes formalin fixation is satisfactory for protein histochemistry, despite the fact that formalin modifies many of the reactive groups in the protein molecules. This does not interfere with most of the protein methods, since adequate washing in water after the formalin fixation will leave enough of the active groups sufficiently unchanged to react normally with the histochemical reagent. However, a non-formalin fixative is preferred for the hydroxy-naphthaldehyde method for amino groups. Barnett and Roth (1958) tested a series of fixatives in certain protein histochemical methods and found that only osmium tetroxide completely inhibited any of the reactions.

In general, freeze dried sections give the best staining intensity and localization in protein histochemistry, although the warm formalin vapour used for fixation tends to interfere with the reactive groups more than routine formalin solutions.

METHOD 36

Amino groups: The Ninhydrin-Schiff method (Yasuma and Itchikawa, 1953)

Reagents required

(1) Ninhydrin
(2) Absolute alcohol
(3) Schiff's reagent

Preparation of solutions

(1) *Ninhydrin 0·5 per cent solution*

Ninhydrin	500 mg
Absolute alcohol	100 ml

(2) *Schiff's reagent*
See Method 20, page 87.

Sections

Freeze dried
Paraffin sections
Cryostat unfixed
Cryostat prefixed

Suitable control tissue

Pancreas

Method

(1) Bring sections down to 70 per cent alcohol
(2) Treat with solution (1), ninhydrin, at 37°C overnight
(3) Wash in running tap water
(4) Place sections in Schiff's reagent, solution (2), for 45 min

(5) Wash well in running tap water
(6) Counterstain if required in haematoxylin
(7) Wash in tap water
(8) Dehydrate through graded alcohols to xylene and mount

Results

α-Amino groups: pink to red

Remarks

(1) 1 per cent Alloxan, also in absolute alcohol, may be used instead of 0·5 per cent ninhydrin.

(2) Control sections may be needed for other PAS-positive material.

METHOD 37

DNFB method for tyrosine, SH and NH_2 groups (Danielli, 1950; Burstone, 1955)

Reagents required

(1) 2–4 Dinitrofluorobenzene
(2) Ethyl alcohol
(3) Sodium hydrogen carbonate
(4) Sodium hydrosulphite
(5) Sodium nitrite
(6) Hydrochloric acid
(7) H-acid (8 amino-1-naphthol 3,6-disulphonic acid)
(8) Veronal acetate buffer pH 9·4

Preparation of solutions

(1) *Dinitrofluorobenzene solution*

2-4 dinitrofluorobenzene saturated in 90 per cent ethyl alcohol saturated with sodium hydrogen carbonate.

(2) *Nitrous acid*

5 per cent sodium nitrite	10 ml
2N hydrochloric acid	40 ml

(3) *'H'-acid*

H-acid saturated in 0·1M veronal acetate buffer pH 9·4 (*see* page 328).

Sections

All types

Suitable control sections

Pancreas

Method

(1) Bring sections to absolute alcohol and allow to dry in air
(2) Place in DNFB solution 2–16 h (overnight is usually ideal)
(3) Rinse in 90 per cent alcohol (3 changes) then tap water
(4) Treat with 5 per cent sodium hydrosulphite at 45°C for 30 min
(5) Wash in distilled water
(6) Treat sections with nitrous acid solution at 4°C for 30 min
(7) Wash in cold distilled water
(8) Treat with H-acid solution at 4°C for 15 min
(9) Wash in tap water
(10) Dehydrate through graded alcohols to xylene
(11) Mount in DPX

Results

A positive reaction is reddish purple

METHOD 38

Hydroxynaphthaldehyde method: NH_2 groups (Weiss, Tsou and Seligman 1954)

Reagents required

(1) 3-Hydroxy-2-naphthaldehyde
(2) Acetone
(3) Veronal acetate buffer pH 7·4, 8·5
(4) Fast Blue B

Preparation of solutions

(1) *Incubating solution*

3-Hydroxy-2-naphthaldehyde 20 mg
Acetone 20 ml
0·1 M veronal acetate buffer (pH 8·5) 30 ml

The 3-hydroxy-2-naphthaldehyde is dissolved in the acetone and the buffer added.

(2) *Diazonium salt solution*

This is prepared during the technique using Fast Blue B and veronal acetate buffer pH 7·4.

Sections

All types (non-formalin fixation preferred).

Suitable control sections

Pancreas

Method

(1) Bring sections to water

(2) Place sections in incubating solution for 1 h at room temperature

(3) Wash well in 3 changes of distilled water

(4) Place sections in 0·1M veronal acetate buffer pH 7·4, add to this solution 25 mg of Fast Blue B and shake solution. Leave sections in this solution for 5 min

(5) Wash well in tap water

(6) Dehydrate through graded alcohols to xylene

(7) Mount in DPX

Result

Reactive NH_2 groups: blue

METHOD 39

Disulphides: DDD reaction (Barrnett and Seligman, 1952; 1954)

Reagents required

(1) 2:2′-Dihydroxy-6:6′-dinaphthyl disulphide (DDD)
(2) Absolute alcohol
(3) Acetic acid
(4) Veronal acetate buffer, pH 8·5 (0·1 M)
(5) Absolute ether
(6) Fast Blue B
(7) Phosphate buffer, pH 7·4 (0·1 M)
(8) 0·5 per cent Celloidin
(9) N-Ethyl-maleimide
(10) Sodium hydroxide (0·1 N)
(11) Potassium cyanide

Preparation of solutions

(1) *Blocking solution*

N-Ethyl-maleimide	1·25 g
0·1 M phosphate buffer, pH 7·4	100 ml

(2) *Reducing agent*

Potassium cyanide	10 ml
Distilled water	90 ml

(3) *Incubating solution*

DDD reagent	25 mg dissolved in
Absolute alcohol	15 ml
0·1 M Veronal acetate buffer	35 ml

(4) *Fast Blue B solution*

Fast Blue B	50 mg
0·1 M Phosphate buffer, pH 7·4	50 ml

This solution must be freshly prepared before use.

Sections

Freeze dried
Paraffin sections
Cryostat sections

Suitable control sections

Pancreas, pituitary, skin

Method

(1) Dewax paraffin sections
(2) Bring all sections to 85 per cent alcohol
(3) Coat sections in 0·5 per cent celloidin
(4) Rinse in 70 per cent alcohol
(5) Wash in tap water
(6) Place sections in blocking agent, solution (1), at 37°C for 4 h
(7) Wash sections in 1 per cent acetic acid for 2 min
(8) Rinse in tap water
(9) Place sections in reducing agent (potassium cyanide), solution (2), for 2 h at 60°C
(10) Wash in tap water
(11) Incubate sections in solution (3), DDD reagent, at 50°C for 1 h
(12) Allow to cool to room temperature
(13) Wash sections in distilled water
(14) Place sections in distilled water, acidified with acetic acid, pH 4·5, 5 min
(15) Place sections in fresh distilled water with acetic acid, pH 4·5, 5 min

(16) Rinse sections in 70 per cent alcohol	2 min
(17) Rinse sections in 90 per cent alcohol	2 min
(18) Rinse sections in absolute alcohol	2 min
(19) Rinse sections in absolute ether	2 min
(20) Rinse sections in absolute alcohol	2 min
(21) Rinse sections in 90 per cent alcohol	2 min
(22) Rinse sections in 70 per cent alcohol	2 min
(23) Rinse sections in distilled water	2 min
(24) Stain sections in solution (4) Fast Blue B	2 min

(25) Wash sections in running tap water.
(26) Dehydrate through graded alcohols to xylene and mount.

Results

Disulphides: bluish-reddish violet

Remarks

This is an indirect result after the sulphydryl groups have been blocked by the first solution. The disulphides are reduced to sulphydryl and then demonstrated. Potassium cyanide is used as the reducing agent to avoid unblocking the sulphydryl groups.

The Fast Blue B solution must be prepared freshly just before use.

METHOD 40

Sulphydryl groups: DDD reaction (Barrnett and Seligman, 1952; 1953/4)

Reagents required

(1) 2:2′-Dihydroxy-6:6′-dinaphthyl disulphide (DDD)
(2) Absolute alcohol
(3) Acetic acid
(4) Veronal acetate buffer, pH 8·5
(5) Ether absolute
(6) Fast Blue B
(7) Phosphate buffer, pH 7·4

Preparation of solutions

(1) *Incubating solution (DDD)*

0·1 M Veronal acetate buffer, pH 8·5	35 ml
DDD reagent	25 mg dissolved in
Absolute alcohol	15 ml

(2) *Fast Blue B solution*

Fast Blue B	50 mg
Phosphate buffer pH 7·4 (0·1 M)	50 ml

This solution is freshly prepared just before use.

Sections

Freeze dried
Paraffin sections
Cryostat sections

Suitable control sections

Pancreas, pituitary, skin, trachea

Method

(1) Bring all sections to water

(2) Incubate sections in solution (1), DDD reagent, at 50°C for 1 h

(3) Allow to cool to room temperature

(4) Wash sections in distilled water

(5) Place sections in distilled water acidified with acetic acid, pH 4·5 for 5 min

(6) Repeat with fresh acidified distilled water 5 min

(7) Rinse sections in 70 per cent alcohol 2 min

(8) Rinse sections in 95 per cent alcohol 2 min

(9) Rinse sections in absolute ether 2 min

(10) Rinse sections in 95 per cent alcohol 2 min

(11) Rinse sections in 70 per cent alcohol 2 min

(12) Rinse sections in distilled water 2 min

(13) Stain section in solution (2), Fast Blue B 2 min

(14) Wash sections in running tap water

(15) Dehydrate through graded alcohols to xylene and mount in DPX

Results

Sulphydryl groups: reddish purple

Remarks

The Fast Blue B solution should be freshly prepared before use each time the method is applied.

METHOD 41

Sulphydryl groups: Mercury Orange method (Bennett and Watts, 1958)

Reagents required

(1) Mercury Orange
(2) N′:N′-Dimethyl formamide

Preparation of solution

Mercury Orange, saturated solution in N′:N′-dimethyl formamide, 40 ml

Sections

Freeze dried
Paraffin sections
Cryostat

Suitable controls

Pancreas, skin, pituitary

Method

(1) Paraffin embed material to absolute alcohol then with
(2) Frozen sections, place directly into Mercury Orange solution, 2 days
(3) Rinse rapidly in 2 changes of absolute alcohol
(4) Place sections in xylene then mount in DPX

Results

Sulphydryl groups: pale orange–orange-red

Remarks

Mercury Orange can also be dissolved in absolute alcohol.

METHOD 42

Disulphides: Performic Acid–Alcian Blue method (Adams and Sloper, 1955/56)

Reagents required

(1) Formic acid
(2) Hydrogen peroxide
(3) Sulphuric acid (conc.)
(4) Alcian Blue
(5) Absolute alcohol

Preparation of solutions

(1) *Oxidizing solution: performic acid (Pearse, 1951)*

98 per cent Formic acid	40 ml
100 vol. Hydrogen peroxide	4 ml
Sulphuric acid	0·5 ml

(2) *Staining solution*

Alcian Blue	1 g
98 per cent Sulphuric acid	2·7 ml
Distilled water	47·2 ml

Sections

Freeze dried
Paraffin
Cryostat

Suitable controls

Pituitary, skin

Method

(1) Bring all sections to water
(2) Remove excess water by blotting

(3) Place sections in oxidizing solution — 5 min
(4) Wash in tap water — 10 min
(5) Dry section by gently heating to 60°C till just dry
(6) Rinse in tap water
(7) Stain in Alcian Blue solution at room temperature for 1 h
(8) Wash in running tap water
(9) Counterstain if required
(10) Wash in tap water
(11) Dehydrate through graded alcohols to xylene and mount in DPX

Results

Disulphides: dark blue
Smaller amounts of disulphides: light blue

Remarks

The oxidizing solution must be prepared fresh daily. After preparation it should be allowed to stand for 1 h before use. The section may tend to lift after the oxidizing solution has been applied.

METHOD 43

Arginine: Sakaguchi method (1925) modified by Baker (1947)

Reagents required

(1) Sodium hypochlorite
(2) α-Naphthol
(3) Sodium hydroxide
(4) Pyridine
(5) Chloroform
(6) 70 per cent Alcohol

Preparation of solutions

Solution (1)

1 per cent Sodium hydroxide

Solution (2)

α-Naphthol	1 g
70 per cent Alcohol	100 ml

Solution (3)

Milton*	1 ml
Distilled water	99 ml

* Milton is the proprietory name of stable sodium hypochlorite.

Incubating solution (4)

Solution (1)	2 ml
Solution (2)	2 drops
Solution (3)	4 drops

Pyridine–chloroform solution (5)

Pyridine	30 ml
Chloroform	10 ml

Sections

Freeze dried
Cryostat
Paraffin sections

Suitable control sections

Testis

Method

(1) Bring all sections to water
(2) Rinse in 70 per cent alcohol
(3) Cover section with incubating solution (4), 15 min
(4) Drain and blot dry
(5) Immerse in pyridine–chloroform, solution (5), 2 min
(6) Mount in pyridine–chloroform mixture and ring coverslip

Result

Arginine: orange-red

Remarks

The slide should be looked at microscopically immediately.

METHOD 44

Tryptophan: DMAB-nitrite method (Adams, 1957)

Reagents required

(1) *p*-Dimethylaminobenzaldehyde
(2) Hydrochloric acid
(3) Sodium nitrite
(4) Acid alcohol (1 per cent)

Preparation of solutions

(1) *p-Dimethylaminobenzaldehyde*

p-Dimethylaminobenzaldehyde	5 g

Hydrochloric acid (conc.)	100 ml

(2) *Sodium nitrite*

Sodium nitrite	1 g
Hydrochloric acid (conc.)	100 ml

(3) *Acid alcohol*

Hydrochloric acid (conc.)	1 ml
70 per cent Alcohol	99 ml

Sections

Freeze dried
Paraffin sections
Cryostat

Suitable control sections

Pancreas, duodenum, pituitary

Method

(1) Bring sections to alcohol	
(2) Celloidinize in 0·5 per cent celloidin	
(3) Place sections in solution (1), DMAB	1 min
(4) Transfer sections to solution (2), sodium nitrite	1 min
(5) Wash carefully in tap water	30 sec
(6) Rinse sections in solution (3), acid alcohol	15 sec
(7) Dehydrate through graded alcohols to xylene and mount.	

Results

Tryptophan: deep blue

Remarks

This method gives good localization.

METHOD 45

Tyrosine: Millon reaction (1849), Baker (1956)

Reagents required

(1) Mercuric sulphate
(2) Sulphuric acid
(3) Sodium nitrite

Preparation of solutions

Solution (1)

Distilled water	90 ml
Sulphuric acid (conc.)	10 ml

To this solution add 10 g mercuric sulphate and heat until dissolved. Cool to room temperature and add 100 ml distilled water.

Solution (2)

Sodium nitrite	250 mg
Distilled water	10 ml

Staining solution (3)

Solution 1	10 ml
Solution 2	1 ml

Sections

Freeze dried
Paraffin sections
Cryostat sections
Celloidin sections

Suitable controls

Pancreas, duodenum

Method

(1) Bring all sections to water
(2) Place sections in a small beaker, add solution (3) and boil gently — 2 min
(3) Allow to cool to room temperature
(4) Wash sections in distilled water — 2 min
(5) Repeat wash in distilled water — 2 min
(6) Repeat wash in distilled water — 2 min
(7) Dehydrate through graded alcohols to xylene and mount in DPX

Result

Tyrosine: red, pink or yellowish red.

METHOD 46

Diazotization-coupling method for tyrosine (Glenner and Lillie 1959)

Reagents required

(1) Sodium nitrite
(2) Acetic acid
(3) 8-Amino-1-naphthol-5-sulphonic acid (S-acid)
(4) Potassium hydroxide

(5) Ammonium sulphamate
(6) Hydrochloric acid

Preparation of solutions

(1) *Incubating solution*

Sodium nitrite	6·9 g
Acetic acid	5·8 ml
Distilled water	94 ml
(2) 8-amino-1-naphthol-5-sulphonic acid	1 g
Potassium hydroxide	1 g
Ammonium sulphamate	1 g
70 per cent alcohol	100 ml

Sections

All types

Suitable control sections

Pancreas

Method

(1) Place sections in incubating medium at 4°C overnight in the dark
(2) Rinse in distilled water at 4°C
(3) Treat with solution (2) at 4°C for 1 h also in the dark
(4) Rinse in 3 changes of 0·1 NHCl 5 min each
(5) Wash in tap water 10 min
(6) Dehydrate through graded alcohols to xylene
(7) Mount in DPX

Results

Tyrosine-containing proteins: purple-red.

REFERENCES

Adams, C. W. M. (1957). *J. clin. Path.* **10,** 56
— (1965). *Neurohistochemistry,* ed. by Adams, C. W. M., netherlands: Elsevier
— and Sloper, J. C. (1955). *Lancet* **1,** 651
— — (1956). *J. Endocrinol.* **13,** 321
Baker, J. R. (1947). *Quart. Jl. microsc. Sci.* **88,** 115
— (1956). *ibid.* **97,** 161
Barka, T. and Anderson, P. J. (1963). *Histochemistry, Theory, Practice and Bibliography,* New York: Hoeber
Barrnett, R. J. and Roth, W. D. (1958). *J. Histochem. Cytochem.* **6,** 406
— and Seligman, A. M. (1952). *J. natn. Cancer Inst.* **13,** 215
— — (1953/54). *J. natn. Cancer Inst.* **14,** 769
Bennett, H. S. and Watts, R. M. (1958). *General Cytochemical Methods,* ed. by J. F. Danielli, New York: Academic Press

BENSLEY, R. R. and GERSH, I. (1933). *Anat. Rec.* **57,** 217
BURSTONE, M. S. (1955). *J. Histochem. Cytochem.* **3,** 32
DANIELLI, J. F. (1950). *Cold. Spr. Harb. Symp. quant. Biol.* **14,** 32
FOLIN, O. and CIOCALTEU, V. (1927). *J. biol. Chem.* **73,** 627
— and MARENZI, A. D. (1929). *ibid.* **83,** 89
GLENNER, G. G. (1957). *J. Histochem. Cytochem.* **5,** 297
— and LILLIE, R. D. (1957). *ibid.* **5,** 279
— — (1959). *ibid.* **7,** 416
LILLIE, R. D. (1957). *ibid.* **5,** 528
— (1965). *Histopathological Technique and Practical Histochemistry*, New York: McGraw Hill
MEYER, L. (1864). *Ann. Chim.* **132,** 156
MILLON, A. N. E. (1849). *C. r. Soc. Biol. Paris* **28,** 40
PEARSE, A. G. E. (1951). *Q. Jl. microsc. sci.* **92,** 393
— (1968). *Histochemistry, Theoretical and Applied* (Third Edition), London, Churchill
SAKAGUCHI, S. (1925). *J. Biochem. Tokyo* **5,** 25
SANGER, F. (1945). *Biochem. J.* **39,** 507
— (1950). *Cold Spr. Harb. Symp. quant. Biol.* **12,** 142
WARREN, T. N. and MCMANUS, J. F. A. (1951). *Exp. Cell Res.* **2,** 703
WEISS, L. P., TSOU, K. C.,and SELIGMAN, A. M. (1954). *J. Histochem. Cytochem.* **2,** 29
YASUMA, A. and ITCHIKAWA, T. (1953). *J. Lab. clin. Med.* **41,** 296

9

Amyloid

Amyloid enters this book under false pretences since the methods for its histological demonstration are not truly histochemical, but are probably the result of the strong affinity of the amyloid fibrils for certain dyes and metachromatic stains. Nevertheless it has become traditional to discuss amyloid in histochemical texts, and I intend to follow tradition. In the first edition of this book amyloid was discussed in the chapter on carbohydrates because at that time it was widely believed that amyloid was a mixture of carbohydrates and protein. Recent research work, mainly by Glenner *et al.* (1968), has shown that amyloid is to be more truly regarded as a protein, in most cases being composed of gamma-globulin 'light' chains arranged in a β-pleated pattern. It would seem therefore that amyloid would be best dealt with in the chapter entitled 'Proteins', but since the methods of identifying and localizing amyloid are different from other protein methods, amyloid is worthy of a small chapter on its own.

Amyloid can be deposited extracellularly in a number of organs, but mostly affects the kidney, liver, spleen and adrenals. At microscopical level amyloid is frequently found in the walls of small vessels, even in organs or tissues which do not appear to have amyloid in them macroscopically. This fact is made use of in the most reliable diagnostic test for amyloidosis, namely rectal biopsy; over 90 per cent of all patients with amyloid affecting other organs will have demonstrable amyloid within the walls of small blood vessels in the rectal mucosa and sub-mucosa. Although amyloid is usually found widespread within the body it can occasionally be confined to one site (e.g. amyloid of the heart, and amyloid confined to the stroma of a type of cancer of the thyroid gland).

Amyloid is classified into two main types:—'*primary*' *amyloid*—in which the amyloid is an isolated finding, and is not associated with the presence of any associated disease, and '*secondary*' *amyloid*—in which the amyloid is found in association with some other disease or condition.

There are many diseases with which amyloid may be associated, but they are conveniently subdivided thus:—

(a) chronic inflammatory conditions, both infective and non-infective e.g. long-standing tuberculosis or rheumatoid arthritis;

(b) tumours, the most notable example being the tumour of plasma cells, myeloma;

(c) hereditary and familial disorders, such as hereditary Portuguese neuropathy and familial Mediterranean fever, and

(d) old age, the heart being particularly frequently involved.

'Secondary' amyloid is much more common than 'primary' amyloid.

The histological demonstration of amyloid

In a formalin-fixed paraffin section amyloid appears as a homogenous material staining pink to red with eosin, and a khaki colour with Van Gieson. On a haematoxylin and eosin stained section small amounts of amyloid can easily be confused with other homogenous pink-staining material such as hyaline and old collagen. Special stains have been developed which emphasize any amyloid present. Although none of the methods is specific for amyloid, when two or three different methods are used any material which is positive by all methods can be assumed to be amyloid. The most useful methods are the following.

(1) Congo Red, viewed with bright field, polarized light and with fluorescence microscopy

(2) Thioflavine T, viewed with fluorescence microscopy

(3) Methyl Violet and Methyl Green methods.

The absolute arbiter as to whether a material is amyloid or not is the electron microscope. Amyloid has a characteristic ultrastructure, being composed of cylindrical fibrils (arranged in bundles of 2–8 fibrils in parallel orientation), each fibril being 75Å in diameter and comprising two 25Å electron dense rods separated by a 25Å wide interspace (*see Figure* 9.1).

Congo Red method (Bennhold, 1922; modified by Highman, 1946) and the Alkaline Congo Red method (Puchtler, Sweat and Levine, 1962)

Congo Red has been used for many years as a histological dye. Bennhold (1922) first described a satisfactory method for demonstrating amyloid with this dye (*see Figure* 9.2). Congo Red has a high affinity for amyloid, but will also stain collagen, elastic fibres,

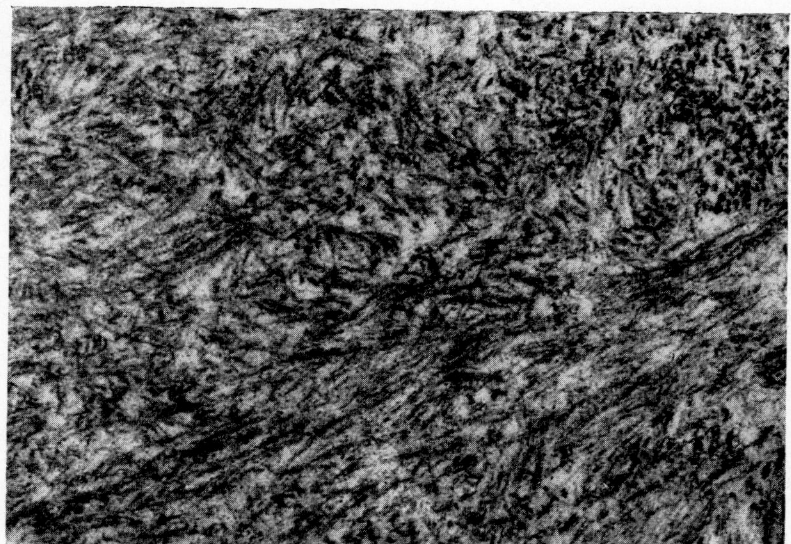

Figure 9.1 Electron micrograph of amyloid from human skin, showing characteristic fibrillary ultrastructure of amyloid. (55,000). Courtesy of Drs G. Robinson and G. Stirling.
(Reduced to two-thirds in reproduction)

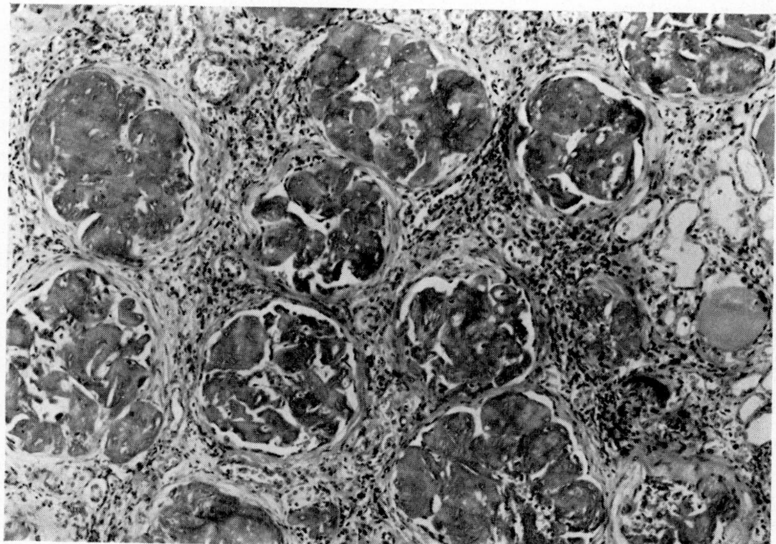

Figure 9.2 Human kidney from a case of advanced amyloidosis. The glomerular amyloid is stained by the Highman Congo Red method. (× 135)
(Reduced to two-thirds in reproduction)

and hyaline material quite strongly. Differentiation is a most important factor with this method. In the Bennhold method differentiation is rapid, sometimes too rapid, and this produces an uneven result, often leaving the dye in collagen whilst removing it from amyloid. Highman, in his modification, uses 0·2 per cent potassium hydroxide in 80 per cent alcohol as the differentiator. This enables a slower differentiation which can be controlled microscopically.

The Alkaline Congo Red method (Puchtler, Sweat and Levine, 1962) is a more time-consuming procedure, but has the advantage that differentiation is unnecessary.

Congo Red and polarized light

Amyloid, when stained with Congo Red, shows birefringence when viewed using polarized light (*see Figure* 9.3). Collagen fibres may also show birefringence, but amyloid is characteristic in that it shows apple green birefringence; collagen shows yellow birefringence. This apple green birefringence is claimed to be a specific feature of amyloid and, while this is probably not absolutely true (some proteins found in plants and insects may also show apple green birefringence),

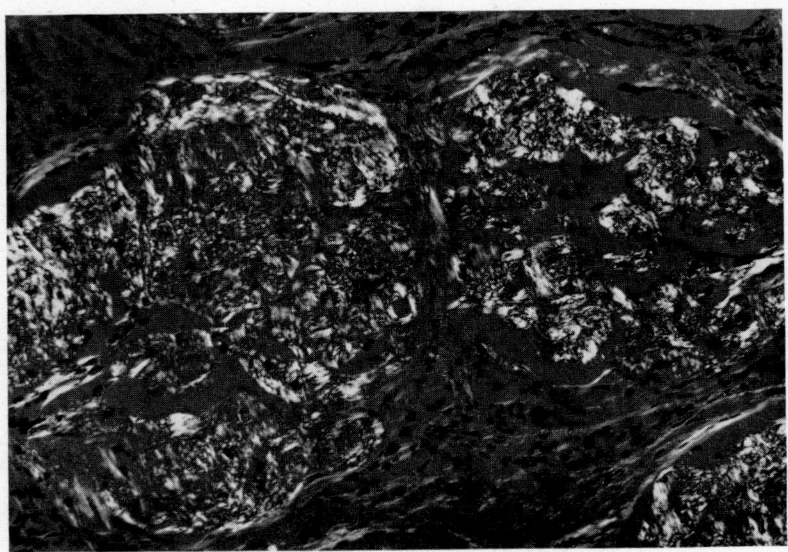

Figure 9.3 Human kidney from a case of amyloid showing amyloid birefringence after Congo Red staining. (× *340*)

(Reduced to two-thirds in reproduction)

it is sufficiently near the truth in human tissues to make this the single most specific method for identifying amyloid by light microscopy.

Congo Red with fluorescence

Amyloid, when stained with Congo Red, fluoresces. Unfortunately other congophilic material such as collagen and arterial elastic laminae, also fluoresces. This non-amyloid fluorescence can be greatly minimized by using a modification of the Congo Red staining method, as suggested by Cohen *et al.* (1959) (*see Figure* 9.4). In this method the section is stained for a very short time in dilute Congo Red and is then over-differentiated in alkaline alcohol until no colour remains, even when the section is viewed under the microscope. When the section is viewed with the fluorescent microscopy any amyloid present will still show obvious fluorescence and the fluorescence of other congophilic material will be barely discernible.

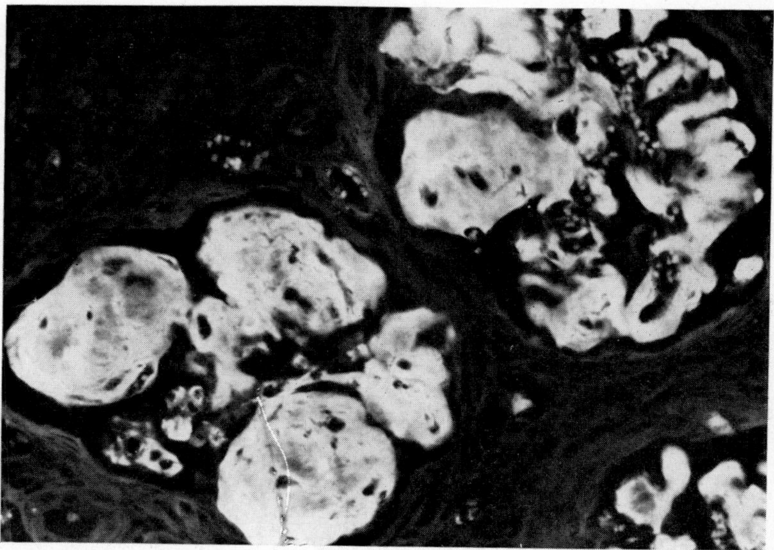

Figure 9.4 Human kidney from a case of amyloid, lightly stained by Congo Red and photographed through a fluorescence microscope. The fluorescence is orange-red. (× *325*)
(Reduced to two-thirds in reproduction)

Thioflavine T

Thioflavine T is a fluorochrome which has a particular affinity for amyloid. It was recommended by Vassar and Culling (1959) as the fluorochrome of choice for the demonstration of amyloid. The tissue section is treated with Thioflavine T and examined by fluorescence microscopy; amyloid shows brilliant silver-blue to yellow fluorescence, the colour depending on the wavelength and filters used (*see Figure* 9.5). Unfortunately there are two problems with this type of technique. First, Thioflavine T has an affinity for other tissue components, such as the juxtaglomerular apparatus in the kidney, and these structures will fluoresce brightly. Cell nuclei have an affinity for Thioflavine T and will therefore show some fluorescence; this effect can be minimized by pretreating the section with haematoxylin for a short time. This effectively masks the fluorescence of the nuclei which normally occurs after treatment with Thioflavine T. Secondly, non-specific fluorescence occurs if the section is dehydrated through alcohols containing traces of eosin, since eosin itself is fluorescent. Clean fresh alcohols and xylene must be used.

The Thioflavine T fluorescent method is probably the most sensitive detector of small amounts of amyloid, and is very useful as a 'scanning' method, but, because of its lack of specificity, it must always be used in conjunction with another method. The amyloid

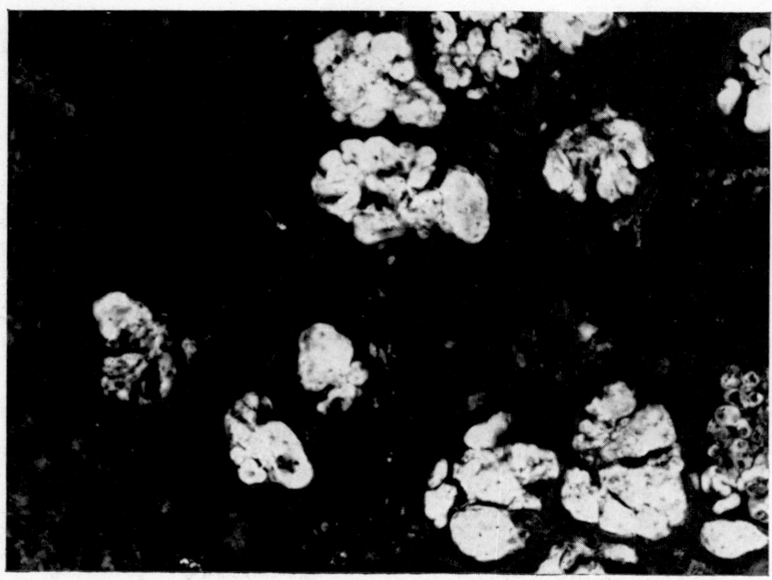

Figure 9.5 Human kidney from a case of amyloid stained by the Thioflavine T method and photographed through a fluorescence microscope. The colour of fluorescence varies according to the filters used. (× *100*)

(Reduced to seven-tenths in reproduction)

nature of any fluorescent material should be confirmed by examining an adjacent section stained with Congo Red under polarized light.

Methyl Violet and Methyl Green methods

The dye, or dye mixture, known as Methyl Violet was one of the earliest means used to stain amyloid; it was said to stain amyloid metachromatically in that it stained the amyloid a colour different from the colour of the stain itself. Methyl Violet, which is a bluish-violet solution, stains amyloid a pinkish-violet colour and the background bluish-violet. The so-called 'metachromasia' is even more apparent if the method is performed on a frozen section, when the amyloid is stained red. Differentiation is carried out with dilute acetic or formic acid. Occasionally it is difficult to obtain satisfactory differentiation without removing much of the dye from the amyloid; this is particularly likely to happen if the tissue has been in formol saline for a long time. The true mechanism of the staining of amyloid by Methyl Violet is in doubt; it is suggested that since Methyl Violet is an impure dye (Kramer and Windrum 1955) containing traces of other dyes, it is one of the impurities which stains the amyloid, and that the dye is not truly metachromatic. Methyl Violet tends to leak out of the amyloid into other tissues and into the mountant ('bleeding'); this can be minimized by using a watery mountant such as glycerin jelly or corn syrup. Even so, diffusion will still occur and sections stained by Methyl Violet must be examined immediately and are not permanent.

The Methyl Green method for amyloid (Bancroft 1967) is a suitable way of demonstrating amyloid in frozen sections and requires no differentiation. If a frozen section containing amyloid is stained with a 2 per cent aqueous Methyl Green solution (*not* chloroform-washed), the Methyl Violet (which is an inevitable contaminant of unwashed Methyl Green) will stain the amyloid pink, whilst the nuclei are stained green (*see Figure* 9.6). The section can be mounted in corn syrup to minimize the diffusion of Methyl Violet. Permanent preparations can be prepared by washing the section in distilled water after staining, allowing it to dry, then immersing it in triethyl phosphate; after soaking in xylol the section can be mounted in DPX (Hamilton 1967). This staining method is usually unsuccessful when applied to paraffin sections.

All the methods so far described give far better results when applied to frozen sections, although all (with the exception of the Methyl Green) can be satisfactorily used with normally processed paraffin sections.

Other methods for the histological demonstration of amyloid are as follows.

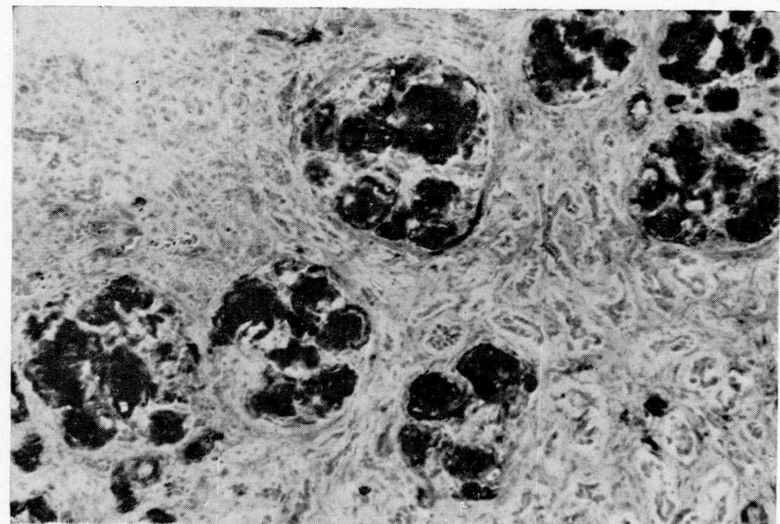

Figure 9.6 Human kidney. Amyloid staining with Methyl Green. (× *150*)
(Reduced to six-tenths in reproduction)

Sirius Red

This dye is related to Congo Red, and demonstrates amyloid in a similar manner; in my opinion it has no advantage over the Congo Red methods. Amyloid stained by Sirius Red also shows apple green birefringence.

Alcian Blue method for amyloid (Lendrum, Slidders and Fraser, 1969)

This modified Alcian Blue method purports to distinguish between old and recently formed amyloid. The method is not specific for amyloid and cannot be used to specifically identify amyloid deposits.

Peptic Digestion

Amyloid is more resistant to proteolytic enzymes than most other material, and retains some of its characteristic staining reactions. The Pepsin Digestion technique makes use of this fact; the section containing amyloid is treated with a pepsin–hydrochloric acid mixture. Control sections are incubated in hydrochloric acid alone. Only amyloid resists the peptic digestion, and can subsequently be demonstrated by eosin or Congo Red. One problem with this method is that it often proves difficult to keep the sections on the slide.

Variability of amyloid staining

Amyloid may show considerable variation in staining intensity with any or all of the staining methods discussed above. Methyl Violet is particularly unreliable in this respect, often failing to stain amyloid which is easily demonstrated by Congo Red and Thioflavine T. For this reason the Methyl Violet technique is now out of favour. In certain circumstances amyloid cannot be demonstrated by any of the staining methods, and has to be diagnosed by electron microscopy. Amyloid of the so-called 'primary' type tends to show more variation in its staining than 'secondary' amyloid, although chemically and ultrastructurally the two types seem to be identical.

METHOD 47

Amyloid: Congo Red (modified by Highman, 1946)

Reagents required

(1) Congo Red
(2) Potassium hydroxide
(3) Absolute alchohol
(4) Distilled water

Staining solutions

(1) *Congo Red*

Congo Red	500 mg
Absolute alcohol	50 ml
Distilled water	50 ml

(2) *Differentiator*

Potassium hydroxide	200 mg
Absolute alcohol	80 ml
Distilled water	20 ml

Sections

All types.

Staining method

(1) Bring all sections down to water	
(2) Stain in solution (1), Congo Red	3 min
(3) Wash off excess Congo Red in tap water	
(4) Differentiate in solution (2), control by microscope	
(5) Wash in tap water	3 min
(6) Counterstain in haematoxylin	3–5 min
(7) Wash in tap water	
(8) Dehydrate through graded alcohols to	
(9) Xylene, and mount in DPX	

Results

Amyloid: orange-red

Nuclei: blue
Elastin: orange

Remarks

The differentiation of the Congo Red with the alcoholic potassium hydroxide is critical. It is possible to obtain false positives with this method as with all Congo Red methods if the differentiation is not complete, or in extreme circumstances if the section is over-differentiated false negatives will occur.

METHOD 48

Amyloid: Alkaline Congo Red (Puchtler, Sweat and Levine, 1962)

Reagents required

(1) Hydrochloric acid
(2) Sodium chloride
(3) Sodium hydroxide
(4) Congo Red
(5) Absolute alcohol
(6) Distilled water

Staining Solution

(1) *Acid alcohol*

Hydrochloric acid	1 ml
70 per cent alcohol	99 ml

(2) *Stock saturated solution of sodium chloride in 80 per cent alcohol*

80 per cent alcohol	100 ml
Add sodium chloride till saturated	

This solution is stable.

(3) *Alkaline alcohol*

Stock solution (above)	50 ml
1 per cent aqueous sodium hydroxide	0·5 ml
Filtered and used within 15 min	

(4) *Stock solution of Congo Red*

Stock solution (2)	100 ml
Saturate with Congo Red	

This keeps for several months. Allow to stand for 24 h before use.

(5) *Working solution of Congo Red*

Stock solution of Congo Red	50 ml
1 per cent aqueous sodium hydroxide	0·5 ml

This solution is then filtered and used within 15 min.

Sections

Cryostat pre-fixed
Cryostat post-fixed
Frozen formalin-fixed
Paraffin sections

Staining method

(1) After fixation, bring all sections down to water	
(2) Stain in Mayer's haematoxylin	10 min
(3) Wash in tap water	
(4) Differentiate in solution (1) acid alcohol	
(5) Wash in tap water	
(6) Wash well in distilled water	
(7) Place in solution (3) alkaline alcohol in closed vessel	20 min
(8) Place in solution (5) working Congo Red solution in closed vessel	20 min
(9) Dehydrate through graded alcohols to	
(10) Xylene, and mount in DPX	

Results

Amyloid: orange-red and dichroic
Nuclei: blue
Elastin: orange-red
Other structures: unstained to yellow

Remarks

(1) The Congo Red stock solution should stand overnight before being used.

(2) This technique may be used as a fluorescent method.

METHOD 49

Congo Red as a fluorescence method for amyloid (Cohen *et al.* 1959; Puchtler and Sweat 1965)

Reagents required

(1) Congo Red
(2) Potassium hydroxide

Preparation of solutions

(1) *Congo Red stain*

Congo Red	100 mg
Absolute alcohol	50 ml
Distilled water	50 ml

(2) *Differentiator*

Potassium hydroxide	200 mg
Absolute alcohol	80 ml
Distilled water	20 ml

Sections

All types (frozen give best result)

Suitable control

Previous known positive control

Method

(1) Bring sections to water
(2) Stain in Congo Red stain 1 min
(3) Wash in tap water
(4) Differentiate in solution (2) until all the section appears colourless
(5) Wash in water
(6) Dehydrate through clear alcohol and clear in fresh xylene
(7) Mount in DPX or fluorofree mountant

Results

Amyloid deposits fluoresce orange to red.

Remarks

It is possible to over-differentiate, but this rarely happens. Known positive control will confirm this.

METHOD 50

Amyloid: Thioflavine T (Vassar and Culling, 1959)

Reagents required

(1) Thioflavine T
(2) Acetic acid
(3) Haematoxylin
(4) Distilled water

Staining solutions

(1) 1 *per cent Thioflavine T*

Thioflavine T	500 mg
Distilled water	50 ml

(2) *Differentiator*

Acetic acid	1 ml
Distilled water	99 ml

Haematoxylin (*see* page 322)

Sections

All types

Staining method

(1) Bring all sections down to water	
(2) Stain sections in solution (3), haematoxylin	2 min
(3) Wash in tap water	3 min
(4) Stain in solution (1), Thioflavine T	3 min
(5) Rinse in tap water	1 min
(6) Differentiate in solution (2), acetic acid	20 min
(7) Wash in water	3 min
(8) Mount in Apathy's medium	
or	
(9) Dehydrate through *fresh* alcohol to	
(10) Fresh xylene and mount in a fluoro-free mountant	

Results

Amyloid: bright yellow
Mast cells: yellow

Remarks

(1) The colour of fluorescence obtained with this method varies with different deposits of amyloid and also depends upon the filters used with the microscope. It is possible for other material to fluoresce also, so one of the other methods given for amyloid should be carried out alongside this technique.

(2) Eosin-free alcohol must be used, eosin being a fluorescent dye.

METHOD 51

Amyloid: Methyl Violet method

Reagents required

(1) Methyl Violet
(2) Acetic acid
(3) Distilled water

Staining solutions

(1) *Methyl Violet 0·25 per cent*

Methyl Violet	250 mg
Distilled water	100 mg

(2) *Differentiator*

Acetic acid	1 ml
Distilled water	99 ml

Sections

All types

Staining method

(1) Bring all sections to water	
(2) Stain in solution (1), Methyl Violet	5–10 min
(3) Wash in tap water	1 min
(4) Differentiate in 1 per cent acetic acid	approx. 1 min
(5) Wash in tap water	1 min
(6) Mount in glycerin jelly	

Results

Amyloid: pink to red
Nuclei: blue
Other tissue: blue

Remarks

The differentiation with 1 per cent acetic acid (4) is carried out with the aid of a microscope, so that as much as possible of the background staining is removed, while the amyloid is left untouched. Stronger solutions of Methyl Violet may be used, but the stronger the solution, the more background staining obtained.

METHOD 52

Amyloid: Methyl Green method (Bancroft, 1967)

Reagents required

(1) Methyl Green
(2) Distilled water
(3) Acetic acid

Staining solution

2 per cent Methyl Green

Methyl Green	2 g
Distilled water	100 ml

Differentiator (for paraffin sections)

Acetic acid	1 ml
Distilled water	99 ml

Sections

Preferably cryostat, but also paraffin

Staining method

(1) Fix cryostat sections in formal saline	2 min
(2) Wash briefly in tap water	
(3) Stain in 2 per cent Methyl Green	2 min
(4) Wash in tap water	30 s
(5) Allow to dry (aid by blotting)	
(6) Rinse in triethyl phosphate	10 s
(7) Place in xylol	
(8) Mount in DPX	

Results

Amyloid deposits: pink
Nuclei: green
Elastic fibres: blue

Remarks

If the technique is applied to paraffin sections it is necessary to extend the staining time in Methyl Green to 5–10 min and then to differentiate in 2 per cent acetic acid after stage (4) in the method. Otherwise, with frozen sections, no differentiation is necessary.

METHOD 53

Pepsin Digestion technique for demonstrating amyloid

Reagents required

(1) Pepsin (porcine)
(2) Hydrochloric acid
(3) Distilled water
(4) Eosin

Preparation of solutions

(1) *Pepsin solution*

Pepsin	200 mg
0·02 N Hydrochloric acid	40 ml
pH of solution, 1·6	

(2) 0·02 N *Hydrochloric acid 40 ml*
See page 325

(3) *1 per cent Eosin*

Sections

All types (two sections required)

Incubating method

(1) Bring all sections to water
(2) Place test section in pepsin solution at 37°C for 4 h
(3) Place control section in hydrochloric acid solution at 37°C for 4 h
(4) Wash both sections very carefully in distilled water
(5) Stain in 1 per cent eosin for 2 min
(6) Wash in tap water very carefully
(7) Dehydrate through graded alcohols to xylene
(8) Mount in DPX

Result

Amyloid: pink
Other tissue: digested
Control section: no digestion should take place of amyloid

REFERENCES

BANCROFT, J. D. (1967). *J. med. Lab. Technol.* **24,** 309
BENNHOLD, E. (1922). *Münch. med. Wschr.* **2,** 1537
COHEN, A. S., CALKINS, E. and LEVINE, C. (1959). *Am. J. Path.* **35,** 971
GLENNER, G. G., KEISER, H. R., BLADEN, H. A., CUATRECASAS, P., EANES, E. D., RAM, J. S., HANFER, J. N. and DELELLIS, R. A. (1968). *J. Histochem. Cytochem.* **16,** 633
HAMILTON, E. G. H. (1967). Personal communication
HIGHMAN, B. (1946). *Archs. Path.* **41,** 559
KRAMER, H. and WINDRUM, G. M. (1955). *J. Histochem. Cytochem.* **3,** 277
LENDRUM, A. C., SLIDDERS, W. and FRASER, D. S. (1969). *Ned. Tijdschr. Geneesk.* **113,** 374
PUCHTLER, H., SWEAT, F. and LEVINE, M. (1962). *J. Histochem. Cytochem.* **10,** 355
VASSAR, P. S. and CULLING, C. F. A. (1959). *Am. Arch. Path.* **68,** 487

10

Lipids

The terminology applied to lipids has been ill-defined and complex; in some instances different names have been used to describe the same substance. The term 'lipid' will be used in this chapter to include all naturally occurring fats and fat-like materials which have formerly been referred to as lipoid, lipin, lipine and lipide. The majority of lipids are soluble or part-soluble in organic solvents and for this reason, many of the histochemical techniques are applied to frozen sections. The means of demonstration of lipid substances includes the use of lipid dyes, microscopy and extraction techniques. The information obtained from histochemical methods cannot be compared to a biochemical classification due to a lack of specificity of the histochemical techniques. This is due in part to the fact that lipids are frequently found in tissue sections as mixtures of several substances. They are often bound to proteins (lipoproteins) or carbohydrates (glycolipids) with the resulting alteration of their chemical and physical properties leading to the failure of techniques such as differential solubility, and the possible misleading result of staining methods for specific lipid substances. Lipids are normal components of all tissues and are usually in the form of stored lipids or as particular lipid structures such as myelin. In certain diseases abnormally large amounts of lipids can be found in cells of different organs of the body and these are known as the lipid storage diseases. There is no agreement on how lipids should be classified, it is probably easiest to make the following subdivisions.

(1) Simple lipids
(2) Compound lipids
(3) Derived lipids

Lipids in general terms can be termed as compounds of long chain fatty acids with an alcohol.

Simple lipids

These are esters of both saturated and unsaturated long chain fatty acids with alcohols. Long chain fatty acids are neutral and therefore this type of lipid is frequently called neutral lipid. The fatty acids can be stearic, palmitic and oleic acids, they will dissolve in organic solvents and are insoluble in water. The neutral lipids can suitably be termed triglycerides. Also included under the heading of simple lipids are ester waxes. They are the esters of different fatty acids combined with the steroid alcohol, cholesterol. Simple lipids are demonstrated by the Sudan dyes depending upon the preferential absorption of Sudan dyes by the simple lipids (Methods 54, 55). The red oxazone component of the Nile Blue sulphate technique (Method 56) will stain them red.

Compound lipids

These contain a non-lipid group, as well as long chain fatty acids and an alcohol. They may be subdivided into the following groups.

(1) Phospholipids
(2) Glycolipids

(1) *Phospholipids*

These on hydrolysis yield a fatty acid, phosphoric acid linked to a nitrogenous base, and an alcohol which is usually glycerol. Phospholipids occur in many tissues, brain, liver and heart muscle being particularly rich. They are regarded as esters of phosphatidic acid and are also known as glycerophosphatides.
They can be subdivided into:—

(i) Lecithins
(ii) Kephalins
(iii) Plasmals
(iv) Sphingomyelin

(i) *Lecithins*—These phospholipids are the major components of the phospholipids demonstrated in tissue sections. The alcohol is glycerol, to which fatty acids and the phosphoryl base are esterified, and the base is choline.

(ii) *Kephalins*—These are of similar chemical composition with the exception that the organic base is either ethanolamine or serine.

(iii) *Plasmals*—These are found in tissues as two types, firstly as acetal phosphatides and secondly as plasmalogens. They are closely related chemically and are often considered together. They consist of aldehydes of fatty acids usually of palmitic or stearic, incorporated into the phosphatidyl ester structure.

(iv) *Sphingomyelin*—Contain a fatty acid, phosphoric acid, choline and the complex alcohol sphingosine. Apart from their lack of a sugar component sphingomyelins are similar to cerebrosides and in some instances are not classed under the broad heading of phospholipids. They can be histochemically differentiated from the cerebrosides by their failure to react with the PAS reaction, and can be demonstrated by the NaOH OTAN method.

(2) *Glycolipids*

Two major groups of glycolipids occur in tissue sections, firstly, cerebrosides, which contain a single fatty acid chain, a complex alcohol (usually sphingosine) and one or more hexose sugars, usually galactose. The second group comprises the gangliosides, which are chemically similar to cerebrosides but also contain neuraminic acid or its derivatives. Histochemically the two glycolipids cannot be separated. They can be shown by the Periodic Acid–Schiff reaction. Whereas the method is negative for phospholipids, glycolipids are found most commonly in nervous tissue.

(3) *Derived lipids*

These contain the fatty acids that are produced by hydrolysis of the simple and compound lipids discussed previously. The fatty acids can be either saturated or unsaturated. Saturated fatty acids include palmitic and stearic acids, and these contain no double bonds in their molecule. Unsaturated fatty acids such as oleic acid contain double bonds. Also classed in this group are the sterols, which are histochemically the more important. They are produced by the hydrolysis of ester waxes, and cholesterol is the most important histochemically.

DEMONSTRATION AND IDENTIFICATION

Lipid material

Lipids usually occur as mixtures and because of this the individual components may not react in their characteristic manner. They usually occur as granules or droplets and in some cases bound to components within the cell. Lipid droplets can be demonstrated by staining methods as well as by extraction with organic solvents. Bound lipids are difficult to demonstrate as they are intermingled with other tissue components, and they form complex groups with other substances, e.g. with proteins to form lipoproteins. The physicochemical state of lipids in cells and tissues is variable. Cain (1950) listed the four following possibilities.

(1) Lipids detectable as such in living or fixed tissues;

(2) Lipids present as such in living tissues but detectable only after fixation;

(3) Lipids not present as such in living tissues but demonstrable only after fixation (fixation unmasks certain lipids);

(4) Lipids that can be detected only after special treatment (unmasking) in addition to fixation.

Fixation

Formaldehyde

In many instances it is preferable to demonstrate lipids in unfixed tissue sections. However this is not usually possible and formaldehyde is the routine fixative of choice. Baker (1944) states that phospholipids may be lost in formol saline and suggests incorporating calcium chloride, as its buffering effect stops the loss of phospholipids. There are grounds for a number of lipids to react chemically with formaldehyde and this should be borne in mind if considering applied lipid histochemistry. As a general rule fixation should be kept as short as possible.

Alcohol

The majority of lipids, including triglycerides and most phospholipids, are soluble in alcohol. Alcohol fixation also makes sectioning difficult and should be avoided.

Mercuric chloride

This fixative reacts with phospholipids, hydrolyzes plasmalogens, and also interferes with sectioning by making the blocks brittle and difficult to cut.

Osmium tetroxide

This fixative will react with the double bonds of unsaturated fatty acids and is involved in a number of histochemical methods for lipids.

Potassium dichromate

Potassium dichromate, like mercuric chloride, will oxidize some lipids and also binds chromium to lipid as in the Weigert Pal technique. It should be avoided as a routine fixative unless essential for the histochemical method.

Embedding

Frozen and cryostat sections are the material of choice, and are best stained free-floating for the lipid soluble dye methods. Paraffin and celloidin processing will remove the majority of lipids. Freeze drying followed by Carbowax embedding is a useful technique; Carbowax embedding of routinely fixed tissue can also be used.

IDENTIFICATION OF LIPIDS

The various lipids can be differentiated from other substances by using a number of techniques. These include physical methods, with and without dyes, and histochemical techniques for some of the complex lipids. A number of points must be considered at this stage. The compound lipids contain some hydrophilic lipids which are water soluble; some of these can be rendered insoluble by fixation in formol calcium. The simple lipids are soluble in many organic solvents and for their demonstration only frozen sections can be used. Many of the lipids found in tissues are bound, usually to carbohydrates or proteins, with the resulting alteration to their chemical and physical properties. A number of lipids are liquid at body temperature but may be solid at room temperature which will affect their staining properties.

Extraction

Pure hydrophobic lipids can be extracted by organic solvents and this technique is used to assist in the identification of lipids. Extraction methods usually fail to demonstrate specific tissue lipids, because of the binding of the lipid to other tissue structures. While the technique is worth attempting, the results must be viewed with caution. The process is carried out on fresh tissue blocks placed in the extraction fluid or fluids for up to 48 hours at 60°C, or in some instances, at the boiling point of the solvent. After extraction, the block is fixed in formol saline for 24 hours, washed in tap water, frozen and suitable sections cut. These are stained alongside unextracted tissue as a suitable control. The extraction technique can also be applied to unfixed frozen sections and with less success on fixed frozen sections. The majority of lipids are extracted by treatment with hot chloroform–methanol 2:1, cerebrosides by hot acetone, triglycerides, cholesterol and cholesterol esters by treatment with cold acetone and the majority of phospholipids are removed after exposure to hot ether (Keilig, 1944). In theory lipid extraction followed by suitable staining methods should be a control for the staining method employed, also extraction should allow for demonstration of specific lipids by their identification on the basis of their differential solubilities. The results must be viewed with caution.

General lipid staining methods

The Sudan dyes (Sudan III, Sudan IV, Sudan Black, Fettrot, and Oil Red O) have long been used to demonstrate lipids. Sudan Black and Oil Red O are the most recent and the most used.

The dyes are suspended in a solvent in which they are only partially soluble, and when the dye solution is applied to lipids (in which the dye is *more* soluble), transfer of the dye into the lipid occurs.

TABLE 10.1

Suggested lipid methods

General lipids	Oil Red O or
Liquid and semi liquid	Sudan Black B
Triglycerides	Calcium lipase
Unsaturated lipids	Performic Acid–Schiff: OTAN
General phospholipid	Sudan Black B; OTAN
Choline-containing phospholipids	Acid haematin; OTAN
Sphingomyelin-containing phospholipids	NaOH OTAN
Plasmalogen-containing phospholipids	Mercuric Chloride–Schiff
Fatty acids	Holczingers: NaOH OTAN
Glycolipids	PAS
Cholesterol and esters	PAN; digitonin

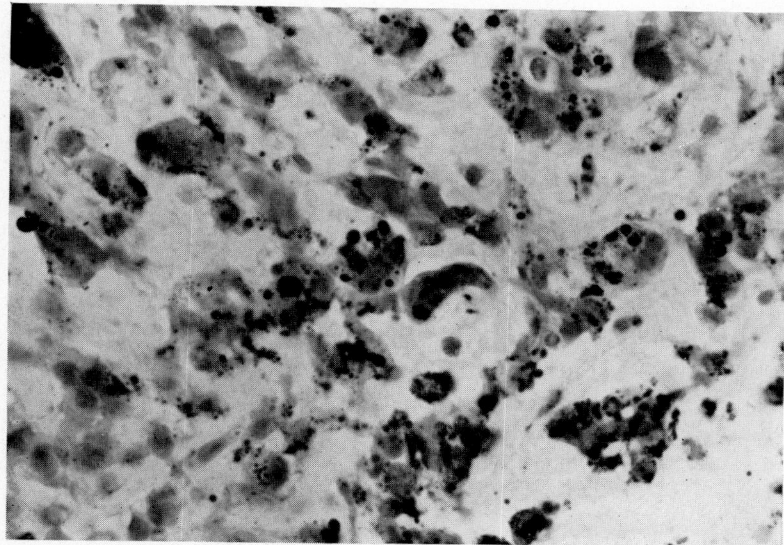

Figure 10.1 Human retroperitoneal sarcoma. Frozen section stained by Oil Red O. Fat droplets within most of the tumour cells enabled a diagnosis of poorly differentiated liposarcoma to be made. ($\times$ *490*)

(Reduced to two-thirds in reproduction)

The original dye solvent must not be capable of dissolving appreciable amounts of the lipid in the tissue section. Therefore staining occurs with these lipid-soluble dyes because the dye is more soluble in the lipid in the tissue section than it is in the original solvent. (Bancroft & Stevens, 1974)

(a) *Oil Red O*

This dye is slightly soluble in organic solvents, is insoluble in water and is preferentially absorbed by lipids from solvents. The coloration obtained by using this dye is more intense than with other Sudan dyes. (*see Figure* 10.1).

(b) *Sudan Black B*

Sudan Black B has a slightly different chemical structure from Oil Red O. Because of its amino groups Sudan Black B is a slightly basic dye and will combine with acidic groups in compound lipids and therefore also stain phospholipids. It has a similar solubility to Oil Red O and stains neutral lipids by preferential absorption.

(c) *Nile Blue*

This method, first introduced by Lorrain Smith (1908), has since been adapted by many others, notably by Cain (1947). The method is usually employed to differentiate between acidic and non-acidic (neutral) lipids. Nile Blue solution contains three components (Barka and Anderson, 1963).

(1) Oxazone salt of Nile Blue, which is dark blue in colour.
(2) The free base of Nile Blue oxazone, which is red in colour.
(3) The oxazone derivative, which is red in colour.

The first is soluble in water and alcohol, but insoluble in lipids. The second is insoluble in water but very soluble in lipids, while the last one is also insoluble in water and soluble in lipids. When a 1 per cent solution of Nile Blue is applied to a section, neutral lipids dissolve the red component (Nile Red) in the same manner as Sudan Black and Oil Red O. Acidic lipids dissolve the oxazone and combine with the free base. The result of this combination is a salt which is lipid-soluble and dark blue in colour.

When carrying out the method, three sections are required. The first section is stained in Sudan Black B or Oil Red O to indicate areas of lipid material. The other two sections are processed through the Nile Blue method. One section is stained in 1 per cent Nile Blue at 60°C–70°C for 5 min, and the other in 0·2 per cent Nile Blue. The weaker solution contains more of the free base. If the two Nile Blue stained sections are the same, the first is discarded. This method is not specific for any lipid group but it is useful in the process of determining whether the lipid is acidic or neutral.

(d) *Osmium tetroxide*

This substance is soluble in all types of lipids; its usefulness is dependent upon its reduction to osmium dioxide by unsaturated fatty acids or choline. It will fail to react with lipids in which all the fatty acids are fully saturated, and those in which the base choline is not present. It is not used as a general lipid method, but is employed in some of the differential methods given at the end of the chapter.

Choice of solvent for lipid-soluble dyes

To obtain a satisfactory staining result, a solvent that will dissolve the dye in sufficient concentration must be used. The dye must also be more soluble in the lipid than in the solvent. If this is not the case, the final staining of the lipid material will be poor and patchy. The solvents normally used are as follows.

(1) 70 per cent Alcohol (Baker, 1956)
(2) 60 per cent Isopropyl alcohol (Lillie and Ashburn, 1943)
(3) 60 per cent Triethylphosphate (Gomori, 1952)
(4) Propylene glycol (Chiffelle and Putt, 1951)
(5) 70 per cent Alcohol/absolute acetone mixture (Herxheimer's, 1903, solvent)

Differential lipid staining methods

Acid Haematein method

This method for phospholipids was introduced by Baker (1947). It is based on the technique of Smith–Dietrich (Dietrich, 1910). It is specific only when used in conjunction with the pyridine extraction technique. Substances other than phospholipids may give a positive result, but only phospholipids are removed by pyridine extraction. The method is carried out on a rigid time scale which includes fixation of the block. The method depends upon the formation of a dye lake by the combination of chrome ions with phospholipids. Differentiation is carried out with a borax–ferricyanide mixture. Components that contain phosphoric acid retain the dye, whereas others do not. Phospholipids are the only group of lipids to contain this acid.

OTAN method

This technique published by Adams (1959) involves the use of osmium tetroxide which is soluble in all types of lipid and is reduced by unsaturated fatty acids. The reduction is in two stages. The product of the first reduction is a colourless substance which is further reduced to produce black osmium dioxide. The addition of sodium perchlorate can prevent this final reduction by some of the lipids. The simple lipids are not water-soluble and therefore are unaffected by the sodium perchlorate; they will continue to reduce the osmium tetroxide until black osmium dioxide is formed. Some compound lipids such as phospholipids are partly water-soluble and the sodium perchlorate will inhibit the final reduction of osmium tetroxide by these types of lipids; the sodium perchlorate stops the reduction at the colourless intermediate substance stage. This colourless substance is chelated with α-naphthylamine to produce an orange-red colour.

The method demonstrates sites of simple lipids (triglycerides, cholesterol and its esters) and fatty acids as black, and phospholipids as orange-red.

NaOH OTAN method

This is a modification of the OTAN technique (Adams and Baylis, 1963) which allows the separation of lecithin from sphingomyelin. The choline-containing phospholipids such as lecithin have ester linkages which will be broken by alkaline hydrolysis, the result being no osmium staining. The linkage of the fatty acid to sphingosine is not affected and is in consequence stained black. The plasmalogen linkage also resists treatment with sodium hydroxide and will also react with osmium tetroxide but it can be blocked by treatment with mercuric chloride.

The Plasmal reaction

The acetal phosphatides (plasmalogens) are phospholipids that contain one molecule of an aldehyde of a fatty acid which combines with the glycerol group, the linkage between the two components being of the acetal type. Feulgen and Voit (1924) introduced a method to demonstrate these lipids. The acetal linkage is split by exposure to mercuric chloride. The aldehydes are released, and these can then be demonstrated by the Periodic Acid–Schiff method. Terner and Hayes (1961) described this method in great detail, but there is doubt regarding its specificity. Their general conclusion was that the plasmalogens were being demonstrated. For further details, readers are referred to the original paper and to Pearse (1968).

Performic Acid–Schiff method

This method depends upon the oxidation of unsaturated bonds (ethylenic bonds) to produce free aldehyde. This is demonstrated by the Schiff's reagent. The oxidation can be carried out using performic acid or peracetic acid. Performic acid is used in preference to peracetic acid. The method is not specific for unsaturated lipids, as keratin and DNA will also react. If blocking is carried out using bromine water (*see* Method 63), staining of the unsaturated lipid is prevented. These two techniques should always be carried out simultaneously when unsaturated lipids are being demonstrated.

PAS reaction for glycolipids

The reaction for glycolipids depends upon their content of D-galactose. This sugar is PAS-positive. All the aldehydes in the section are first blocked, using Method 31. This technique will distinguish between glycolipids and other lipid groups, but not between the two members of the glycolipid group: cerebrosides and gangliosides.

The Perchloric Acid–Naphthoquinone method

The standard method for the demonstration of cholesterol was, at one time, the Schultz method (1924; 1925). This has been replaced by a more sensitive method introduced by Adams (1961). His technique is known as the Perchloric Acid–Naphthoquinone method (PAN). The basis of the reaction is that perchloric acid first forms an insoluble perchlorate with cholesterol. This is then converted to cholesta-3:5-diene by the elimination of water, (Adams, 1965), and this subsequently reacts with 1:2-naphthoquinone-4-sulphonic acid to form a dark blue pigment. The pigment is stable for a few hours, but the section should be examined immediately.

Digitonin method

This technique is used to distinguish between cholesterol and cholesterol esters. Windaus (1910) introduced the technique which requires two formalin-fixed frozen sections. The first section is stained by the Oil Red O method for lipid material. The second section is placed in a solution of digitonin. Free cholesterol forms a complex with the digitonin, and characteristic birefringent crystals are precipitated from this solution. The section is examined under a polarizing microscope. Birefringent needle-like crystals indicate free cholesterol. The control section stained in Oil Red O will also exhibit birefringence of free cholesterol, whereas esters will be stained by Oil Red O and will not be birefringent.

The Copper–Rubeanic Acid method

Methods suitable for the demonstration of free fatty acids are restricted to modifications of the technique introduced by Fischler (1904). Holczinger (1959) reviewed a number of these methods and recommended the Copper–Rubeanic Acid method as the best available technique. Sections are exposed to copper acetate for 2–5 hours, followed by treatment in ethylenediamine tetra-acetic acid (EDTA) to remove non-specific absorbed copper. Dilute rubeanic acid is applied to the sections and copper soaps are produced indicating the presence of fatty acid deposits.

Identifying a lipid

The process of identifying a lipid is complicated, and may involve using four or more staining methods as well as extraction techniques. When lipid material is suspected, two sections of fixed frozen material are used. The first is stained by a lipid-soluble dye method, which will reveal the presence of any lipid material. The second section

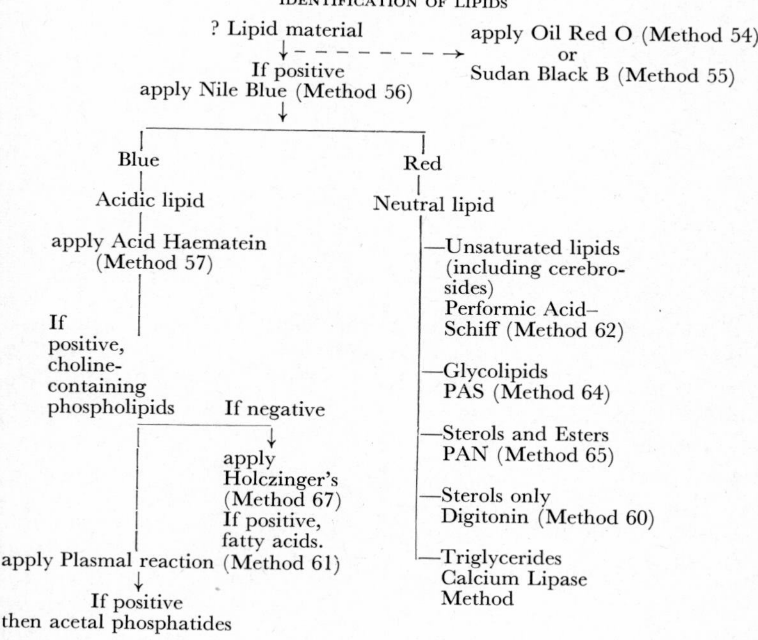

is looked at unstained. In this state, refractile droplets indicate lipid material. The section is then viewed by a polarizing microscope, for if the lipid material is cholesterol or cholesterol esters these can be detected by their birefringence. Once lipid material has been confirmed, it is necessary to test whether it is acidic or non-acidic (neutral). This is done by applying the Nile Blue technique Acidic lipids are stained blue, and the non-acidic (neutral) droplets, red. If the lipid material is acidic, this indicates that it is either a phospholipid or a fatty acid. If it is non-acidic, it may be one of the following: an unsaturated lipid, a glycolipid, cholesterol and cholesterol esters, or a simple lipid. The procedure outlined above should be undertaken in order to complete identification. The extraction of lipids plays an important role in their identification, and should be used in conjunction with the various staining methods.

METHOD 54

Lipid material: Oil Red O (Lillie and Ashburn, modified 1943)

Reagents required

(1) Oil Red O
(2) Triethyl phosphate
(3) Distilled water

Preparation of staining solution

Oil Red O	1 g
Triethyl phosphate	60 ml
Distilled water	40 ml

The distilled water is added to the triethyl phosphate, the dye is then added, the mixture is heated to 100°C for 5 min and is stirred constantly. The mixture is filtered when hot and again when cool. This solution will keep as a stock solution but must be filtered before use.

Sections

Formalin-fixed frozen sections, free-floating
Cryostat post-fixed, preferably free-floating

Method

(1) Wash sections in distilled water
(2) Place sections in 60 per cent triethyl phosphate
(3) Stain sections in Oil Red O solution at 20°C for 15 min
(4) Wash sections in 60 per cent triethyl phosphate for 30 sec
(5) Wash sections in distilled water
(6) Stain sections in haematoxylin for 1 min
(7) Wash sections in tap water for 5 min
(8) Mount in glycerin jelly

Results

Lipid material: red
Nuclei: blue

Remarks

This method can be employed at 37°C or 60°C if required.

METHOD 55

Lipid material: Sudan Black B (Lison and Dagnelie, 1935)

Reagents required

(1) Sudan Black B
(2) Triethyl phosphate
(3) Distilled water

Preparation of staining solution

Sudan Black B	1 g
Triethyl phosphate	60 ml
Distilled water	40 ml

The distilled water is added to the triethyl phosphate, the stain is added to this solution and the mixture is heated to 100°C for 5 min and stirred constantly. The mixture is filtered when hot and once again immediately before use. The solution will keep well as a stock solution, but must be filtered each time it is used.

Sections

Formalin-fixed frozen sections, free-floating
Cryostat post-fixed, preferably free-floating

Method

(1) Wash sections in distilled water
(2) Place sections in 60 per cent triethyl phosphate
(3) Stain sections in Sudan Black B solution at 20°C for 10 min
(4) Place sections in 60 per cent triethyl phosphate for 30 sec
(5) Wash in distilled water
(6) Stain in Mayer's Carmalum for 3 min
(7) Wash in distilled water
(8) Mount in glycerin jelly

Results

Lipid material, including phospholipids: black
Nuclei: red

Remarks

This technique using triethyl phosphate can be carried out at 37°C or 60°C as required.

METHOD 56

Acidic lipids: Nile Blue (Smith-Dietrich, modified by Cain, 1947)

Reagents required

(1) Nile Blue
(2) Acetic acid
(3) Distilled water

Preparation of solutions

(1) *Nile Blue 1 per cent*

Nile Blue	500 mg
Distilled water	50 ml

(2) *Nile Blue 0·02 per cent*

Nile Blue	10 mg
Distilled water	50 ml

(3) *Differentiator*

Acetic acid, conc.	0·5 ml
Distilled	50 ml

Sections

Formalin-fixed frozen sections
Cryostat pre-fixed
Cryostat post-fixed

Method

It is necessary to stain one section by the Oil Red O or Sudan Black methods (*see* Methods 54, 55, pp. 152-153). This slide is numbered 3. Two sections are required for the following technique.

(1) Bring both sections to water
(2) Stain sections 1 and 2 in 1 per cent Nile Blue for 5m in at 60°C (solution 1)
(3) Differentiate at 60°C in solution (3) for 30 s
(4) Wash in tap water
(5) Mount section 1 in glycerin jelly
(6) Place section 2 in solution (2) (0·02 per cent Nile Blue) for 5 min at 60°C
(7) Wash in tap water
(8) Differentiate section 2 in solution (3) at 60°C for 30 s

(9) Wash in tap water
(10) Mount in glycerin jelly

Results

Section 1. Any blue staining that can be compared with a positive section 3 is taken to be acidic lipid material.

Section 2. Any red staining that can be compared with a positive result in section 3 is taken to be a non-acidic lipid.

Section 3. Control for above.

Remarks

This method has caused much controversy in the literature, and its specificity is doubtful, it is however well worth applying when trying to identify an unknown lipid.

METHOD 57

Phospholipids: Acid Haematein method (Baker, 1946)

Reagents required

(1) Formalin
(2) Calcium chloride
(3) Potassium dichromate
(4) Haematoxylin
(5) Sodium iodate
(6) Glacial acetic acid
(7) Sodium tetraborate (borax)
(8) Potassium ferricyanide
(9) Distilled water

Preparation of solutions

(1) *Fixative*

Formalin	10 ml
Calcium chloride (anhydrous)	1 g
Distilled water	90 ml

(2) *Post-chroming solution*

Potassium dichromate	5 g
Calcium chloride	1 g
Distilled water	100 ml

(3) *Acid Haematein solution*

Haematein	50 mg
1 per cent Sodium iodate	1 ml
Distilled water	49 ml

Heat the solution to boiling point, allow to cool and add 1 ml of glacial acetic acid.

(4) *Differentiator*

Potassium ferricyanide	250 mg
Sodium tetraborate (borax)	250 mg
Distilled water	100 ml

Sections

For this method unfixed pieces of tissue are recommended

Method

(1) Place blocks in fixative, solution (1) at 22°C, for 6–12 h
(2) Transfer tissue (no washing) to post-chroming solution (2) at 22°C for 18 h
(3) Transfer tissue to fresh post-chroming solution (2) at 60°C, for 24 h
(4) Wash in running tap water for 6 h
(5) Cut frozen sections 10 μm thick
(6) Place sections in post-chroming solution (2) at 37°C, for 1 h
(7) Wash well in distilled water for 5 min
(8) Stain in acid haematein, solution (3), at 60°C, for 5 h
(9) Rinse well in distilled water
(10) Transfer sections to differentiating solution (4) at 37°C for 18 h
(11) Wash in tap water for 10 min
(12) Mount in glycerin jelly

Results

Phospholipids: dark blue
Other material may be blue (*see Remarks*)

Remarks

This method is only specific when a control is submitted to the pyridine extraction method (*see* Method 58).

METHOD 58

Phospholipids: Pyridine Extraction (Baker, 1946)

Reagents required

(1) Picric acid
(2) Formalin
(3) Glacial acetic acid
(4) Distilled water

(5) 70 per cent Alcohol
(6) 50 per cent Alcohol
(7) Pyridine
(8) Distilled water

Preparation of solutions

Fixative (*Bouin's*)

Saturated aqueous picric acid	50 ml
Formaldehyde	10 ml
Glacial acetic acid	5 ml
Distilled water	35 ml

Sections

To act as a control for Method 57 a comparable block must be used.

Method

(1) Fix the block in the dilute Bouin's fixative	20 h
(2) Wash in 70 per cent alcohol	1 h
(3) Wash in 50 per cent alcohol	30 min
(4) Wash in running tap water	30 min
(5) Place in pyridine at 22°C	1 h
(6) Transfer block to fresh pyridine at 22°C	1 h
(7) Transfer block to fresh pyridine at 60°C	24 h
(8) Wash in running tap water	2 h
(9) Transfer to stage (2) of Method 57	

Results

After the haematein method has been applied to the blocks processed by the above technique, phospholipids are negative.

METHOD 59

OTAN method (Adams, 1959)

Reagents required

(1) Osmium tetroxide
(2) Potassium perchlorate
(3) α-naphthylamine

Preparation of solutions

(1) *Osmium tetroxide solution*

1 per cent osmium tetroxide	1 part
1 per cent potassium perchlorate	3 parts

(2) *α-naphthylamine solution.* Saturated solution in warm distilled water, β-naphthylamine may be a contaminant and is a carcinogen.

Sections

Frozen sections (formol-calcium-fixed)

Method

(1) Treat free-floating sections with osmium solution in suitable container filled with fluid and tightly stoppered for 18 h
(2) Wash in distilled water for 10 min
(3) Pick up on slides
(4) Treat with α-naphthylamine solution at 37°C for 20 min
(5) Wash sections in distilled water for 5 min
(6) Mount in glycerin jelly

Results

Phospholipids: orange-red
Cholesterol esters: black
Triglycerides: black

Remarks

Sections may be counterstained after stage (5) if required.

METHOD 60

Sodium Hydroxide OTAN method (Adams and Bayliss, 1963)

Reagents required

(1) Osmium tetroxide
(2) Potassium perchlorate
(3) α-naphthylamine
(4) Sodium hydroxide

Preparation of solutions

(1) *Osmium tetroxide* (*see* Method 59)
(2) *α-napthylamine* (*see* Method 59)
(3) *Sodium hydroxide*

Sodium hydroxide	8 g
Distilled water	100 ml

Sections

Frozen sections (formol-calcium-fixed)

Method

(1) Treat free-floating sections with sodium hydroxide solution at 37°C for 1 h

(2) Wash in distilled water

(3) Treat sections in 1 per cent acetic acid

(4) Continue from step (1) in previous method

Results

Sphingomyelin: orange-red

Other alkali resistant lipids will stain black—alkali labile lipids will be destroyed.

METHOD 61

Acetal phosphatides: the Plasmal reaction (Feulgen–Voit, 1924, modified by Terner and Hayes, 1961)

Reagents required

(1) Sodium chloride
(2) Mercuric chloride
(3) Hydrochloric acid
(4) Schiff's reagent (*see* Method 20)
(5) Sodium metabisulphite

Preparation of solutions

(1) *Sodium chloride solution*

Sodium chloride	900 mg
Distilled water	100 ml

(2) *Mercuric chloride solution*

Mercuric chloride	1 g
Distilled water	100 ml

(3) *Schiff's reagent*

See Method 20, page 87

(4) *Sulphurous acid rinse*

Sodium bisulphite	500 mg
Distilled water	99·5 ml
Conc. hydrochloric acid	0·5 ml

Sections

Frozen formalin-fixed
Frozen unfixed
Cryostat post-fixed
Cryostat pre-fixed

Method

With this technique it is necessary to have a control section that is not placed in solution (2), the mercuric chloride.

(1) If section is unfixed, place in three changes of solution (1) *otherwise*

(2) Wash fixed sections in distilled water.

All sections:

(3)	Place section in solution (2) mercuric chloride	7 min
(4)	Transfer sections to Schiff's reagent, solution (3)	10 min
(5)	Transfer sections to sulphurous acid rinse 1	2 min
(6)	Transfer sections to sulphurous acid rinse 2	2 min
(7)	Transfer sections to sulphurous acid rinse 3	2 min
(8)	Wash in tap water	2 min
(9)	Counterstain in 2 per cent Methyl Green	3 min
(10)	Wash in running tap water	
(11)	Mount in glycerin jelly	

Results

Acetal phosphatides: Schiff-positive, reddish-pink. The control section should be negative.

Remarks

It is possible that aldehydes are present in the section, in which case a false positive may be obtained.

METHOD 62

Unsaturated lipids: Performic Acid–Schiff (Lillie, 1951)

Reagents required

(1) Formic acid
(2) Hydrogen peroxide
(3) Sulphuric acid
(4) Schiff's reagent

Solutions

(1) *Performic acid*

90 per cent Formic acid,	40 ml
100 vol. or 30 per cent Hydrogen peroxide	4 ml
Sulphuric acid (conc.)	0·5 ml

Allow to stand for 1 h before use

(2) *Schiff's reagent*

See Method 20, page 87

Sections

Cryostat post-fixed
Cryostat pre-fixed
Formalin-fixed frozen sections
Freeze dried paraffin sections

Method

(1) Bring all sections down to tap water
(2) Treat sections with solution (1) for 30 min
(3) Wash in tap water for 15 min
(4) Immerse in Schiff's reagent (solution 2) for 40 min
(5) Wash in running tap water
(6) Dehydrate through alcohols to xylene
(7) Wash and mount in DPX

Results

Unsaturated lipids including cerebrosides: red

Remarks

(1) The performic acid solution must be allowed to stand for 1 h before use, and can only be used on the day it is prepared.

(2) For control method see bromination technique (Method 63).

METHOD 63

Unsaturated lipids: Bromination (Lillie, 1954)

Reagents required

(1) Carbon tetrachloride
(2) Bromine water
(3) Sodium metabisulphite
(4) Absolute alcohol

(a) FROZEN SECTIONS

Solutions required

(1) *2·5 per cent Bromine water*

Bromine water	1 ml
Distilled water	39 ml

(2) *0·5 per cent Sodium metabisulphite*

Sodium metabisulphite	500 mg
Distilled water	50 ml

Method

(1) Attach sections to slides and allow to dry

(2) Immerse sections in 2·5 per cent bromine water 1-6 h
(3) Wash in tap water
(4) Treat sections with 0·5 per cent sodium metabisulphite 2 min
(5) Wash in running tap water
(6) Apply method

(b) Paraffin Sections

Solution

Carbon tetrachloride	39 ml
Bromine water	1 ml

Method

(1) Dewax sections in xylol
(2) Immerse sections in carbon tetrachloride, 2 changes 4 min
(3) Immerse sections in bromine solution 1 h
(4) Immerse sections in carbon tetrachloride, 2 changes 4 min
(5) Rinse sections in 90 per cent alcohol 1 min
(6) Rinse sections in 60 per cent alcohol 1 min
(7) Rinse sections in water
(8) Apply method

METHOD 64

Glycolipids: PAS reaction

Reagents required

(1) Periodic acid
(2) Schiff's reagent
(3) Distilled water

Preparation of solutions

(1) *Periodic acid*

Periodic acid	500 mg
Distilled water	100 ml

(2) *Schiff's reagent*
(*See* Method 20, page 87)

Sections

Cryostat post-fixed
Cryostat pre-fixed
Formalin-fixed frozen sections
Freeze dried paraffin sections

Method

(1)	Bring sections down to water	
(2)	Transfer sections to solution (2)	5 min
(3)	Wash in tap water	3 min
(4)	Place in Schiff's reagent	20 min
(5)	Wash in tap water	20 min
(6)	Counterstain in haemalum	5 min
(7)	Wash in tap water	
(8)	Differentiate in 1 per cent acid alcohol	5 s
(9)	Wash in tap water	
(10)	Mount in glycerin jelly	

Results

Glycolipids, mucins, etc.: red
Nuclei: blue

Remarks

It is necessary to use the following controls when applying this method for glycolipids.

(1) Oil Red O or Sudan Black to confirm site of possible glycolipid.

(2) Aldehydes to be blocked (*see* page 96).

Note: If formalin-fixed frozen sections are used, they must be well washed in several changes of distilled water to remove any free aldehydes. If cryostat sections are used, alcohol should be used as a fixative.

METHOD 65

Cholesterol and related substances: Perchloric Acid–Naphthoquinone reaction (Adams, 1961)

Reagents required

(1) 1:2-Naphthoquinone-4-sulphonic acid
(2) Ethanol
(3) Perchloric acid
(4) Formaldehyde
(5) Distilled water

Preparation of solution

1:2-Naphthoquinone-4-sulphonic acid	12 mg
Ethanol	6 ml
60 per cent Perchloric acid	3 ml
Conc. formaldehyde	0·3 ml
Distilled water	2·7 ml

The ethanol–perchloric acid–formaldehyde—water solution is prepared first and the reagent dissolved in it.

Sections

Formol saline-fixed, frozen sections, free-floating
Formol calcium-fixed, frozen sections, free-floating

Suitable sections for controls

Adrenal gland

Method

(1) Cut frozen sections and float into formalin. Leave for 7 days
(2) Mount sections on slides and dry at room temperature
(3) Soak sections in reagent
(4) Heat sections in reagent to 60–70°C for 10 min
(5) Mount section in 60 per cent perchloric acid

Results

Cholesterol and its esters: dark blue

Remarks

(1) The dark blue colour is stable for a few hours.

(2) During the heating, the section should change colour from red to dark blue.

METHOD 66

Free cholesterol: Digitonin method (Windaus, 1910)

Reagents required

(1) Ethyl alcohol
(2) Digitonin
(3) Distilled water

Preparation of solutions

(1) *Ethyl alcohol 50 per cent*

Ethyl alcohol	100 ml
Distilled water	100 ml

(2) *Digitonin solution*

Digitonin	500 mg
Solution (1)	100 ml

Sections

Formalin-fixed frozen sections free-floating. A control section is stained by the Oil Red O method.

Method

(1) Incubate sections for 3 h in solution (2) at room temperature
(2) Rinse sections in solution (1)
(3) Float sections onto slides
(4) Mount in glycerin jelly

Results

Digitonin section: free cholesterol, birefringent.

Oil Red O section: free cholesterol, birefringent. Cholesterol ester, stained by Oil Red O.

METHOD 67

Fatty acids: Copper–Rubeanic Acid method (Holczinger 1959)

Reagents required

(1) Copper acetate
(2) Rubeanic acid
(3) Ethanol
(4) Distilled water
(5) Ethylenediamine tetra-acetic acid (Disodium), EDTA

Preparation of solutions

(1) *0·005 per cent Copper acetate*

Copper acetate	5 mg
Distilled water	100 ml

(2) *0·1 per cent EDTA*

Ethylenediamine tetra-acetic acid	50 mg
Distilled water	50 ml

(3) *0·1 per cent Rubeanic acid*

Rubeanic acid	50 mg
Absolute alcohol	35 ml
Distilled water	15 ml

Dissolve the rubeanic acid in the absolute alcohol by warming slightly then add the distilled water.

Sections

Cryostat unfixed
Cryostat pre-fixed
Formalin-fixed frozen sections

Method

(1)	Place sections in copper acetate solution	3–5 h
(2)	Wash sections in EDTA solution	10 sec
(3)	Wash sections again in EDTA solution	10 sec
(4)	Wash sections in distilled water	10 min
(5)	Immerse sections in rubeanic acid solution	30 min
(6)	Wash sections in 70 per cent alcohol	3 min
(7)	Wash sections in running tap water	
(8)	Mount sections in glycerin jelly or dehydrate through graded alcohols and mount in DPX	

Results

Fatty acids: greenish black

REFERENCES

ADAMS, C. W. M. (1959). *J. Path. Bact.* **77,** 648

— (1961). *Nature, Lond.* **192,** 331

— (1965). *Neurohistochemistry,* Ed. by C. W. M. Adams, London: Elsevier

— BAYLISS, O. (1963). *J. Path. Bact.* **85,** 113

BANCROFT, J. D. and STEVENS, A. (1975). *Histopathological Techniques and their Diagnostic Uses.* London: Churchill Livingstone

BAKER, J. R. (1944). *Q. Jl Miscrosc. Sci.* **85,** 1

— (1946). *Q. Jl Microsc. Sci.* **87,** 441

— (1947). *Q. Jl Microsc. Sci.* **88,** 463

— (1956). *Q. Jl Microsc. Sci.* **97,** 621

BARKA, T. and ANDERSON, P. J. (1963). *Histochemistry Theory Practice and Bibliography,* New York: Hoeber

CAIN, A. J. (1947). *Q. Jl. Microsc. Sci.* **88,** 467

— (1950). *Biol. Rev.* **25,** 73

CHIFFELLE, T. L. and PUTT, F. A. (1951). *Stain Technol.* **26,** 51

DIETRICH, A. (1910). *Verh. dt. path. Ges.* **14,** 263

FEULGEN, R. and VOIT, K. (1924). *Pflüger's Arch. ges. Physiol.* **206,** 389

FISCHLER, C. (1904). *Zbl. allg. Path. anat.* **15,** 913

GOMORI, G. (1952). *Microscopical Histochemistry,* University of Chicago Prcss

HERXHEIMER, G. W. (1903). *Zbl. Allg. Path. anat.* **14,** 491

HOLCZINGER, L. (1959). *Acta. histochem.* **8,** 167

KEILIG, I. (1944). *Virchows Arch. path. Anat. Physiol* **312,** 405

— (1954). *Histopathological Technique and Practical Histochemistry,* New York: York: Blakiston

LILLIE, R. D. (1954). *Histopathological Technique and Practical Histochemistry,* New Blakiston

— and ASHBURN, L. L. (1943). *Archs. Path.* **36,** 432

LISON, L. and DAGNELIE, J. (1935). *Bull Histol. appl. Physiol Path.* **12,** 85

LORRAIN SMITH, J. (1908). *J. Path. Bact.* **12,** 1

PEARSE, A. G. E. (1968). *Histochemistry Theoretical and Applied,* Vol. 1, 3rd Edn., London: Churchill-Livingstone

SCHULTZ, A. (1924). *Zbl. allg. Path. anat.* **35,** 314
— (1925). *Verch. Dtsch. Path. Ges.* **20,** 120
TERNER, G. Y. and HAYES, E. R. (1961). *Stain Technol.* **36,** 265
WINDAUS, T. (1910). *Z. phys. Chem.* **65,** 110

11

Nucleic Acids

The nucleic acids deoxyribonucleic acid (DNA) and ribosenucleic acid (RNA), are found in all animal and plant tissues, and are usually combined with basic proteins to form so-called nucleoprotein. DNA is mainly found in the nucleus, and RNA in the cytoplasm. Hydrolysis of nucleic acids yields the following components: (i) phosphate groups, (ii) five-carbon sugars, and (iii) nitrogenous bases, purines and pyrimidines. The structure is in the form of a ladder, the side-arms of which are composed of alternate sugar and phosphate groups. The transverse struts are formed by the nitrogenous bases linked to each other and to the sugar groups of the side arms of the ladder. The nitrogenous bases are of four types, two of which are purines and two are pyrimidines; in the cross-struts a purine is always linked to a pyrimidine. The arrangement can be diagrammatically represented thus:—

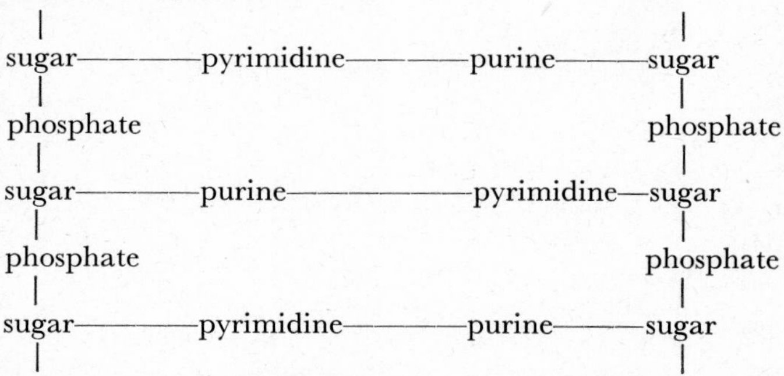

The final structure is this ladder arrangement twisted into a spiral.

Both DNA and RNA have this basic structure, but differ in two important respects. These are:—

(i) *Sugar content.* In DNA the 5-carbon sugar is deoxyribose, but in RNA it is ribose.

(ii) *Purine and pyrimidine content.* In DNA the purines are adenine and guanine, and the pyrimidines are thymine and cytosine. In RNA the purines are the same as in DNA, but the pyrimidines are uracil and cytosine.

Demonstration of DNA and RNA

The large number of phosphate radicals in the nucleic acid molecule ensure that nucleic acids will take up basic dyes such as haematoxylin. Thus the nucleus, with a high DNA content, will stain blue-black with haematoxylin. The cytoplasm of most cells do not contain enough RNA for the haematoxyphilia to overcome the eosinophilia of the large amount of protein present in the rest of the cytoplasm. In some cells however, e.g. plasma cells, there is such a large amount of RNA present that the haematoxyphilia almost overcomes the red staining of the cytoplasm, and the final staining colour of the cytoplasm is purplish.

The following histochemical methods are used for the identification of DNA and RNA.

Feulgen method for	DNA	Method 68
Methyl Green–Pyronin methods for	RNA, DNA	Method 69,70
Gallocyanin–Chrome Alum method for	RNA, DNA	Method 71
NAH–Feulgen method for	DNA	Method 72
Acridine Orange method for	RNA, DNA	Method 73
Deoxyribonuclease extraction for	DNA	Method 74
Ribonuclease extraction for	RNA	Method 76

Feulgen nucleal method

This technique, first introduced by Feulgen and Rossenbeck (1924), is considered to be specific for deoxyribonucleic acid (DNA) since only nucleic acids containing the sugar deoxyribose will show the reaction. It is the most reliable method available for the demonstration of DNA. The reaction involves mild hydrolysis of deoxyribose sugars with warm hydrochloric acid; ribose sugar is not hydrolyzed by NHCl and therefore RNA does not show the Feulgen reaction. Hydrolysis releases free aldehydes and Schiff's reagent is then applied, to produce a coloured compound indicating the presence of DNA. Two most important factors contributing to the outcome of the Feulgen reaction are (a) the means of fixation of the tissue and (b) the duration of hydrolysis in dilute acid. The hydrolysis time, which varies with the type of fixative used, is critical. Each fixative has its own optimum. By prolonging the hydrolysis, a stronger result is produced until the optimal time is reached. If this is exceeded, the intensity of staining becomes weaker and may eventually disappear altogether. Excessive hydrolysis results in total extraction of DNA from the section. Bauer (1932) published a paper dealing with optimal hydrolysis times for different fixatives. These figures are reproduced in Table 11.1, together with some additional data. Formol saline buffered to pH 7.2 or Carnoy's are recommended fixatives. Bouin's fixative should not be used, as this causes over-hydrolysis of the nucleic acid during fixation.

Control sections are incubated in deoxyribonuclease before hydrolysis (Method 74) after which the technique will prove negative.

Methyl Green-Pyronin

The Methyl Green–Pyronin technique is able to demonstrate both DNA and RNA. The method was first published by Pappenheim (1899) and modified by Unna (1902). It is often referred to as the Unna Pappenheim Stain. Several attempts have since been made to render the method more specific (Kurnick, 1955; Taft, 1951; Brachet, 1953; and Trevan and Sharrock, 1951).

Methyl Green is an impure dye containing Methyl Violet. To obtain satisfactory results with this method it is necessary to wash the Methyl Green (2 per cent aqueous solution) several times with equal parts of chloroform. Six or more washings may be required before all the violet is removed. When treated in this way, Methyl Green seems to be specific for DNA at a slightly acid pH. Methyl Green is a basic dye, and its affinity for DNA is not fully understood. However, Kurnick (1955) has suggested that binding of Methyl Green to DNA involves two sites, two amino groups on the dye combining with two phosphoric acid groups of the DNA. If the dye is used at a slightly acid pH, protein material does not stain.

Pyronin Y, used in the method, is less specific and must be used under carefully regulated conditions. Precisely-controlled staining times must be used, and the pH of the staining solution is critical. When using pyronin solutions, it is always advisable to use a control section which has been subjected to ribonuclease digestion. Pyronin Y obtained commercially varies, and certain batches fail to give satisfactory results. Because of this, it is necessary to compare each batch on its arrival against a known good batch of dye. The chemical basis of the method is not fully understood. It is discussed in considerable detail by Pearse (1968).

Gallocyanin-Chrome Alum method

This method, first introduced by Einarson (1932) for Nissl granules, was later adapted (Einarson, 1951) to demonstrate nucleic acids. The method does not distinguish between DNA and RNA, but with suitable extraction methods it is possible to identify one or the other when required. The method is simple to perform and is a progressive stain. The mechanism is due to the combination at an acid pH of the phosphoric acid residue of the nucleic acid with gallocyanin. The reaction must be carried out at a pH of 1 because at higher values (pH 2, or above), other tissue components will stain.

Feulgen-Naphthoic Acid-Hydrazide reaction

This method is recommended as a control method for the Feulgen nucleal technique (Method 68), because material giving a possible positive Schiff result (i.e., some lipoproteins) will not be stained by this method. The sections are hydrolyzed in the manner described earlier, using normal hydrochloric acid. The free aldehydes produced on hydrolysis combine with 2-hydroxy-3-naphthoic acid hydrazide (Pearse, 1951). This is then coupled to Fast Blue B. producing a purplish blue colour at the site of coupling. The localization is identical to that shown by the true Feulgen reaction. Danielli (1947) originally used 2:4-dinitrophenylhydrazine, but better results are obtained using 2-hydroxy-3-naphthoic acid hydrazide.

Acridine Orange

This fluorescent technique was introduced by Von Bertalanffy and Bickis (1956) and is widely used in exfoliative cytology. The technique is for DNA and RNA. Nuclear DNA fluoresces apple green while RNA fluoresces red, as do the mucins. The successful application of this method depends upon the concentration of Acridine Orange, the pH of the staining solution and the fixative applied to the fresh frozen sections or to the smears. In the recommended method (Bertalanffy and Nagy, 1962), the strength of Acridine Orange is 0·1 per cent in phosphate buffer, pH 6·0. If the Acridine Orange is too concentrated the red coloration masks the green. Formalin and Bouin fixation must be avoided as these both prevent differential staining. Acetic ethanol or 70 per cent alcohol are recommended for use.

DIGESTION METHODS

The two enzyme techniques for the digestion of nucleic acids are invaluable as controls for the methods discussed. Deoxyribonuclease is specific for the removal of DNA in sections, while not affecting the RNA content.

When ribonuclease is applied to tissue sections, all the RNA is removed whilst the DNA is unaltered. The digestion methods were introduced by Brachet (1940) as controls for the Methyl Pyronin method. Great care must be taken that the enzymes are of a high purity, for impure enzymes will remove all nucleic acids. Both ribosenuclease and deoxyribosenuclease are expensive reagents. A useful digestion method which is not so specific as the enzyme digestion methods, is that which uses perchloric acid. It will either remove RNA alone or both RNA and DNA according to the conditions under which the extractions are controlled.

TABLE 11.1

Hydrolysis in N-HCl at 60°C

Fixative	*Time (min)*
Bouin	not recommended
Carnoy	6
Flemming's	8
Formalin	8–10
Newcomer's	20
Susa	18
Zenker	5

METHOD 68

DNA: Feulgen nucleal reaction (Feulgen and Rossenbeck, 1924)

Reagents required

(1) Hydrochloric acid
(2) Schiff's reagent
(3) Potassium metabisulphite
(4) Light green, 1 per cent aqueous

Preparation of solutions

(1) *N-HCl*

Hydrochloric acid, (conc.)	8·5 ml
Distilled water	91·5 ml

(2) *Schiff's reagent* (*See Method 20, page* 87)

(3) *Bisulphite solution*

10 per cent Potassium metabisulphite	5 ml
N-Hydrochloric acid	5 ml
Distilled water	90 ml

Sections

All types

Suitable control sections

Pancreas

Method

(1)	Bring all sections to water	
(2)	Rinse sections in N-HCl at room temperature	1 min
(3)	Place sections in N-HCl at 60°C, *see* page 172	
(4)	Rinse sections in N-HCl at room temperature	1 min
(5)	Transfer sections to Schiff's reagent	45 min
(6)	Rinse sections in bisulphite, solution (3)	2 min
(7)	Repeat wash in bisulphite, solution (3)	2 min
(8)	Repeat wash in bisulphite, solution (3)	2 min
(9)	Rinse well in distilled water	
(10)	Counterstain if required in 1 per cent Light Green	2 min
(11)	Wash in water	
(12)	Dehydrate through graded alcohols to xylene and mount	

Results

DNA: red-purple
Cytoplasm: green

Remarks

(1) The hydrolysis time is important (*see* text), and the correct time for the fixative must be used.

(2) The N-HCl should be preheated to 60°C.

METHOD 69

RNA, DNA: Methyl Green-Pyronin method. (Modified by Kurnick, 1955)

Reagents required

(1) Methyl Green
(2) Chloroform
(3) Pyronin Y
(4) 0·1 M Acetate buffer, pH 4·8 (*see* page 326)

Preparation of solutions

(1) *Methyl Green*

Methyl green	2 g
Distilled water	100 ml

Dissolve the Methyl Green in the distilled water by stirring well,

Pour the solution into a separating funnel. Add 100 ml chloroform and shake well; pour off contaminated chloroform and repeat until no more violet is extracted (about 6–8 washes).

(2) *Pyronin Y*

Pyronin Y	2 g
Distilled water	100 ml

(3) *Staining solution*

Methyl Green	7·5 ml
Pyronin Y	12·5 ml
Acetate buffer, pH 4·8	30·0 ml

Sections

All types, freeze dried recommended

Suitable control section

Pancreas

Method

(1) Bring all sections to water
(2) Stain in Methyl Green–Pyronin solution, 4–10 min
(3) Blot dry
(4) Rinse rapidly in absolute acetone
(5) Rinse rapidly in 10 per cent acetone in xylene
(6) Rinse rapidly in 50 per cent acetone in xylene
(7) Rinse in xylene
(8) Place sections in fresh xylene and mount in DPX

Results

DNA: green
RNA: red

Remarks

(1) This method can be unreliable, the main causes being that some samples of Pyronin Y will not work satisfactorily, or that the Methyl Green is not pure enough.

(2) The dehydration through acetone and xylene should be rapid.

(3) Triethyl phosphate may be used for dehydration instead of acetone.

(4) Methyl Green alone may be used in the manner described above to demonstrate DNA.

METHOD 70

Methyl Green-Pyronin method for RNA, DNA (Trevan and Sharrock, 1951) (modified)

Reagents required

(1) 2 per cent Methyl Green. *See* previous method
(2) 5 per cent Pyronin Y
(3) Acetate buffer pH 4·8. *See* page 326.

Solution A

2 per cent Methyl Green (chloroform-washed)	10 ml
5 per cent Pyronin Y	17·5 ml
Distilled water	250 ml

Solution B

Acetate buffer pH 4·8

Working solution

Solution A	25 ml
Solution B	25 ml

Method

(1) Bring sections to water
(2) Rinse in distilled water and blot dry
(3) Stain in working solution 20–30 min
(4) Rinse rapidly in distilled water and blot dry
(5) Dehydrate in acetone
(6) Rinse in acetone xylene 50:50, clear in xylene
(7) Mount in DPX

Results

DNA: green–bluish green
RNA: red

Remarks

(1) Fixation should be in neutral fixatives

METHOD 71

RNA, DNA: Gallocyanin–Chrome Alum method (Einarson, 1932, 1951)

Reagents required

(1) Chrome alum
(2) Gallocyanin
(3) Distilled water

Preparation of solution

Chrome alum	5 g
Distilled water	100 ml
Gallocyanin	150 mg

The chrome alum is dissolved in the distilled water, the gallocyanin added and the solution slowly heated until it boils. It is allowed to boil for 5 min. When the solution has cooled to room temperature, the volume is adjusted to 100 ml. The solution is filtered before use.

Sections

All types

Suitable control sections

Pancreas

Method

(1) Bring sections down to water
(2) Stain in gallocyanin–chrome alum solution 18–48 h
(3) Wash in tap water
(4) Dehydrate through graded alcohols and mount in DPX

Results

RNA, DNA: blue

Remarks

This method does not distinguish between RNA and DNA but is specific for nucleic acids.

METHOD 72

DNA: Naphthoic Acid Hydrazine–Feulgen method (Pearse, 1951)

Reagents required

(1) 2-Hydroxy-3-naphthoic acid hydrazine
(2) Absolute alcohol
(3) Acetic acid
(4) Fast Blue B
(5) Veronal acetate buffer, pH 7·4
(6) N-Hydrochloric acid

Preparation of solutions

(1) *N-Hydrochloric acid*

Hydrochloric acid, (conc.)	8·5 ml
Distilled water	91·5 ml

(2) *NAH solution*

2-Hydroxy-3-naphthoic acid hydrazide	50 mg
Absolute alcohol	47 ml
Acetic acid (conc.)	3 ml

(3) *Fast Blue B solution*

Fast Blue B	50 mg
Veronal acetate buffer, pH 7·4	50 ml (*see* page 328)

This solution must be freshly prepared.

Sections

All types

Suitable control sections

Pancreas

Method

(1) Bring all sections to water	
(2) Rinse briefly in N-HCl	
(3) Place sections in N-HCl at 60°C, *see* Table 11.1, p. 172	
(4) Rinse sections in N-HCl at room temperature	1 min
(5) Rinse sections in distilled water	1 min
(6) Rinse sections in 50 per cent alcohol	1 min
(7) Place sections in NAH solution at room temperature	3–6 h
(8) Rinse sections in 50 per cent alcohol	10 min
(9) Rinse sections in 50 per cent alcohol	10 min
(10) Rinse sections in 50 per cent alcohol	10 min
(11) Rinse sections in distilled water	1 min
(12) Place sections in fresh Fast Blue B solution	3 min
(13) Dehydrate through graded alcohols to xylene and mount in DPX	

Result

DNA: blue to bluish purple
Protein material: possibly purplish red

METHOD 73

RNA, DNA: Acridine Orange (Bertalanffy and Nagy, 1962)

Reagents required

(1) Acridine Orange

(2) 0·2 M Phosphate buffer
(3) Calcium chloride
(4) Distilled water
(5) Acetic acid

Preparation of solutions

Acridine Orange solution

Acridine Orange	50 mg
Distilled water	40 ml

The pH of the solution is adjusted to 6·0 with phosphate buffer. The volume is then made up to 50 ml.

(1) *Phosphate buffer, pH* 6·0
See Buffer Tables, p. 327

(2) *Calcium chloride*

Calcium chloride	11 g
Distilled water	50 ml

Sections

Frozen sections
Cryostat sections
Paraffin sections
Freeze dried sections } Not formalin-fixed
Smears

Suitable control sections

Pancreas

Staining method

(1) Bring all sections to distilled water	
(2) Rinse briefly in 1 per cent acetic acid	15 s
(3) Rinse sections in distilled water	15 s
(4) Stain in Acridine Orange solution	10 s—2 min
(5) Transfer sections to phosphate buffer, pH 6·0	1 min
(6) Differentiate sections in calcium chloride solution	20 s
(7) Transfer sections to phosphate buffer, pH 6·0	10 s

(8) Mount sections wet and examine under fluorescent microscope

Results

RNA: red
DNA: light green

Remarks

The authors state that formalin fixation should not be employed.

METHOD 74

DNA: Extraction (Brachet, 1940)

Reagents required

(1) Deoxyribonuclease
(2) 0·2 M Tris buffer, pH 7·6 (*see* Buffer Tables, p. 328)

Preparation of solution

Extraction of solution

0·2 M Tris buffer, pH 7·6	10 ml
Distilled water	50 ml
Deoxyribonuclease	10 mg

Method

(1) Bring test and control sections to water
(2) Place test section in extraction solution, control in tris buffer, pH 7·6 at 37°C, for 4 h
(3) Wash in running tap water
(4) Stain by method (Feulgen method) both sections

Results

Test section: DNA negative
Control section: DNA red

METHOD 75

RNA: Extraction (Brachet, 1940)

Reagents required

(1) Ribonuclease
(2) Distilled water

Preparation of solution

Ribonuclease	8 mg
Distilled water	10 ml

Method

(1) Bring test and control slides to water
(2) Place test slide in ribonuclease solution, control slide in distilled water at 37°C for 1 h
(3) Wash in distilled water
(4) Apply Method 69, Methyl Green–Pyronin

Results

Test slide: RNA negative, DNA green
Controlled slide: RNA red, DNA green

Remarks

Nucleic acids may also be extracted by using perchloric acid. This is not as specific as enzyme digestion, but is a reliable technique and may be used on many occasions where extraction is required as considerable reduction is compared with enzyme digestion, the technique is given below.

METHOD 76

Extraction of nucleic acids with perchloric acid

Reagents required

Perchloric acid
Sodium carbonate

Preparation of solutions

(1)	Perchloric acid	2·5 ml
	Distilled water	47·5 ml
(2)	Perchloric acid	5 ml
	Distilled water	45 ml
(3)	Sodium carbonate	1 g
	Distilled water	100 ml

Method

To remove RNA only

(1) Bring sections down to water
(2) Place sections in 10 per cent perchloric acid (solution 2) at 4°C overnight
(3) Briefly rinse in distilled water
(4) Transfer to the sodium carbonate 5 min
(5) Wash in tap water
(6) Employ nucleic acid method

Remarks

To remove both RNA and DNA place sections in 5 per cent perchloric acid (solution 1) at 60°C for 30 min at stage (2) then continue method.

REFERENCES

Bauer, H. (1932). *Z. Zellforsch* **15,** 225
Bertalanffy, F. D., von and Bickis, I. (1956). *J. Histochem. Cytochem.* **4,** 481
— and Nagy, I. (1962). *Med. Radiophotogr. Phot.* **38,** 82

REFERENCES

BRACHET, J. (1940). *c.r. Soc. Biol.* Paris **133**, 88
— (1953). *Q. Jl microsc. Sci.* **94**, 1
DANIELLI, J. F. (1947). *Sympos. Soc. exp. Biol.* **1,** 101
EINARSON, L. (1932). *Am. J. Path.* **8,** 295
— (1951). *Acta. path. microbiol. scand.* **28,** 82
FEULGEN, R. and ROSSENBECK, H. (1924). *Z. Physiol. Chem.* **135,** 203
KURNICK, N. B. (1955). *Inte. Rev. Cytol.* **4,** 221
PAPPENHEIM, A. (1899). *Virchows Arch. path. Anat. Physiol.* **157,** 19
PEARSE, A. G. E. (1951). *J. clin. Path.* **4,** 1
— (1968). *Histochemistry Theoretical and Applied,* 3rd Edn., vol. 1, London Churchill Livingstone
TAFT, E. B. (1951). *Expl Cell Res.* **2,** 322
TREVAN, D. J. and SHARROCK, A. (1951). *J. Path Bact.* **63,** 326
UNNA, P. G. (1902). *Mh. prakt. Derm.* **35,** 76

12

Pigments

A considerable number of different types of pigments can be found in tissue sections. They may be seen in normal tissue and in pathological conditions. These pigments may be classed as follows:

(1) Artefactual
(2) Endogenous, including haematogenous
(3) Exogenous

ARTEFACT PIGMENTS

These are seen in sections usually as a result of a chemical reaction between the fixative and a tissue component.

(a) *Formalin pigment*

The most common artefact pigment is formalin pigment which is seen as a brownish black granular deposit formed as a result of formaldehyde at an acid pH reacting with haemoglobin to form acid formaldehyde haematin. The formation of this pigment can be reduced or eliminated by using formaldehyde at neutral pH. This pigment is often seen in the spleen and other areas containing a large amount of blood, such as in haemorrhages. Treatment with saturated alcoholic picric acid for two hours or longer will remove the pigment. For some techniques a lengthy wash is required before staining.

(b) *Malarial pigment* ('*haemazoin*')

Also seen in tissue sections as an intracellular brownish black granular deposit which is seen over red blood cells that contain malarial parasites. It looks identical to formalin pigment in sections. It is removed by treatment with saturated alcoholic picric acid.

(c) *Mercury pigment*

Seen in tissue sections from blocks fixed in any fixative which contains mercuric chloride. The pigment is seen as coarse brown-black granules which are soluble in iodine.

TABLE 12.1

Artefact pigments

Pigment	*Birefringent*	*Removed by*	*Features*
Formalin	Yes	Sat. alcoholic picric acid	Dark brown granules
Malarial (haemazoin)	Yes	Sat. alcoholic picric acid	Dark brown granules
Mercury	No	Iodine–alcohol	Intracellular coarse black crystals
Dichromates	No	Acid alcohol	Fine yellow deposit

(d) *Dichromate deposit*

May be seen in sections as a fine yellow deposit, though it is often missed. Potassium dichromate fixatives are responsible. The pigment is removed by treatment with acid alcohol.

ENDOGENOUS PIGMENTS
(including Haematogenous)

These pigments are produced normally by the body. In pathological conditions their site and quantities may be changed.

(a) *Haemoglobin*

Haemoglobin is seen stained red by eosin after formaldehyde fixation. Haemoglobin consists of two basic parts, haem (to which iron and oxygen attach) and globin, a colourless protein. Haemoglobin may be seen as a yellow-brown pigment in renal casts in the kidney. A number of methods are available to demonstrate haemoglobin, by one of the peroxidase methods (e.g. using benzidine or Leuco-Patent Blue) or by the Dunn–Thompson method which is a modified Van Gieson stain. For the rare occasions that haemoglobin is required to be shown in tissue sections, the modified Van Gieson gives acceptable results. In the first edition of this text the benzidine method to demonstrate peroxidase was given. This chemical is now accepted to be carcinogenic and the method is rarely used today.

(b) *Haemosiderin*

Iron is stored in the bone marrow in the form of the golden-brown pigment, haemosiderin. Where there has been excessive breakdown of blood, or at the site of destruction of red cells, haemosiderin may be found in the area. Haemosiderin contains ferric iron which can be satisfactorily demonstrated by Perl's Prussian Blue reaction. Ferrous iron is only occasionally found in tissue sections, and when required can be demonstrated by the Tirmann–Schmelzer Turnbull Blue reaction.

(c) *Bile pigments*

These consist of a number of different pigments, the two main constituents being bilirubin and haematoidin. The pigments are seen as golden brown globules, which are non-fluorescent. The existing methods for their demonstration are the Gmelin technique, Stein's method and Fouchet's method, all of which are either time-consuming or damaging to the tissue, and not permanent. A standard Van Gieson stain, however, will often demonstrate bile a bright green colour.

The three types of pigments described above are derived from haemoglobin and are often called the haemotogenous pigments. The next group are naturally occurring pigments found normally in human tissues.

TABLE 12.2

Histochemical reactions of autogenous pigments

Method	*Haemoglobin*	*Haemosiderin*	*Bile*	*Lipofuscin*	*Ceroid*	*Melanin*	*Chromaffin cells*	*Argentaffin cells*
Schmorl	NEG	NEG	NEG	POS	weak POS	POS	POS	POS
Periodic Acid–Schiff	NEG	NEG	NEG	POS	POS	NEG	NEG	NEG
Perl's Prussian Blue	NEG	POS	NEG	NEG	NEG	Occ. weak POS	NEG	NEG
Sudan Black	NEG	NEG	NEG	some POS	POS	NEG	NEG	NEG
Alkaline Diaz.	NEG	NEG	NEG	NEG	NEG	NEG	NEG	POS
Gmelin	NEG	NEG	POS	NEG	NEG	NEG	NEG	NEG
Silver Methods	NEG	NEG	NEG	POS	POS	POS	POS	POS
Fluorescence	NEG	NEG	NEG	POS	POS	NEG	POS*	POS*

* after formalin fixation

(d) *Lipofuscin*

This term covers a number of pigments found throughout the body. It is seen as golden brown droplets that have a variable composition. The pigment is often found in liver cells and in cardiac muscle cells, usually concentrated around the nucleus. As the pigment appears to increase in amount with ageing it is often termed a 'wear and tear' pigment. The nature and production of lipofuscin is not known, but it is probably a breakdown product of lipid and lipoproteins. Most of the lipofuscins fluoresce, but the colour of the fluorescence appears to depend upon the organ in which the pigment is located. The pigments are mostly insoluble with the possible exception of some which are partly soluble in chloroform. A considerable number of staining reactions will demonstrate lipofuscins; they sometimes give a strong coloration with Sudan Black and are well demonstrated by a long Ziehl–Neelsen method. Lipofuscins are capable of reducing silver and the Masson Fontana silver solution is slowly reduced. The Schmorl reaction gives a positive result after reduction of ferric ferricyanide (*see Figure* 12.1). The PAS reaction is often positive.

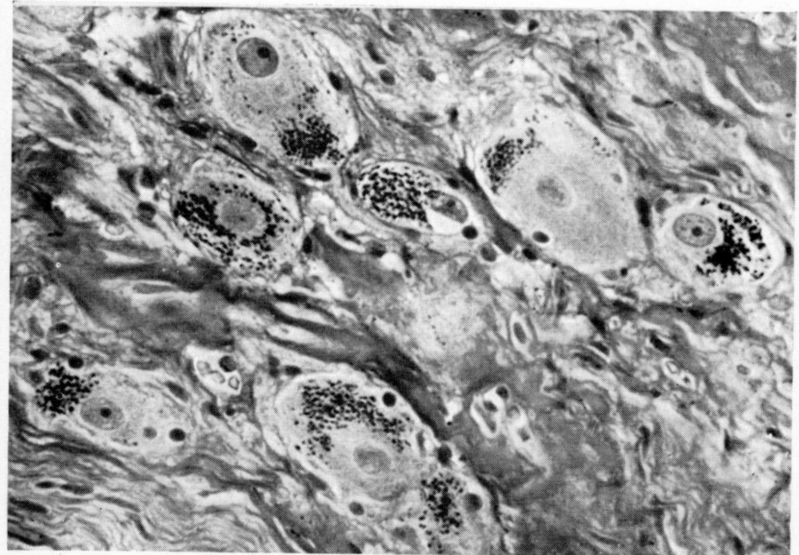

Figure 12.1 Human nerve ganglion. Lipofuscin demonstrated as fine granules. Schmorl reaction. (× 600)

(Reduce to six-tenths in reproduction)

Ceroid—This is probably a type of lipofuscin that is seen in liver. It appears as yellow globules and is localized in phagocytes or in the liver cells. It exhibits a greenish yellow fluorescence, which fades whilst being exposed to ultra violet light. Ceroid is insoluble except in strong acids. It can be demonstrated by using the oil-soluble dyes (Lillie, 1965). The PAS reaction is usually positive and on occasions Perls' method or Schmorl's reaction will be positive; not all the pigment stains. The variation of the staining reactions suggests that 'ceroid' varies in composition, and that it may be a lipofuscin variant.

(e) *Melanin*

Melanin is a normal tissue pigment and is seen in the melanocytes of the skin. In fixed tissue sections melanin is seen as yellow-brown granules; when seen in large concentrations it appears as black granules. Melanin is commonly found in the skin and in the eyes, but is also found in tumours of melanin-containing cells such as benign naevi ('moles') and malignant melanoma. Melanin is not markedly fluorescent and mainly insoluble. It is capable of reducing silver and is well demonstrated by the Masson Fontana method (*see Figure* 12.2). It will also reduce ferric ferricyanide to

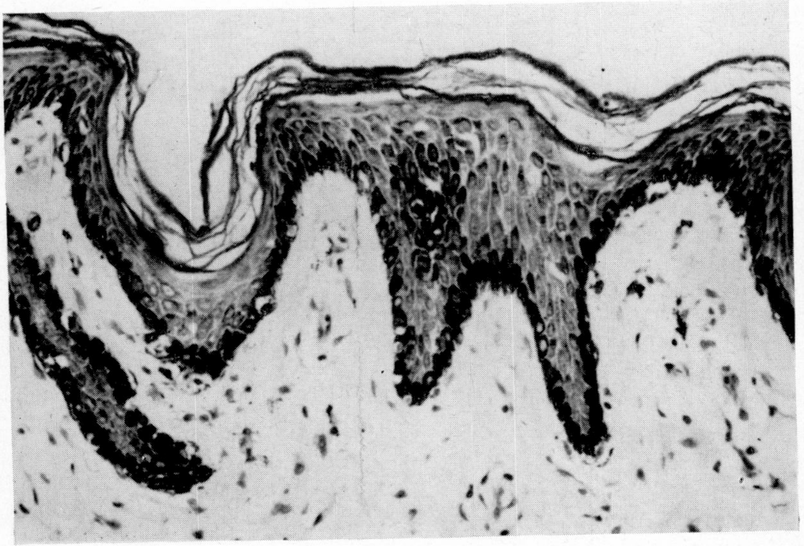

Figure 12.2 Human skin from a Negro. The large amounts of melanin in the basal layer of the epidermis are demonstrated by the Masson Fontana technique. (× *350*)
(Reproduced to two-thirds in reproduction)

give a positive Schmorl reaction. Melanin is produced from tyrosine which is converted into di-hydroxyphenylalanine (DOPA) by the enzyme tyrosinase, which also converts DOPA into melanin. The cells which produce melanin possess the enzyme tyrosinase, and these cells can be demonstrated by the DOPA Oxidase reaction (*see* page 273).

(f) *Chromaffin and argentaffin cells*

The nomenclature applied to this group of cells and substances is confusing to say the least. A number of terms are often used to describe the same cells. The majority of the names were given to the cells on account of their staining characteristics.

True chromaffin cells—These cells, which are mostly found in the adrenal medulla, contain granules which react with chromates, and when fixed in a chromate-containing fixative, the granules become brown. These granules remain uncoloured after fixation with other fixatives, including formol saline. This 'chromaffin reaction' is often weakly positive in sections which are post-fixed in dichromate after initial formalin fixation. The granules in the chromaffin cells contain adrenalin, noradrenalin and their precursors. The histochemical reactions of chromaffin cells are due to the presence of this high level of catechol amine. The chromaffin cells when fixed in formalin have the ability to reduce silver and ferric ferricyanide. Fixation in chromate destroys this reducing activity. To demonstrate chromaffin granules after chromate fixation, a dilute Giemsa should be used; the granules stain bottle-green.

'*Argentaffin*' *cells*—Certain cells in the alimentary tract have the ability to directly reduce silver solutions without the aid of an external reducing agent, This is known as the 'argentaffin reaction', and the cells which have this ability are called argentaffin cells. These cells, particularly concentrated at the base of the intestinal glands of the small bowel and appendix, contain large amounts of the active amine 5-hydroxy tryptamine (5HT, serotonin) and it is this high amine content which is probably responsible for this spontaneous reduction of silver salts. Sometimes these cells form a tumour called a carcinoid or argentaffinoma, and these tumours will also usually show the argentaffin reaction. Because of their high amine content these special cells also show other chemical reactions; for example they will demonstrate a modified chromaffin reaction, providing that the tissue has been fixed in formaldehyde and post-fixed in dichromate. For this reason they are sometimes known as 'enterochromaffin cells'. They do not show the true chromaffin reaction. Argentaffin cells are also capable of reducing ferric ferricyanide (Schmorl-positive) and diazonium salts at an alkaline pH (Alkaline Diazo) (*see Figure* 12.3).

If a silver method which includes an extrinsic reducing agent (e.g. Bodian's Silver Protargol and Gomori's Hexamine Silver) is applied to sections of alimentary tract the argentaffin cells will stain black. In addition many other cells will be demonstrated which are not shown by the true argentaffin reaction. This second group of

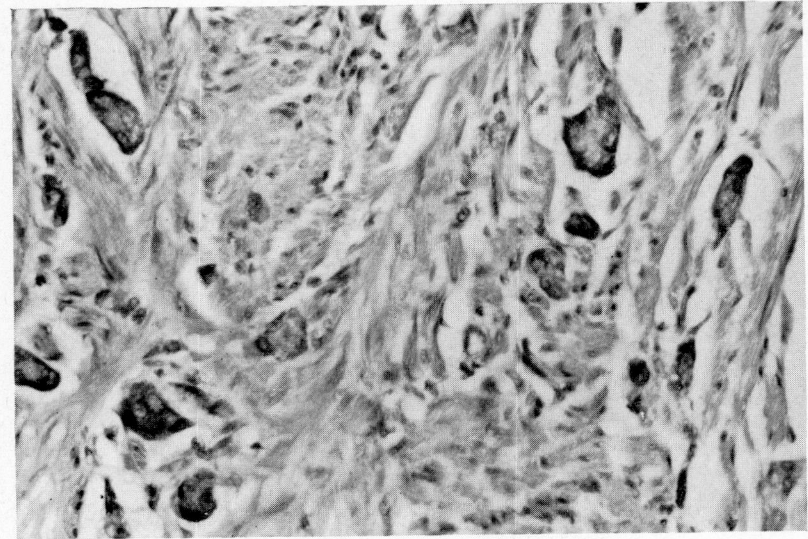

Figure 12.3 Carcinoid tumour infiltrating muscle. The islands of carcinoid tumour show argentaffin granules demonstrated by the Alkaline Diazo method. ($\times$ *525*)
(Reduced to two-thirds in reproduction)

cells, which require the assistance of an external reducing agent are called 'argyrophil cells' and are much more numerous than true argentaffin cells.

TABLE 12.3

Cells	*Other names*	*Substance stored in granules*	*Histochemical methods*
Chromaffin cells		Noradrenalin Adrenalin	Chromaffin reaction after dichromate fixation. Giemsa, Masson Fontana, Schmorl.
Argentaffin	(1) Enterochromaffin (2) Kultschitsky cells	5HT (Serotonin)	Masson Fontana (48 h) Schmorl Alkaline Diazo
'Argyrophil' cells			Bodian Silver (incorporating external reducing agent)

TABLE 12.4
Effects of fixation

Cells	*Fixation*	*Result*
Chromaffin cells	Dichromate only	Brown granules seen in cells
Chromaffin cells	Formalin only	Granules unstained
Chromaffin cells	Formalin, post-fixed in dichromate	Weakly yellow-brown
Argentaffin	Formalin	Silver reduction, fluorescence
Argentaffin	Formalin, post-fixed dichromate	Weak chromaffin reaction
Argentaffin	Dichromate only	No chromaffin reaction

EXOGENOUS PIGMENTS

The 'pigments' considered under this heading in most books (including the first edition of this book) are in fact minerals, most of which are not pigmented. These exogenous minerals are dealt with in Chapter 13.

METHODS FOR PIGMENTS

Dunn–Thompson modified Van Gieson for haemoglobin

A quick reliable method for haemoglobin; whilst not being specific it produces acceptable results. Acid fixatives should be avoided. It is a modified Van Gieson method.

Leuco–Patent Blue method for haemoglobin

This method stains haemoglobin dark green-blue. It is based upon the demonstration of haemoglobin peroxidase and has replaced similar peroxidase methods which used carcinogenic reagents such as benzidine. Since it is a peroxidase method, other peroxidase-containing elements (e.g. the granules of neutrophils and eosinophils) will also be demonstrated.

Prussian Blue reaction for iron

This technique, first introduced by Perls (1867), is one of the classical methods of histochemistry. The method can be applied to either paraffin sections or frozen sections. A solution of potassium ferrocyanide and dilute hydrochloric acid is applied to the section. The acid liberates loosely bound iron and the ferric ions then react with potassium ferrocyanide to form ferric ferrocyanide. This is an insoluble blue compound and is located at the site of the reaction. The concentrations of the two constituents are not critical and many workers use concentrations widely different from those given in Method 80, with equally satisfactory results.

Gmelin method for bile pigment

This technique, with which deposits of haematoidin and bilirubin may be demonstrated, has been in use for very many years. The reaction works best when applied to formalin-fixed paraffin sections. Sections thought to contain either haematoidin or bilirubin are treated with alcoholic nitric acid. This is a severe procedure and invariably causes damage to the sections. The oxidation of the bile pigments goes through three or more stages, each of these stages producing a colour which is visible under the light microscope. The colour change should be from red through purple to the final colour of green. An alternative reagent used is nitrous acid (HNO_2). This is prepared as a 2 per cent nitrous acid solution in nitric acid. In this case, the colour change observed during the oxidation is green to red and finally to blue. The preparations are not permanent and they should be examined and then discarded.

Long Ziehl–Neelsen for lipofuscin

This usually demonstrates lipofuscin well. Because of its lipid nature lipofuscin has the property of acid-fastness shown by tubercle bacilli. The section requires a long staining time. The lipofuscins retain their red colour after differentiation in acid alcohol. If the nuclear counterstain is too heavy the lipofuscins will appear dark purple.

Sudan Black method for lipofuscin and ceroid

Some lipofuscins and all ceroids are sudanophilic, and can sometimes be demonstrated by the Sudan Black B method in paraffin sections. Pearse (1972) believes that only early lipofuscins, produced recently from triglyceride and phosphatide oxidation, are sudanophilic. The method given in Chapter 10, page 153, can be used to demonstrate these lipofuscins.

The Schmorl reaction

This technique, which is capable of demonstrating lipofuscins, melanins, argentaffin granules, chromaffin cells and sulphydryl groups, is a much used method in the identification of pigments in tissue sections. The solution applied to the section contains potassium ferricyanide and ferric chloride. Components of these pigments reduce the ferric ferricyanide to ferric ferrocyanide, which is then seen as a blue precipitate. Substances less able to reduce the ferric ferricyanide solution often give a greenish blue colour. The staining time is important. Adams (1956) suggests that 90 seconds is long

Remarks

Fixation should be in formaldehyde; tissue blocks should be small and the fixation time kept to a minimum.

METHOD 80

Iron: Prussian Blue reaction (Perls, 1867)

Reagents required

(1) Potassium ferrocyanide
(2) Hydrochloric acid
(3) Distilled water
(4) Neutral Red or Mayer's Carmalum

Preparation of solutions

(1) *Potassium ferrocyanide, 2 per cent*

Prepare fresh before use

Potassium ferrocyanide	1 g
Distilled water	50 ml

(2) *Hydrochloric acid, 2 per cent*

Hydrochloric acid	1 ml
Distilled water	49 ml

Staining solution

2 per cent Hydrochloric acid	25 ml
2 per cent Potassium ferrocyanide	25 ml

Sections

All types

Suitable control sections

Previously known controls

Staining methods

(1) Bring all sections to water	
(2) Place in staining solution (freshly prepared)	5–30 min
(3) Wash in tap water	
(4) Counterstain in 1 per cent Neutral Red	20 s
(5) Wash rapidly in water	
(6) Dehydrate through graded alcohols to xylene	
(7) Mount in DPX	

Result

Ferric iron: blue
Nuclei: red

Remarks

(1) Use iron-free reagents
(2) Solution (1) should be freshly prepared
(3) In some cases, after Neutral Red has been used, it is necessary to blot the section lightly and dehydrate through the alcohols.

METHOD 81

Bile pigment: Gmelin method (Stein, 1935)

Reagents required

(1) Nitric acid (conc.)
(2) Absolute alcohol

Preparation of solution

Nitric acid (conc.)	5 ml
Absolute alcohol	5 ml

Sections

Paraffin sections (formalin-fixed)

Suitable control sections

Known positive section

Method

(1) Bring all sections to water
(2) Apply freshly prepared solution (a few drops to cover section)
(3) Place coverslip over the section
(4) Remove excess reagent with filter paper
(5) Ring coverslip with paraffin wax
(6) Examine under microscope

Result

Bile pigment and haematoidin crystals change colour from red through to green.

METHOD 82

Long Ziehl–Neelsen method for lipofuscin

Reagents required

(1) Basic fuchsin

(2) Phenol
(3) Absolute alcohol
(4) Distilled water
(5) Acid alcohol
(6) Haematoxylin

Preparation of solutions

(1) *Carbol fuchsin solution*

Basic fuchsin	1 g
Phenol	0·5 g
Absolute alcohol	10 ml
Distilled water	100 ml

Sections

All types

Suitable control sections

Previously known positive control

Staining method

(1) Bring sections to water
(2) Stain sections in carbol fuchsin solution at 60°C for 3 h
(3) Wash well in tap water
(4) Differentiate in acid alcohol
(5) Wash well in tap water
(6) Counterstain in haematoxylin if required
(7) Wash in tap water
(8) Dehydrate, clear and mount

Results

Some lipofuscins: red
Nuclei: blue

METHOD 83

Melanin, lipofuscin, argentaffin: Schmorl method

Reagents required

(1) Ferric chloride
(2) Potassium ferricyanide
(3) Acetic acid
(4) Neutral Red
(5) Distilled water

Preparation of solutions

(1)	Ferric chloride	500 mg
	Distilled water	50 ml
(2)	Potassium ferricyanide	500 mg
	Distilled water	50 ml

Staining solution

Ferric chloride solution	37·5 ml
Potassium ferricyanide	5 ml
Distilled water	7·5 ml

Sections

All types

Suitable control sections

Skin

Staining method

(1) Bring all sections to water

(2) Immerse in staining solution. Examine under microscope after 30 s to see if any colour has developed. When a deep blue colour is observed, remove the section from the solution. Leave the sections in the staining solution, for a maximum of 5 min.

(3) Wash in 1 per cent acetic acid

(4) Wash in tap water

(5) Dehydrate through graded alcohols to xylene

(6) Mount in DPX

Result

Melanin, lipofuscin or argentaffin granules produce a deep blue colour.

Remarks

(1) As can be seen from above, the method will show more than one pigment.

(2) The time in the ferric ferrocyanide solution should be kept to a minimum as the background will stain after a few minutes.

METHOD 84

Melanin and argentaffin cells: Masson Fontana method

Reagents required

(1) Silver nitrate

(2) Ammonia

(3) Distilled water

(4) Sodium thiosulphate

Preparation of silver solution

To 20 ml of 10 per cent silver nitrate add concentrated ammonia drop by drop. The first few drops will cause a precipitate to form. Add ammonia to the silver solution until this precipitate has almost disappeared and a faint opalescence remains, then add 20 ml of distilled water to the solution. Then store the solution for one day, and after storage filter the solution into a dark bottle and keep in the dark. The solution must be filtered before use and not used repeatedly.

Note: If too much ammonia is added and the precipitate is completely removed, further silver nitrate may be added until the faint opalescence returns.

Sections

All types (formalin-fixed)

Suitable control sections

Skin

Staining method

(1) Bring all sections to distilled water, two changes
(2) Transfer sections to silver solution in the dark overnight (*See Remarks*)
(3) Rinse in distilled water
(4) Transfer sections to 5 per cent thiosulphate for 2 min
(5) Wash in tap water
(6) Counterstain if required
(7) Wash in tap water
(8) Dehydrate through graded alcohols to xylene
(9) Mount in DPX

Result

Melanin: black

Remarks

Melanin is well demonstrated after 18–24 h
Argentaffin cells usually need up to 48 h

METHOD 85

Chromaffin reaction

Reagents required

(1) Regaud's fixative or Orth's fluid

Method

(1) Thin slices of fresh tissue are fixed in Regaud's fixative for two days

(2) Rinse tissues in distilled water

(3) Cut frozen sections or dehydrate, clear and embed in paraffin wax

(4) Sections from either type of preparation will show chromaffin cells yellow-brown in an unstained state

Suitable control tissue

Adrenal medulla

METHOD 86

Modified Giemsa for chromaffin cell granules

Reagents required

(1) Standard Giemsa stain
(2) Buffered distilled water pH 6·8
(3) 0·5 per cent acetic acid

Preparation of Giemsa stain

Standard Giemsa stain	2 ml
Buffered distilled water pH 6·8	48 ml

Sections

All types after chromate fixation

Suitable control sections

Adrenal medulla

Staining method

(1) Bring sections to water
(2) Rinse in distilled water
(3) Stain in dilute Giemsa stain overnight
(4) Rinse in distilled water
(5) Wash in 0·5 per cent acetic acid until section is pink 2 min
(6) Wash in distilled water
(7) Dehydrate rapidly through graded alcohols to xylene
(8) Mount in DPX

Results

Chromaffin cell granules: greenish yellow
Nuclei: blue

METHOD 87

Argentaffin cell granules: Alkaline Diazo method

Reagents required

(1) Diazonium salt Fast Red B (diazotate of 5-nitro-anisidine)
(2) 0·1 M Veronal acetate buffer, pH 9·2
(3) Distilled water
(4) Haematoxylin

Preparation of staining solution

Fast Red B salt	50 mg	
0·1 M Veronal acetate buffer, pH 9·2	50 ml	(*see* page 328)

Sections

All types (formalin fixation)

Suitable control sections

Adrenal medulla

Staining method

(1) Bring all sections to water	
(2) Transfer sections to staining solution at 4°C	30 s
(3) Wash well in tap water	
(4) Stain nuclei in haematoxylin	5 min
(5) Wash in tap water	5–10 min
(6) Dehydrate through graded alcohols to xylene	
(7) Mount in DPX	

Result

Argentaffin (enterochromaffin granules): orange-red
Nuclei: blue-black

Remarks

According to Pearse (1960) other stable diazotates may be used instead of Fast Red B, and those giving reddish azo dyes are preferred.

METHOD 88

Noradrenaline: Fluorescence technique (Eränkö, etc.)

The Fluorescence technique can be applied to either formalin-fixed frozen sections or to freeze dried, formalin-vapour-fixed sections. Both methods are given. However, vastly superior results are obtained with the latter method.

Formalin-Fixed Frozen Sections

(1) Fix tissue for 24 h in formol saline
(2) Cut frozen sections (10 microns thick)
(3) Mount in glycerin
(4) Examine under fluorescence microscope

Result

Noradrenaline: strong fluorescence (colour depends upon filters used)

Freeze Dried Sections

(1) Freeze dry piece of tissue (*see* Method 10)
(2) Fix in formalin vapour (*see* Method 12)
(3) Embed in paraffin wax
(4) Cut sections 8 microns thick
(5) Mount in light petroleum
(6) Examine under fluorescence microscope

Result

Noradrenaline: strong fluorescence (colour depends upon filters used)

Remarks

The fluorescence method is probably the most specific of the techniques used to demonstrate noradrenaline.

METHOD 89

Melanin and lipofuscin: Bleaching techniques

No one bleaching agent is recommended in the literature to give satisfactory results. This is due in part to the difference in the composition of the melanins and lipofuscins. Below are given the solutions most commonly used along with the average time of exposure to bleach the pigments.

(1) Hydrogen peroxide, 10 vol., 3–36 h (McManus and Mowry, 1964)

(2) Hydrogen peroxide, 30 vol., 24–48 h (Pearse, 1960)

(3) 0·1 per cent Potassium permanganate, 1 per cent oxalic acid, 12–24 h (Pearse, 1972)

(4) 5 per cent Chromic acid (sometimes patchy), 1–3 h (Lillie, 1965)

(5) Peracetic acid 40 per cent, 2–16 h (Pearse, 1960)

The methods of choice appear to be numbers (3) and (5). Pearse (1972) felt that peracetic acid was probably the best. The permanganate and oxalic acid technique will bleach all pigments. Lipofuscins (according to Pearse) should not be bleached after 16 h with the peracetic method, but will be after 24 h.

Method

(1) Bring all sections to water

(2) Place duplicate slides in distilled water

(3) Transfer sections to 40 per cent peracetic acid until bleached, 2–16 h

(4) Apply required melanin technique to both sections

Result

Test slide: melanin, negative
Control slide: melanin, positive

REFERENCES

ADAMS, C. W. M. (1956). *J. Histochem. Cytochem.* **4,** 23

DUNN, R. C. and THOMPSON, E. C. (1945). *Arch. Path.* **39,** 49

— — (1946). *Stain Technol.* **21,** 65

ERANKO, O. (1955). *Nature, Lond.* **175,** 88

LILLIE, R. D. (1965). *Histopathological Technique and Practical Histochemistry,* New York: McGraw-Hill

MASSON, P. (1928). *Amal. J. Path.* **4,** 181

MCMANUS, J. F. A. and MOWRY, R. W. (1964). *Staining Methods, Histological and Histochemical,* New York: Hoeber

PEARSE, A. G. E. (1960). *Histochemistry, Theoretical and Applied,* 2nd edition. London: Churchill

— (1972). *Histochemistry, Theoretical and Applied,* 3rd edition. Vol. 2. London: Churchill Livingstone

PERLS, M. (1867). *Virchows Arch. Path. Anat.,* **39,** 42

STEIN, J. (1935). *C.r. Soc. Biol.,* **120,** 1136

13

Minerals

Iron and calcium are the most important minerals which are capable of being demonstrated histochemically in human tissues. Other metallic ions, such as potassium and sodium, are present in greater concentrations in tissues, but cannot yet be satisfactorily demonstrated by histochemical means. Other minerals are normally present in such small quantities that they cannot be demonstrated either histologically or histochemically. Iron, calcium and copper are important endogenous minerals; the others dealt with in this chapter are largely exogenous and usually gain access to the body by inhalation into the lungs or by implantation into the skin as foreign material. The most common cause of this illegal entry is as a result of industrial exposure in the mining and metal industries.

Iron

Iron can be found in the body in many forms, most of which can be demonstrated histochemically (*see Figure 13.1*). Some of the stored iron in the body is found in loose combination with protein in the form of a golden brown pigment called haemosiderin. This has been dealt with in some detail in the chapter on pigments, and will not be considered further here. Another storage form of iron is ferritin, in which iron is bound to a protein called apoferritin. The iron can be separated from the protein by reducing agents such as hydrosulphite. Other iron in the tissues is much more strongly bound to protein (e.g. in haemoglobin, myoglobin) and the iron is not available for demonstration; treatment for a short time by 100 vol hydrogen peroxide may release sufficient iron for demonstration by the Perls' reaction.

Particulate iron, usually in the form of an inert iron oxide, may be found in the lungs in industrial disease such as 'haematite (iron oxide)-miners lung' and 'mirror polisher's lung' where fine iron oxide particles are inhaled over many years. Iron in this form is

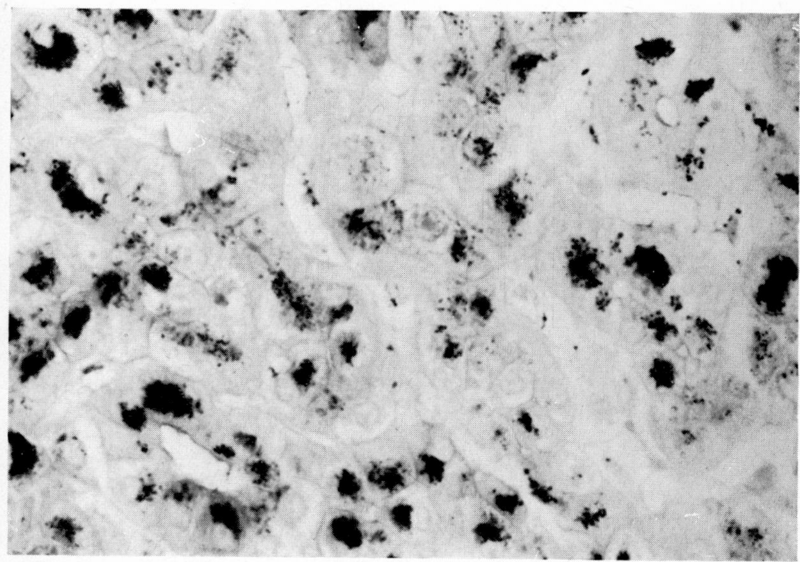

Figure 13.1 Human liver from a patient with excessive iron storage. The iron in the liver cells is demonstrated by the Perls' reaction. (× *220*)

(Reduced to two-thirds in reproduction)

not directly demonstrable by Perls' or related methods, but haemosiderin and ferritin are invariably found in association with the iron oxide.

Calcium

Calcium is the most important cation in bone, and exists there in the form of bone salts, mainly crystalline hydroxy apatite (hydrated calcium phosphate, with traces of carbonate, citrate and other ions). Methods to demonstrate calcium are widely applied to sections of undecalcified bone in the diagnosis of some types of bone disease, particularly in distinguishing between the two bone diseases, osteoporosis and osteomalacia (*see Figure 13.2*). In certain disorders of calcium metabolism, excessive calcium is deposited in insoluble form in tissues which normally do not contain calcium, and the deposition of calcium is common in many degenerative and chronic inflammatory diseases (e.g. atherosclerosis and tuberculosis). Calcium in its insoluble form produces a blue-black calcium lake with haematoxylin, and therefore is easily seen in a routine haematoxylin and eosin section. Unfortunately this is not specific for calcium but serves to draw attention to the possible presence of calcium in a

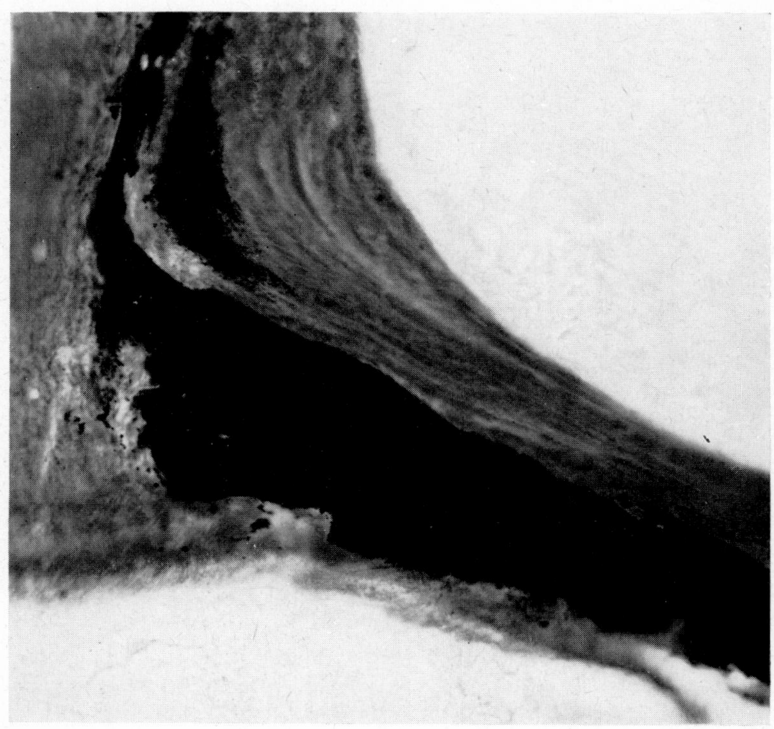

Figure 13.2 Human bone from a case of osteomalacia. The reduced calcium content of the bone trabeculae is shown by the Von Kossa method; counterstained by Van Gieson. (× *520*)
(Reduced to nine-tenths in reproduction)

section. Calcium also forms an orange-red dye-lake with the dye Alizarin Red S; this can be used to identify calcium in tissue sections but is not specific for calcium, since other cations produce coloured lakes with Alizarin Red S. The specificity can be increased by performing the reaction within the pH range 6·3–8·5 (Dahl, 1952). A traditional way of demonstrating calcium is by the Von Kossa silver reduction method (*see Figures 13.2 and 13.3*). This method in fact demonstrates phosphates and carbonates, and not calcium; since most of the phosphates and carbonates present are those of calcium, the method is usually regarded as a fairly specific demonstrator of sites of calcium.

Calcium also exists in the body as soluble salts (e.g. calcium chloride) and as ionized calcium in combination with proteins. Calcium in these forms rarely requires demonstration.

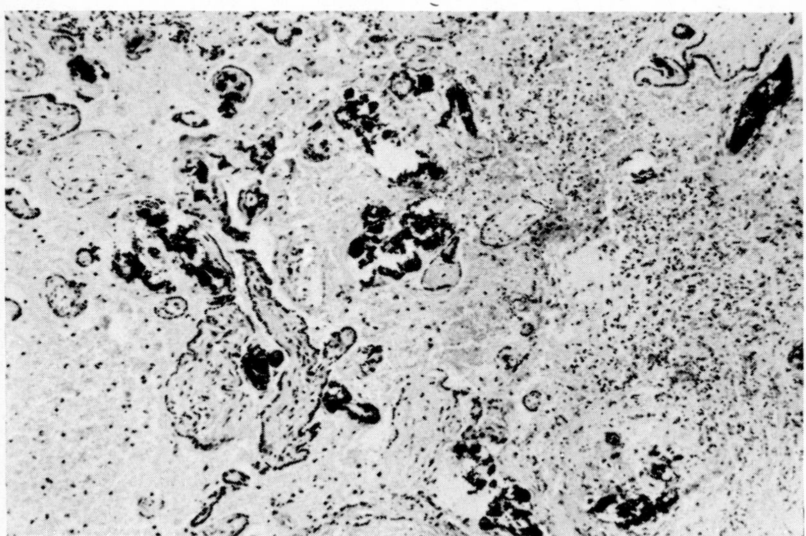

Figure 13.3. Human placenta. Calcium deposits being shown by the Von Kossa method. (×*150*)

(Reduced to six-tenths in reproduction)

Copper

Copper is present in many tissues in concentrations too small to be detectable by histochemical means. In the disease called Wilson's disease ('hepato-lenticular degeneration') there is a disorder of copper metabolism leading to excessive deposition of copper in liver and in the basal ganglia region of the brain. The diagnosis can be established in life by demonstrating excessive copper in a needle biopsy of the liver. The method of choice is the Rubeanic Acid technique (*see Figure 13.4*). Early methods for copper used fresh solutions of haematoxylin (Mallory and Parker, 1939); copper forms a blue lake with haematoxylin. Unfortunately many other metals form lakes with haematoxylin and so the method lacks specificity.

Silica

Silica particles are commonly inhaled by miners of coal and many metal ores, since most ores co-exist with silicaceous rocks. The inhaled silica dust excites a marked fibrous reaction in the lung tissue, leading to the crippling industrial disease, silicosis. The silica

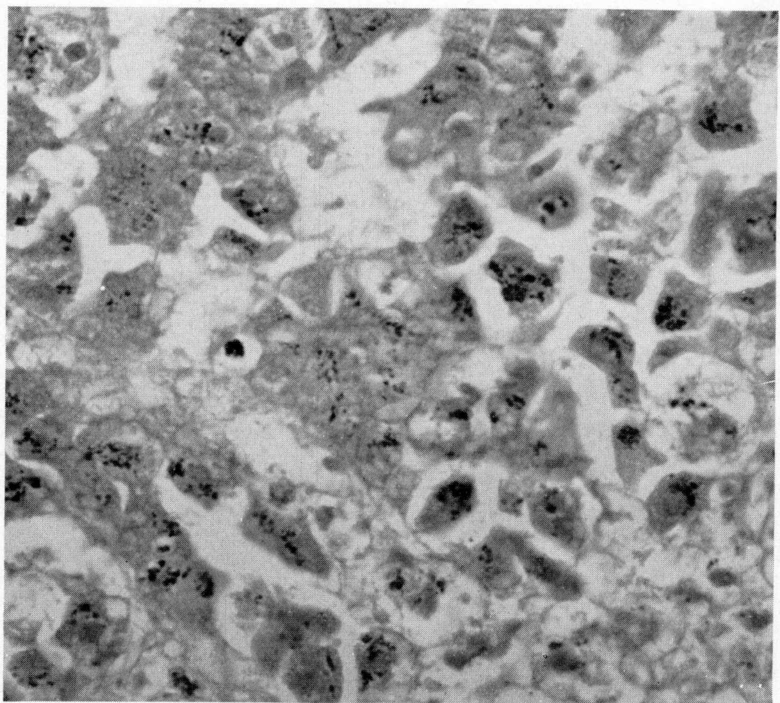

Figure 13.4 Human liver from a patient with excessive copper storage (Wilson's disease). The copper in the degenerate liver cells is demonstrated by the Rubeanic Acid method. (× 525)

particles are often mixed with other particles, for example coal dust in coal miner's pneumoconiosis and red iron oxide in haematite miner's lung. There is no histochemical method for the positive identification of silica, but the particles can be demonstrated by their birefringence in polarized light, and by microincineration methods (*see* page 304).

A special form of silica is asbestos, which exists in the form of long thin crystalline fibres. Asbestos fibres may be inhaled by workers in asbestos mines and factories, and by workers in any of the many industries which use asbestos. Prolonged exposure to asbestos can lead to crippling fibrosis of the lung ('asbestosis'), and even slight exposure to certain types of asbestos may eventually induce a type of cancer in the pleural lining of the lung. Asbestos fibres themselves cannot be demonstrated histochemically, but once in the lung the fibres become coated with a smooth protein sheath which contains iron. The 'asbestos body' so formed appears brown in unstained and in haematoxylin-and eosin-stained sections (*see Figure 13.5*), and the iron in the protein sheath can be well demonstrated by the Perls reaction.

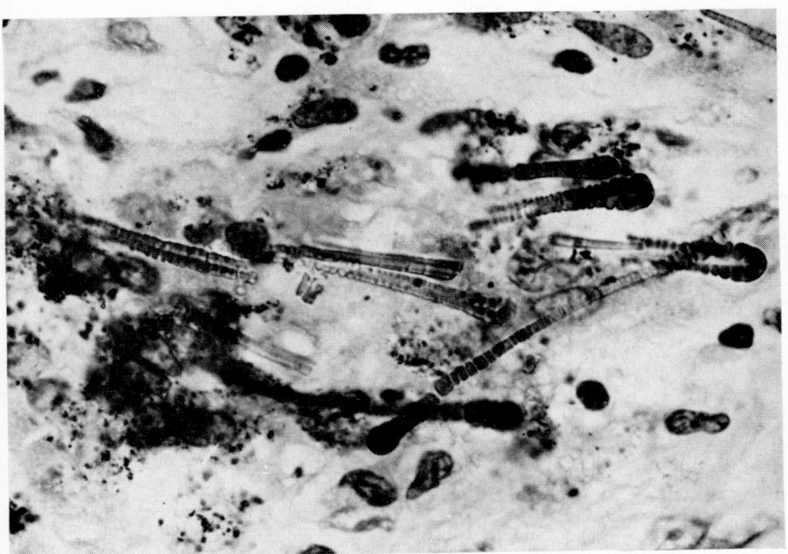

Figure 13.5 *Human lung from a case of asbestosis. The characteristic morphology of asbestos bodies is clearly seen in an H & E stained preparation.* (× *1200*)
(Reduced to two-thirds in reproduction)

Lead

Lead poisoning is now uncommon but used to occur following the ingestion of lead-based paints, usually in children who gnawed toys and cots painted with lead-based paints. Adults working in industries involving lead e.g. the battery industry, occasionally developed lead poisoning. In such cases the excessive lead content of the body can be confirmed by the chemical estimation of lead in the serum, and can be demonstrated histochemically within the tissues, particularly bone. Lead can be demonstrated in tissues by the Sulphide-Silver method (Timm, 1958) and by the Rhodizonate method. The Sulphide-Silver method has low specificity since many other heavy metals will show the positive reaction. The Rhodizonate method is probably more specific.

Beryllium

Beryllium can gain access to the body as a result of industrial exposure. Engineers working with beryllium may get minute beryllium particles implanted in the skin, but a more common route of entry is by inhalation into the lung. Beryllium can be identified in tissues by the Naphthochrome Green B method, and the Solochrome Azurine method. Many beryllium salts fluoresce and it is often worth examining an unstained section in ultra-violet light; beryllium deposits often emit a characteristic bluish white fluorescence (Pearse, 1972).

Aluminium

Aluminium usually gains entry to the body by inhalation of particles in industrial exposure. It can be identified by the Naphthochrome Green B method, although this is not specific (*see* also Beryllium).

Silver

This metal may be found in the skin, alimentary tract and other organs in silver workers; it gives the skin a peculiar slate-grey appearance ('argyria'). In sections the particles appear as dark brown to black granules. Silver can be removed from sections by 1–2 hours treatment in Lugol's iodine followed by sodium thiosulphate. Ammonium sulphide converts silver deposits into the black sulphide; this can be removed by 5 per cent aqueous KCN. Silver can be demonstrated in tissues by the Dimethylaminobenzylidene-Rhodanine method.

Carbon

Carbon is the most common exogenous element found in human tissues. It is inhaled in particulate form in large amounts by coal miners, smokers and city dwellers. It is phagocytosed by macrophages in the lung alveoli, and is then carried to the regional lymph nodes. Carbon is very inert and cannot be demonstrated histochemically.

Urates

Urates are deposited in the tissues in large amounts in the condition known as 'gout'. In the early stages of the disease the urate crystals are deposited in the tissues lining the joints, and crystals also float freely in the lubricating (synovial) fluid of the joint.

When the disease is of long standing, urates may be deposited elsewhere in the body; the kidney is a particularly important site.

HISTOCHEMICAL METHODS

Perls' Prussian Blue reaction for iron

Loosely bound iron is demonstrated by the Perls reaction which is described in Chapter 12.

Alizarin Red S

This technique used by Dahl (1952) and McGee-Russell (1958) is a dye-lake reaction. This means that the dye has the ability to form a lake with the calcium. This type of reaction is not specific for calcium, as other metals may also form a lake with the dye. Haematoxylin, Nuclear Fast Red and Alizarin Red S are all capable of forming lakes with calcium at a suitable pH. The best results are obtained with Alizarin Red S. This dye forms a dye-lake with calcium phosphates and carbonates. The length of the staining time is critical, for if the stain is left too long, the orange-red precipitate diffuses over the section and it is difficult to see the true deposits. If large amounts of calcium are present, the staining time must be greatly reduced. When this technique has been mastered, excellent results can be obtained by also using counterstains, but not at an acid pH.

Von Kossa method for calcium salts

This technique, first described in 1901, is a metal substitution technique, the calcium in the calcium salt being replaced by a different metal. The method is essentially a means of demonstrating insoluble carbonates and phosphates, but since most of the insoluble carbonates and phosphates in the body are their calcium salts, the method can be regarded as demonstrating sites of calcium. The basis of the reaction is that when a solution containing silver nitrate is applied to a section containing one of these insoluble calcium salts, the calcium is replaced by silver. The resultant silver salt in bright light e.g. sunlight or ultra-violet light, undergoes reduction to metallic silver. The section is then removed from the silver solution, washed and placed in 'hypo' (sodium thiosulphate). Sites of calcium salts are marked by a dense black precipitate. Fixation for this technique should be with fixatives containing no free acids and at a neutral pH. McGee-Russell (1958) suggests that for the demonstration of small amounts of calcium, alcohol is a better fixative than formol saline.

Rubeanic Acid method for copper

The Rubeanic Acid method was first introduced by Okamoto and Utamura (1938), and modified by Uzman (1956) and again by Howell (1959). Howell's modification is given in Method 92. This method can be used to demonstrate copper when the metal is found in excessive amounts in tissue sections. The original method was described for tissue blocks but Howell's modification allows it to be applied to sections. A dilute rubeanic acid solution in alcohol will give a dark green precipitate of copper rubeanate when applied to sections containing copper. Rubeanic acid also combines with cobalt and nickel, but according to Uzman (1956), if the staining solution is acid and acetate ions are also present, then these metals will not react.

Methods for silica and asbestos

No histochemical methods exist for the demonstration of these inert substances. Silica particles can often be identified in tissues because of their birefringence, and asbestosis can be detected because of the iron content of the protein sheath which asbestos fibres rapidly acquire on gaining entry into the tissues.

Rhodizonate method for lead salts

The method is based upon the reaction between lead and the chelating agent, sodium rhodizonate. Lead salts appear red. The method is applicable to decalcified bone (*see* Pearse (1972)).

Solochrome Azurine method for aluminium and beryllium

This metal chelation technique demonstrates aluminium and beryllium; both stain deep blue. The two metals can be differentiated, if necessary, by pretreatment of the section with an alkali which removes aluminium salts but leaves beryllium unaffected.

Naphthochrome B method for aluminium and beryllium

The compound Naphthochrome Green B was used to demonstrate beryllium in tissue sections by Denz (1949). Pearse (1960) modified the technique, which is capable of demonstrating aluminium, iron and calcium as well as beryllium. These metals will react with Naphthochrome Green B to produce a dye-lake. The pH of the dye solution is extremely critical. Beryllium and Naphthochrome Green B produce a deep apple-green colour at pH 5·0. At this pH, calcium is soluble and consequently will not be shown, while iron and aluminium are only lightly stained. If Naphthochrome Green B is used at a slightly alkaline pH, 7·2–7·4, beryllium will stain weakly, while aluminium will produce a deep-green colour.

Paradimethylaminobenzylidene-Rhodanine method for silver

This metal chelation technique leads to the production of a reddish brown deposit of silver rhodanate. The main disadvantage in this technique is that the silver rhodanate is not absolutely insoluble and some diffusion is almost inevitable.

Demonstration of carbon

Carbon is inert and cannot be demonstrated histochemically. It is sometimes necessary to distinguish between carbon and other black pigments such as melanin in a tissue section. Carbon is resistant to the action of Mallory bleach and acids; other black pigments are removed by this treatment.

Demonstration of urates

Urates and uric acid are soluble in aqueous solutions. For the specific demonstrations of urates alcohol should be used as a fixative. The crystals of uric acid are birefringent and slightly soluble in dilute alkalis. They are argentaffin pigments and can be demonstrated by silver methods of which Gomori's Methenamine Silver is probably the best.

TABLE 13.1

Inorganic constituents staining methods

Constituent	*Staining method*	*Birefringence*	*Site*
Iron	Perls	No	Many possible
Calcium	Von Kossa, Alizarin Red S etc.	No	Many possible
Copper	Rubeanic acid	No	Liver
Silica		Yes	Lungs, lymph glands, skin
Lead	Rhodizonate	No	Bone; many other possible sites
Beryllium	Naphthochrome B	No	Lungs, liver, skin
Aluminium	Naphthochrome B	No	Lungs, skin
Silver	Rhodanine	Yes	Intestine, skin

METHOD 90

Calcium salts: Alizarin Red S method (Dahl, 1952)

Reagents required

(1) Sodium alizarin sulphonate
(2) Ammonia
(3) Distilled water
(4) Absolute alcohol
(5) Hydrochloric acid

Preparation of solutions

(1) *Alizarin Red S*

Sodium alizarin sulphonate	500 mg
Distilled water	45 ml

This solution is thoroughly mixed, then 5 ml of ammonia (28 per cent ammonia, 1 part; distilled water, 99 parts) is added slowly whilst the solution is being stirred. The pH of the solution should be between 6·3 and 6·5; if it is not it must be adjusted by the use of buffers.

(2) *Differentiator*

Hydrochloric acid	0·1 ml
95 per cent Alcohol	99·9 ml

Sections

All types, but fixed in neutral fixatives

Suitable control sections

Sections known to contain calcium

Staining method

(1) Bring all sections to water	
(2) Place sections in Alizarin Red S solution	2 min
(3) Wash in distilled water	10 s
(4) Rinse in acid alcohol solution	10 s
(5) Rinse in 95 per cent alcohol	
(6) Rinse in absolute alcohol	
(7) Place sections in xylene	
(8) Mount in cedarwood oil	

Result

Calcium deposits: orange-red

Remarks

(1) If large amounts of calcium are in the section, the staining time should be reduced by half.

(2) The rinse in the acid alcohol solution gives a sharper result. The rinsing should be kept to a minimum because of the danger of removing the calcium. Pearse (1960) thought it improbable that any calcium is removed by a short rinse.

(3) Fixatives containing acid should be avoided.

METHOD 91

Calcium salts: Metal Substitution method (Von Kossa, 1901) (modified)

Reagents required

(1) Silver nitrate
(2) Sodium thiosulphate
(3) Neutral red
(4) Distilled water

Preparation of solutions

(1) *Silver nitrate* 1·5 *per cent*

Silver nitrate	750 mg
Distilled water	50 ml

(2) *'Hypo' solution*

Sodium thiosulphate	2·5 g
Distilled water	50 ml

Sections

All types fixed in neutral fixatives

Suitable control sections

Sections known to contain calcium

Method

(1) Bring all sections to distilled water. Wash well	
(2) Place sections in 1·5 per cent silver nitrate (*see Remarks* (1)	15–30 min
(3) Wash very well in distilled water	
(4) Place sections in 'hypo' solution	1 min
(5) Wash well in distilled water	
(6) Counterstain in 2 per cent Neutral Red	30 s
(7) Wash in tap water, rapidly	
(8) Dehydrate through alcohols to xylene	
(9) Mount in DPX	

Results

Calcium salts: brown to black
Nuclei: red

Remarks

(1) The silver nitrate solution should be used in direct sunlight, or under an ultra-violet source.

(2) Distilled water should be used before and after the silver solution.

(3) No fixatives containing acid should be used.

METHOD 92

Copper: Rubeanic Acid method (Howell, 1959, after Okamoto and Utamura)

Reagents required

(1) Rubeanic acid
(2) Absolute alcohol
(3) Sodium acetate
(4) Distilled water

Preparation of solutions

(1) *Rubeanic acid stock solution*

Rubeanic acid	50 mg
Absolute alcohol	50 ml

(2) *Sodium acetate solution*

Sodium acetate	10 g
Distilled water	100 ml

Staining solution

Rubeanic acid stock solution	2·5 ml
Sodium acetate solution	50 ml

Sections

All types

Suitable control sections

Previously known positive section

Staining method

(1) Bring all sections to water
(2) Place sections in staining solution at 37°C overnight
(3) Place sections in 70 per cent alcohol for 15 min
(4) Transfer sections to absolute alcohol for 6 h
(5) Place sections in xylene
(6) Mount in DPX

Result

Copper: greenish black granules

Remarks

(1) Copper will only be demonstrated when present in above normal quantities.

(2) Howell (1959) found that the sections tended to lift off the slides.

METHOD 93

Rhodizonate method for lead salts

Reagents required

Sodium rhodizonate
Acetic acid

Preparation of solution

Sodium rhodizonate	200 mg
Distilled water	99 ml
Acetic acid	1 ml

Sections

All types

Suitable control sections

Known positive control sections

Staining method

(1) Bring sections to water
(2) Place in rhodizonate solution for 1 h
(3) Rinse in tap water
(4) Stain in 0·1 per cent Light Green in 1 per cent acetic acid
(5) Rinse briefly in water
(6) Mount in glycerin jelly

Results

Lead salts: red
Background: green

METHOD 94

Solochrome Azurine method for aluminium and beryllium

Reagents required

Solochrome azurine

Preparation of solution

Solochrome azurine	200 mg
Distilled water	100 ml

Sections

All types

Suitable control sections

Known control section

Staining method

(1) Bring sections to water
(2) Stain in solochrome azurine
(3) Rinse in distilled water
(4) Dehydrate through graded alcohols to xylene
(5) Mount in DPX

Results

Aluminium: deep blue
Beryllium: deep blue

Remarks

If it is necessary to differentiate between the aluminium and beryllium please refer to page 212.

METHOD 95

Beryllium: Naphthochrome Green B method (Denz, 1949; Pearse, 1960)

Reagents required

(1) Naphthochrome Green B
(2) 0·1 M Phosphate buffer, pH 5·0
(3) Absolute alcohol
(4) Distilled water

Preparation of solution

Naphthochrome Green B	50 mg
0·1 M Phosphate buffer, pH 5·0	50 ml

Sections

All types

Suitable control sections

Previously known positive section

Staining method

(1) Bring all sections to water
(2) Transfer sections to Naphthochrome Green B at 37°C — 30 min
(3) Wash sections in distilled water
(4) Wash sections in 70 per cent alcohol rapidly
(5) Place sections in absolute alcohol — 5–30 min
(6) Transfer sections to xylene
(7) Mount in DPX

Result

Beryllium: light green

METHOD 96

Aluminium and calcium: Naphthochrome Green B method (Denz, 1949; Pearse, 1960)

Reagents required

(1) Naphthochrome Green B
(2) Distilled water

Staining solution

Naphthochrome Green B	150 mg
Distilled water	100 ml

Sections

All types

Suitable control sections

Previously known control

Staining method

(1) Bring all sections to water
(2) Stain sections in Naphthochrome Green B solution — 5–10 min
(3) Wash in distilled water
(4) Dehydrate through graded alcohols to xylene
(5) Mount in DPX

Results

Aluminium: deep green
Calcium: brown, brownish red

METHOD 97

p–Dimethylaminobenzylidene Rhodanine method for silver (Okamoto and Utamura, 1938)

Reagents required

p–Dimethylaminobenzylidene rhodanine
10 per cent Ethanol
Nitric acid

Preparation of solution for use with frozen sections

p–Dimethylaminobenzylidene rhodanine	200 mg
Distilled water	90 ml
Ethanol	10 ml
Nitric acid (conc.)	0·1 ml

Sections

All types (*see Method*)

Suitable control sections

Known control section

Staining method: free-floating sections

(1) Cut frozen sections 15–20 μm thick and float into staining solution for 2 h at 37°C
(2) Rinse free-floating sections in 70 per cent alcohol
(3) Rinse in distilled water and mount in glycerin jelly

Staining method: paraffin sections

(1) Bring sections to water
(2) Stain in sat. alcoholic reagent, 3·5 ml; N-HNO_3, 3 ml; distilled water, 93·5 ml; for 24 h at 37°C
(3) Wash in distilled water
(4) Mount in glycerin jelly

Results

Silver: red-violet or red-brown

Remarks

The method gives best results with frozen sections.

METHOD 98

Methenamine Silver for urates (Gomori, 1951)

Reagents required

(1) Methenamine
(2) Silver nitrate

(3) Boric acid
(4) Sodium tetraborate
(5) Sodium thiosulphate

Preparation of solutions

(1) *Methenamine Silver stock*

Add 5 ml of 5 per cent silver nitrate (aqueous) to 100 ml of 3 per cent methenamine. A white precipitate forms. Continue shaking until precipitate dissolves. Store at 4°C. The solution keeps for three months

(2) *Buffer solution*

Boric acid	800 mg
Sodium tetraborate	650 mg
Distilled water	100 ml

Store at 4°C.

(3) *Working solution*

Methenamine stock (solution 1)	25 ml
Buffer stock (solution 2)	5 ml
Distilled water	20 ml

Sections

All types alcohol fixation preferred

Method

(1) Remove wax with xylene
(2) Transfer to absolute alcohol
(3) Place sections in working solution at 37°C for 1 h
(4) Rinse in distilled water
(5) Treat with 2 per cent sodium thiosulphate for 5 min
(6) Rinse in tap water
(7) Counterstain if required
(8) Dehydrate clear and mount

Results

Urate deposit: black

Remarks

(1) Staining time may need to be extended. Working solution should be preheated to 37°C

(2) Calcium salts should not be visible. 0·5 per cent hydrochloric acid can be used as a control for calcium

(3) Urates will be dissolved by treatment with lithium carbonate aqueous

(4) Neutral Red is a satisfactory counterstain

REFERENCES

DAHL, L. K. (1952). *Proc. Soc. exp. Biol. N.Y.* **80,** 474

DENZ. F. A. (1949). *Q. Jl microsc. Sci.* **90,** 317

GOMORI, G. (1951). Methods in medical research, **4,** 1, Chicago

HOWELL, J. S. (1959). *J. Path. Bact.* **77,** 473

MCGEE-RUSSELL, (1958). *J. Histochem. Cytochem.* **6,** 22

MALLORY, F. B. and PARKER, F. (1939). *Am. J. Path.* **15,** 517

OKAMOTO, K. and UTAMURA, M. (1938). *Trans. Soc. Path. Japan* **32,** 99

PEARSE, A. G. E. (1972). *Histochemistry, Theoretical and Applied,* 3rd Edn, Vol. 2, London: Churchill Livingstone

TIMM, F. (1958). *Dtsch Z. ges. Gerichtl. Med.* **46,** 706

UZMAN, L. L. (1956). *Lab. invest.* **5,** 299

VON KÓSSA, J. (1901). *Beitre path. anat.* **29,** 163

14

Principles of Enzyme Histochemistry

Histochemistry is expanding very rapidly; it is no longer considered to be an insignificant part of histopathology but a subject in its own right with deep roots in both histology and biochemistry.

The expansion of the subject has been most marked in the histochemical demonstration of enzyme activity. Enzymes are protein catalysts for the chemical reactions that occur in biological systems. The enzymes are necessary for the normal metabolic processes within the tissues.

Enzymes have long been assayed biochemically but when Pearse (1953) published his first edition he stated that methods existed for at least eighteen enzymes to be demonstrated histochemically. In the last twenty years or so this number has increased to about eighty. Many of the early methods were to demonstrate hydrolytic enzymes; the largest expansion in recent years has been in the demonstration of the group of enzymes known as oxidative enzymes, i.e. enzymes which oxidize the substrate. The first major group, hydrolytic enzymes, hydrolyze the various substrates.

TABLE 14.1

Histochemical classification of enzymes

Oxidoreductases	*Hydrolases*
Oxidative (transfer of electrons)	*Hydrolytic* (addition or removal of *water*)
examples:—	examples:—
Dehydrogenases	Acid phosphatases
Peroxidase	Alkaline phosphatases
Monoamine oxidase	Esterases
	Sulphatases
	β-glucuronidase
Transferases (transfer of radicals)	*Proteolytic enzymes*
example:—	example:—
Phosphorylase	Leucine aminopeptidase

Preservation

Due to the labile nature of the enzymes, preservation is a problem. The different enzymes react in various ways to outside influences. Mitochondria, which contain many of the oxidative enzymes, are damaged rapidly when denied a supply of blood. The membranes become damaged and a loss of enzyme activity occurs, so as little time as possible must be wasted in preparing tissue for this type of histochemical technique. Lysosomes, which contain many of the hydrolytic enzymes, are damaged by the freezing and thawing of the tissue blocks and sections, and the enzymes will diffuse from the damaged organelles. This is the main cause of the gross diffusion seen in post-fixed sections of, say, acid phosphatase. Careful fixation of the tissue, and treatment in gum sucrose before incubation does help to retard this diffusion, but at the same time a loss of demonstrable enzyme activity must take place. Most mitochondrial enzymes are removed or destroyed by normal histochemical fixation but are much less sensitive to the effects of freezing and thawing, since the freezing and thawing appears not to rupture the mitochondrial membrane. A loss of enzyme activity occurs when tissue is left at room temperature, so in enzyme histochemistry the rapid handling of tissue is important. The damage caused to some of the mitochondrial enzymes can possibly be avoided by the use of hypertonic protection media such as polyvinyl pyrrolidone (PVP) first described by Novikoff (1956), now usually used with sucrose. The different enzymes react in varying degrees to the damaging agents discussed. Some of the enzymes are more resistant than others to damage; alkaline phosphatase is more able to withstand the effects of fixation than acid phosphatase. Often a choice has to be made in the case of hydrolytic enzymes as to whether fixation, leading to some enzyme loss but very good localization, is to be preferred to post-fixation or no fixation, with little or no loss of enzyme activity but considerable enzyme diffusion. The dehydrogenases have to be demonstrated on unfixed sections but a choice remains as to whether a protection solution is used.

Factors affecting enzyme activity

Temperature

The optimal temperature for the majority of enzyme reactions is 37°C. At higher temperatures enzymes are rapidly denatured due to their protein nature. Lower temperatures, between 4°C and 30°C, can be usefully employed in histochemistry, for the rate of the enzymic reaction is slowed and, in the case of active enzymes, a better localization can be demonstrated.

pH

The majority of enzymes have a pH at which the rate of the reaction is optimal. For a large number of enzymes this is about pH 7·0. Alkaline phosphatase at pH 9·2 and acid phosphatase at pH 5·0 are outstanding exceptions.

Inhibitors

Enzyme activity in sections can be destroyed by using chemical substances known as inhibitors. There are three main types of inhibitors:

(1) specific inhibitors, e.g. eserine for the cholinesterases;
(2) non-specific inhibitors, e.g. heat for all enzymes;
(3) competitive inhibitors

The specific inhibitor affects the reactive site of the enzyme molecule. Non-specific inhibitors destroy the enzyme reaction by denaturing the protein enzyme. The competitive inhibitors are chemicals which compete with the substrate for the active enzyme sites.

Activators

These are chemicals that are used to promote enzyme activity. An example is magnesium ions, used in the Gomori Metal Precipitation technique for alkaline phosphatase.

Techniques of demonstration

The essential basic principle in most enzyme histochemistry techniques is that any enzyme in the tissue is presented with its own specific substrate in the incubating medium and a reaction takes place. Unfortunately the immediate product of this reaction (the primary reaction product) is frequently invisible and must therefore be allowed to couple with another substance so that an insoluble and visible final reaction product is produced at the site of the enzyme activity. The coupling substance used varies from method to method; for example, diazonium salts in the demonstration of the phosphatases ('Azo-dye methods'), tetrazolium salts in the demonstration of dehydrogenases, and inorganic chemicals like ammonium sulphide in the metal precipitation techniques.

Four basic techniques are available for the demonstration of enzymes.

(1) Metal precipitation techniques
(2) Simultaneous coupling using diazonium salts

(3) Post-incubation coupling using diazonium salts
(4) Self-coloured substrate.

Metal precipitation

This technique is commonly applied to the demonstration of phosphatases (*see* Chapter 15). The phosphate ions released as a result of enzyme activity on the substrate combine with a suitable metallic cation to produce an insoluble precipitate of metal phosphate. The phosphates produced are usually invisible but can be rendered visible by converting them to black sulphides by treatment with ammonium sulphide. The metallic cations most frequently used for combining with the released phosphate are calcium and lead. This technique may be regarded as a type of simultaneous coupling, but using metallic ions instead of diazonium salts.

Simultaneous coupling

This occurs when an incubation mixture containing a substrate and a diazonium salt are applied to suitable sections in a buffered solution. The enzyme present in the section hydrolyzes the substrate to form an invisible primary reaction product (PRP). This complex is immediately coupled with the diazonium salt to produce the final reaction product (FRP) which is seen as a visible, often coloured, deposit under the microscope. This type of method (*Figure*

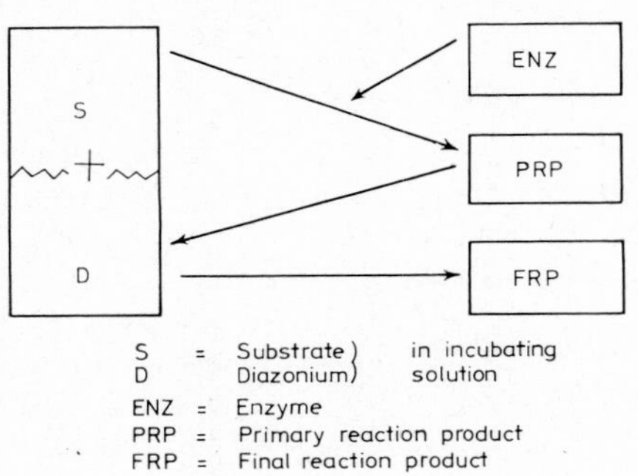

Figure 14.1

14.1) is exemplified by the azo dye methods for phosphatases. The PRP is colourless whereas the FRP should always be coloured. The substrate must be soluble in water or in the buffer medium to an extent that there is sufficient substrate available in solution for the enzyme to hydrolyze. The histochemical method must be performed at a pH at which the enzyme shows maximal activity and the substrate adequate solubility. The diazonium salt also has an optimal pH for its most efficient rate of coupling, and this must be considered when the pH at which the method is to be performed is chosen. The PRP must be fairly insoluble; if it is too soluble then not all the PRP will couple with the diazonium salt. The quantity of the substrate and diazonium salt in the incubating medium is also important; too much of either will cause inhibition of the rate of hydrolysis of the substrate on one hand, and inhibition of the formation of the FRP on the other.

Post-incubation coupling

In this procedure the enzyme hydrolyzes the substrate and produces a reasonably insoluble PRP. The subsequent coupling is carried out in a separate solution. This type of method relies upon the PRP remaining at the initial site of the hydrolysis. It is also necessary that diffusion of the PRP does not occur during the coupling process. Post-incubation coupling has many theoretical advantages. The optimal pH for the initial substrate enzyme reaction can be attained in the first incubation, and a possibly different optimal pH for the coupling can be produced in the second (coupling) stage. The method avoids the deleterious effects that diazonium salts may have upon the initial reaction, and also avoids the effects of these diazonium salts when the incubation time is long, for many workers consider that these salts tend to inactivate enzymes or interfere with hydrolysis. Long exposure of tissue to diazonium salts in acid and alkaline solutions produces non-specific staining. The serious drawback to this type of method results from the solubility of the PRP leading to excessive diffusion between the two stages. Localization may be poor unless the PRP is extremely insoluble.

Self-coloured substrate

There are few methods using this type of procedure. The substrate is a coloured but soluble substance, and the effect of the enzyme to be demonstrated is to remove the solubilizing group without interfering with the colour. The PRP is therefore coloured and insoluble, and no coupling stage is necessary. The insoluble coloured reaction product is precipitated at the site of enzyme activity.

Diazonium salts

Diazonium salts are prepared by treating primary aromatic amines with an acid solution of sodium nitrite. The resulting salt, generally a chloride, will react readily with phenols or with aryl amines to produce the corresponding intensely coloured insoluble azo dye. There are about 30 stabilized diazonium salts in current usage. A list of the 17 most popular appears on page 323. Stabilized diazonium salts cannot be kept indefinitely; they must be stored in a cool dark place and renewed at 6-monthly intervals. During incubation it is important to choose conditions carefully so that combination of the reactants takes place as rapidly as possible, and so that the product so formed remains insoluble through subsequent processing. Failure in either of these respects reduces the accuracy of localization of the enzyme activity.

The rate of coupling of diazonium salt depends not only on the chemical nature of the diazonium salt used, but also on the pH of the incubating medium, and the optimal pH for enzyme activity therefore determines to a large extent the choice of diazonium salt. Precision in locating the sites of enzyme activity also depends upon the concentration of diazonium salt used. There is an average optimal concentration for diazonium salts in the incubating solution. If the concentration is less than optimal, diffusion of the PRP may be a problem. If the concentration is much greater than optimal then inhibition of enzyme activity may occur and the risk of non-specific background staining becomes increased.

Tetrazolium salts

These coupling agents are discussed in the chapter on dehydrogenases.

The use of controls

Controls are a necessary part of enzyme histochemistry. Substrates, diazonium salts and some other chemical solutions used, will deteriorate with time, leading to the possible failure of the method; occasionally false positives may be produced. A positive control should be carried through when incubating test sections, to show that all the chemical solutions are working.

Omission of the substrate from the incubating medium and the inclusion of specific enzyme inhibitors (if available) afford adequate control measures. If further controls are deemed necessary, competitive inhibitors may be added to the incubating solution. Sections may also be pre-treated by immersing them in boiling water for a few minutes, and then processing through the rest of the method, or by 'incubating' in distilled water. In each case, the absence of reaction product indicates that the positive results obtained with the authentic techniques are yielding useful information about the distribution of the enzyme. Non-specific background staining is also excluded as a possible source of error if control sections give negative results. Any activity indicated in control sections must be regarded as a false result.

REFERENCES

Pearse, A. G. E. (1953). *Histochemistry, Theoretical and Applied*, London: Churchill
Novikoff, A. B. (1956). *J. Biophys. Biochem. Cytol.* **2,** 65

15

Phosphatases

INTRODUCTION

Phosphatases are present in a wide variety of animal and plant tissues. They are responsible for the hydrolysis of organic phosphate esters. Some phosphatases act specifically on a single substrate and are known as specific phosphatases. Of these, a number can be demonstrated by reliable histochemical techniques. An example of a specific phosphatase is adenosine triphosphatase which specifically hydrolyzes adenosine triphosphate. The remainder, whose substrate specificity is less limited, are divided into two groups: those exhibiting optimal activity at high pH values (alkaline phosphatases) and those exhibiting optimal activity at low pH values (acid phosphatases).

Reliable histochemical methods are available for the demonstration of the following five phosphatases.

(1) Alkaline phosphatases (*see* Methods 100, 101, 102)
(2) Acid phosphatases (*see* Methods 103, 104, 105)
(3) 5′-Nucleotidase (*see* Method 107)
(4) Glucose-6-phosphatase (*see* Method 108)
(5) Adenosinetriphosphatase (*see* Method 109)

The hydrolysis of organic phosphate esters during incubation provides the basis for the histochemical reactions. The released phosphate ions or the remaining organic residue is made visible by a variety of means. Phosphate ions are generally precipitated as insoluble salts, such as lead or calcium phosphate and then converted to coloured sulphides which are visible under the microscope. This is the basis of the many Gomori-type metal precipitation techniques. Alternatively, the alcoholic residue of the substrate, after enzymatic hydrolysis, may be made to react with a suitable diazonium salt to produce a highly coloured insoluble azo dye. The phosphate esters of α-naphthol or its derivatives are the most commonly used substrates in the azo dye techniques.

Coupling may take place during incubation (simultaneous coupling) or after incubation (post-coupling). The relative merits of each method have been discussed in Chapter 14 and are also considered in relation to the enzymes concerned.

In the demonstration of the phosphatases Pearse (1960) states that the average optimal concentration of the diazonium salt is 1 mg per 1 ml of incubating solution. If the concentration is less, diffusion of the primary reaction product, α-naphthol, may occur. On the other hand if the concentration is much greater, say 5 mg per ml of incubating medium, inhibition of PRP formation may occur, and non-specific background staining may be seen.

Adequate controls should be used to eliminate the possibility of failure of the method, and of producing false positives. In phosphatase histochemistry the general points made on page 228 should be considered. In addition false positive reactions can be obtained if calcium or iron is already present in the tissues.

The pH of the final incubating solution is critical. As mentioned earlier, acid phosphatases and alkaline phosphatases exhibit optimal activity at pH 5·0 and pH 9·2, respectively. The optimal pH values for glucose-6-phosphatase and 5′-nucleotidase occur at pH 6·5 and 7·5–8·5. Adenosine triphosphatase has an optimal pH of 7·2. The importance of pH in determining the choice of diazonium salt has already been mentioned.

ALKALINE PHOSPHATASES

These enzymes exhibit optimum activity at alkaline pH in the region of 9·0–9·6 and are widely distributed throughout many tissues. They are activated by magnesium, manganese and cobalt ions. Cyanide and cysteine inhibit alkaline phosphatase activity and may be incorporated in the incubating medium to provide a control.

There are two types of histochemical methods available for the demonstration of alkaline phosphatases. They are: (1) Gomori Calcium Phosphate method (metal substitution), (2) Azo-Dye Coupling methods, using either simultaneous coupling or post-coupling (*see* page 226).

Gomori Calcium Phosphate method

The original method for the demonstration of alkaline phosphatases was described by two people, quite independently, in 1939. These two workers, Gomori of the United States, and Takamatsu of Japan, provided the incentive for further study with the publication of their methods. A variation of the original Gomori technique, published in 1952, is still in common use today. The incubating medium includes sodium β-glycerophosphate, calcium nitrate and magnesium chloride (*see Figure 15.1*).

If a section is placed in an incubating solution containing a substrate (i.e. sodium β-glycerophosphate) and calcium ions (i.e. calcium nitrate), plus an activator for the phosphatase (i.e. magnesium chloride), a precipitate of calcium phosphate is formed at the sites of enzyme activity. The alkaline phosphatase liberates phosphate from the sodium β-glycerophosphate and this then combines with calcium ions to form calcium phosphate. The precipitate of calcium phosphate is treated with cobalt nitrate to produce cobalt phosphate. This is then treated with dilute ammonium sulphide to form cobalt sulphide, which is visible with the light microscope as a black deposit. The reactions can be summarized in the following flow diagram.

$$\text{Sodium } \beta\text{-glycerophosphate} \xrightarrow{\text{Alkaline phosphatase}} \text{Phosphate ions}$$

$$\text{Phosphate ions} + \text{calcium ions} \longrightarrow \text{Calcium phosphate}$$

$$\text{Calcium phosphate} + \text{cobalt ions} \longrightarrow \text{Cobalt phosphate}$$

$$\text{Cobalt phosphate} + \text{sulphide ions} \longrightarrow \text{Cobalt sulphide (black fine precipitate)}$$

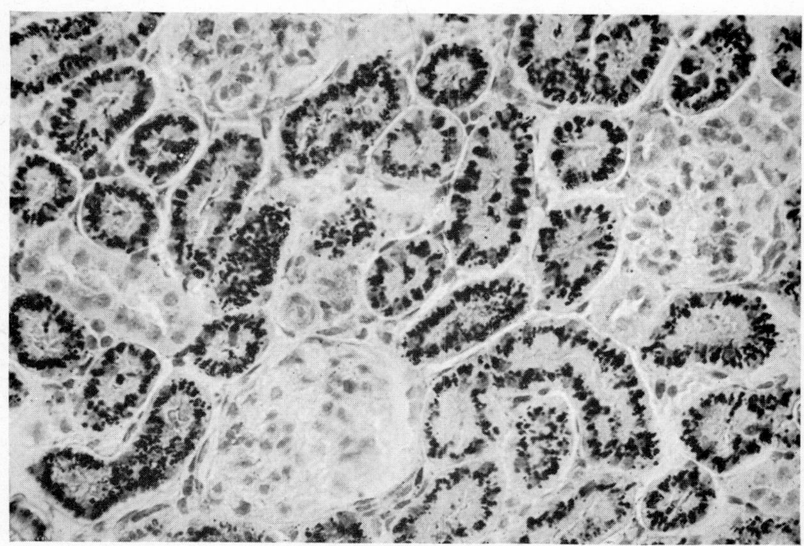

Figure 15.1 Rat kidney—distribution of alkaline phosphatase activity shown by a metal substitution technique (Gomori). (× 340)
(Reduced to two-thirds in reproduction)

The incubating medium does not keep and it is advisable to make up fresh solutions immediately before use. The final pH of the solution is critical. If pH values less than 9·0 are employed, enzyme activity is impaired and the intensity of the final reaction product is reduced. Furthermore, localization is adversely affected owing to the greater solubility of calcium phosphate at lower pH.

Incubation is carried out at 37°C. The duration of incubation must be determined by experiment, and varies with the type of tissue used. Unnecessarily long incubation times should be avoided, as this favours diffusion of the enzyme, especially in unfixed sections. In general, shorter times are necessary for cryostat sections, and the longest for fixed and paraffin processed material.

Azo Dye methods

Simultaneous Coupling method

This method was first described by Menton, Junge and Green in 1944. The original technique has been modified and improved upon by a number of people, notably by Gomori (1951). The method employs sodium α-naphthyl phosphate as the substrate, together with a suitable diazonium salt. The incubating medium is buffered to pH 9·2. The enzyme liberates α-naphthol from the substrate and this is subsequently coupled to the diazonium salt to produce an insoluble azo dye at the sites of enzyme activity.

Best results are obtained when coupling between the α-naphthol and the diazonium salt occurs as rapidly as possible. This depends to a great extent on the choice of diazonium salt and upon the pH of the incubating solution.

$$\text{sodium } \alpha\text{-naphthyl phosphate} \xrightarrow{\text{Alkaline phosphatase}} \text{Primary reaction product } (\alpha\text{-naphthol})$$

$$\text{(PRP) } \alpha\text{-naphthol} + \text{diazonium salt} \longrightarrow \text{Final reaction product coloured precipitate}$$

Azo Dye Simultaneous Coupling method using substituted naphthols

The introduction of substituted naphthols for use in the demonstration of alkaline phosphatases is due to Gomori (1952a) but much of the recent developmental work was carried out by Burstone (1958, 1961). He studied four substituted naphthol esters: Naphthol AS-BI phosphate, Naphthol AS-MX phosphate, Naphthol AS-CL phosphate and Naphthol AS-TR phosphate. These esters are hydrolyzed rapidly by alkaline phosphatases yielding extremely insoluble naphthol derivatives. These are then made to react with a diazonium salt to produce an insoluble azo dye at the sites of enzyme activity.

Many workers agree that the localization with substituted naphthols is superior to that obtained using alternative methods.

Substituted naphthols will also couple with diazonium salts over wider pH ranges. Against these advantages must be mentioned the higher cost of the substituted naphthol substrates.

Stock solutions of substituted naphthol phosphates may be made by dissolving the compound in dimethylformamide (DMF) and adding distilled water and buffer to pH 8·3 (*see* Method 102, page 243). These solutions will keep in a refrigerator for several months. To carry out the reaction it is simply necessary to add a suitable diazonium salt (e.g. Fast Red TR, Fast Blue RR) to the required amount of incubating solution in the ratio of 1 mg/ml. The incubating solution should be prepared immediately before use. Incubation is carried out for 30 minutes at 37°C.

Azo Dye Post-Coupling method

This technique varies from the above methods in that coupling with the diazonium salt takes place separately after incubation. It is therefore of great importance that the product of enzyme hydrolysis be insoluble and that it should remain at the site of activity during the washing that follows incubation. This one requirement dictates the type of substrate to be used. The section is transferred from the incubating solution, washed in distilled water and transferred to a solution of the diazonium salt. Coupling of the two reactants produces an azo dye precipitate at the sites of enzyme activity.

The method has obvious theoretical advantages. The inhibitory effect of the diazonium salt on the enzyme is avoided. The optimal pH for coupling between the salt and the α-naphthol may be used without reference to the optimal pH for enzyme activity. Sections can also be incubated for longer periods without the risk of diffusion of the final reaction product. The main disadvantage of the method, and the reason why it is not in common use today, is the problem of finding a suitable substrate that will be hydrolyzed rapidly by the enzymes, and which produces sufficiently insoluble precipitates.

ACID PHOSPHATASES

These enzymes had, until quite recently, received much less attention than alkaline phosphatases. This is doubtless connected with the fact that only in recent years have the methods for their demonstration become reliable. The specific problems involved are connected with the relatively high solubility of acid phosphatases, and with the difficulty of obtaining accurate localization of the final reaction product. Simultaneous coupling azo dye methods were also beset by the difficulty of finding diazonium salts that could couple efficiently under the acid conditions necessary for optimal enzyme activity.

The enzymes are distributed widely throughout the body; kidney, liver and spleen being particularly rich. Fluoride ions inhibit these enzymes, and the inclusion of sodium fluoride in the incubating medium affords a reliable control measure.

As with the alkaline phosphatases, there are now two reliable techniques for the demonstration of these enzymes: (1) Gomori Lead Phosphate method, and (2) Azo Dye coupling methods using simultaneous coupling or post-coupling methods.

Gomori Lead Phosphate method

This method was first introduced by Gomori (1941) and resembles his method for alkaline phosphatases. Calcium phosphate, which is formed at the site of activity in the alkaline phosphatase technique (*see* page 241), cannot be used in this instance because of its solubility at acid pH levels. Lead nitrate is therefore used to precipitate the phosphate ions.

The section is incubated in a medium containing sodium-β-glycerophosphate as the substrate, and lead nitrate; no activator is required. The enzyme splits phosphate ions from the substrate and these form an insoluble precipitate of lead phosphate at the site of enzyme activity. The sections are treated with a dilute solution of ammonium sulphide and the precipitate converted to lead sulphide. This is visible under the microscope as a dense brown deposit. The deposit is granular, and if the optimal conditions for the method have been fulfilled, the granules should be small.

$$\text{Sodium } \beta\text{-glycerophosphate} \xrightarrow{\text{Acid phosphatase}} \text{Phosphate ions}^-$$

$$\text{Phosphate ions} + \text{lead ions} \longrightarrow \text{Lead phosphate (precipitate)}$$

$$\text{Lead phosphate} + \text{sulphide ions} \longrightarrow \text{Lead sulphide (fine brown black precipitate)}$$

The incubating medium must be made up fresh for each batch of sections to be incubated. It is convenient, however, to keep the individual reagents in stock solutions and stored at 4°C. The preparation of the incubating solution is important. It is necessary to use reagents of a high grade to obtain satisfactory results. As with the Gomori Alkaline Phosphatase method, the pH of the final incubating solution is important. The method works best at a pH of 4·8–5·0. If the pH is increased much above 5·5, it is possible to demonstrate phosphatases other than acid phosphatases. Incubation is carried out at 37°C for 30 min to 6 h, depending on the method of preparation of the material and the tissue used.

Azo Dye methods

Azo Dye Simultaneous Coupling method

The principle employed in the corresponding technique for alkaline phosphatase is again used for the demonstration of acid phosphatases. The substrate used is sodium α-naphthyl phosphate (1-naphthyl phosphoric acid) dissolved in 0·1 M veronal acetate buffer at pH 5·0. α-Naphthol is released at the site of enzyme activity and is then coupled with a suitable diazonium salt.

As mentioned earlier, the problem with azo dye methods for the demonstration of acid phosphatases is to find a diazonium salt that will couple satisfactorily at a low pH. Grogg and Pearse (1952) carried out a comprehensive study of different diazonium salts and their performance when used in the acid phosphatase technique. They concluded that Fast Garnet GBC gave the best results, and it is recommended that this salt be used when applying this method. The localization obtained with this method is considerably inferior to that obtained using a substituted naphthol as substrate and hexazonium pararosanilin as coupler.

Simultaneous Azo Dye Coupling method using substituted naphthols

This method is also applicable to the demonstration of acid phosphatases, and was explored by Burstone (1958). All the substituted naphthols he studied coupled efficiently at an acid pH, but he recommended naphthol AS-BI phosphate as the substrate of choice for the acid phosphatase technique because of the extreme insolubility of the reaction product.

Barka (1960) recommended the use of hexazonium pararosanilin as the diazonium salt in the simultaneous coupling method for acid phosphatase. This salt was first used by Davis and Ornstein (1959) for the demonstration of alkaline phosphatases and esterases. According to Barka, hexazonium pararosanilin does not inhibit the enzyme at an acid pH, and he attributed the improved localization obtained using this salt to the extreme insolubility and substantivity of the azo dye produced. The combination of hexazonium pararosanilin and naphthol AS-BI phosphate allows accurate localization of the reaction product and is recommended for use with this method.

The diazonium salt is prepared in two stages (*see* Method 106, page 248). In the first, pararosanilin hydrochloride is dissolved in distilled water and acidified with concentrated hydrochloric acid. The solution is filtered and stored at room temperature where it is stable for several months. Diazotization is achieved by the addition of a 4 per cent solution of sodium nitrite in distilled water. *It is*

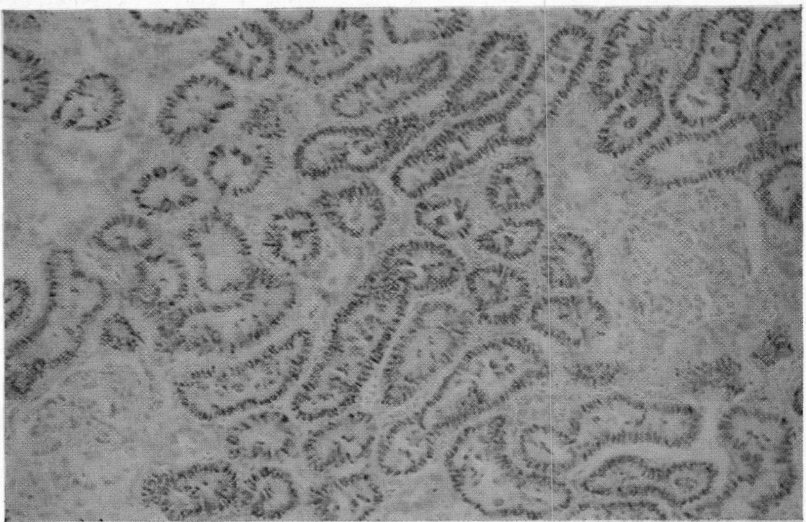

Plate 3 Rat kidney showing the distribution of acid phosphatase activity demonstrated by the azo-dye technique using a substituted naphthol (AS-B1). Note the fine granular localization of the reaction product. (Method 106, Magnification × 225)

(Reduced to nine-tenths in reproduction)

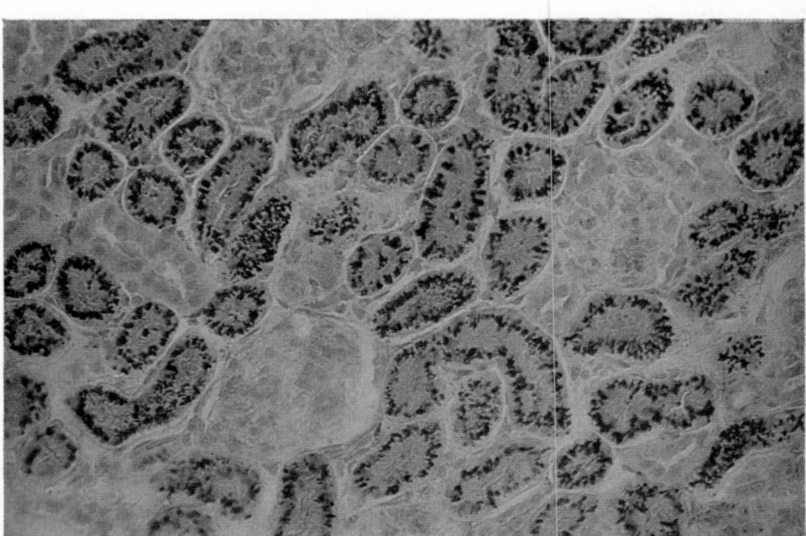

Plate 4 Rat kidney showing the distribution of alkaline phosphatase demonstrated by a metal precipitation technique (Gomori) using calcium and cobalt salts. (Method 101, Magnification × 225)

(Reduced to nine-tenths in reproduction)

Sigma London Chemical Company Ltd. have kindly contributed towards the cost of these colour plates.

SPECIFIC PHOSPHATASES

5′-NUCLEOTIDASE

This enzyme is found in liver, thyroid and certain types of muscle. It exhibits optimal activity at pH 7·5–8·5. This enzyme is not absolutely specific since it effects the hydrolysis of phosphate esters on the carbon 5 of some ribosenucleosides and of deoxyribose nucleosides. It is however much more specific than acid and alkaline phosphatases. The usual substrate used in its demonstration is adenosine 5-phosphate. There are two methods available for the demonstration of 5′-nucleotidase; the Calcium method of Pearse and Reis (1952) and the Lead method of Wachstein and Meisel (1957).

Lead method of Wachstein and Meisel

Adenosine-5-phosphate buffered to pH 7·5 is used as the substrate. Magnesium ions are added to activate the enzyme, and lead nitrate is added to precipitate the phosphate. The reaction is similar to that taking place with the Gomori method for acid and alkaline phosphatases. 5′-Nucleotidase in the section hydrolyzes the substrate and releases phosphate ions. This is precipitated as lead phosphate at the site of enzyme activity and is later converted to a black-brown deposit of lead sulphide by treatment of the sections with dilute ammonium sulphide.

Care must be taken with the preparation of the incubating medium, which must be filtered immediately before use. Incubation is for 30 min to 2 h at 37°C. After incubation, the sections must be washed carefully, twice or more in distilled water. The total time taken for the washing should be kept as short as possible.

The interpretation of the results is complicated by the difficulty of distinguishing between 5′-nucleotidase and alkaline phosphatases, both of which may be demonstrated by the method. The use of control sections incubated under similar conditions and at pH 9·0 and 7·5 but with sodium β-glycerophosphate as substrate, may indicate whether or not phosphatases other than 5′-nucleotidase are contributing to the final reaction product. The method is not quantitative, and the proportion of the total reaction product attributable to 5′-nucleotidase activity cannot be determined with accuracy. If any nuclear staining is observed this must be regarded as artefactual, and under these circumstances it is advisable to repeat the method. In the calcium method, the lead ions are replaced by calcium ions and the pH increased to 8·3.

GLUCOSE-6-PHOSPHATASE

This is a specific enzyme found in large amounts in the liver and also in kidney, colon and rectum. It exhibits optimal activity at pH 6·5. The enzyme hydrolyzes glucose-6-phosphate to glucose.

Lead method for glucose-6-phosphatase

The histochemical method in use at the present time was first introduced by Chiquoine (1954) and further modified by him in 1955. The technique, which is of the Gomori type, was introduced in its present form by Wachstein and Meisel (1956).

The potassium salt of glucose-6-phosphate is used as the substrate. Lead nitrate is included in the incubating medium to precipitate the phosphate produced during incubation. The incubating medium is buffered to pH 6·7. A precipitate of lead phosphate is formed which is later converted to a dense black-brown precipitate of lead sulphide by treatment of the sections with a dilute solution of ammonium sulphide. Incubation is carried out at 37°C for 10 minutes.

Glucose-6-phosphatase is a very sensitive enzyme that is damaged or lost during fixation with formol saline. It is therefore necessary to carry out the method on unfixed cryostat sections and to post-fix the sections after incubation. As both acid and alkaline phosphatases may be demonstrated by the method, control sections incubated for these enzymes must be employed in order to assess the contribution each makes to the final reaction product.

ADENOSINE TRIPHOSPHATASE

This enzyme is one of a complicated group concerned with the hydrolysis of adenosine triphosphate (ATP). The enzyme is found in heart muscle, skeletal muscle, liver and other tissues. The method is carried out at pH 7·2 and the most acceptable techniques for the demonstration of adenosine triphosphatase are the Lead method of Wachstein and Meisel (1957, 1960) and the Calcium technique of Padykula and Herman (1955).

Lead method for adenosine triphosphatase

The principles involved in this technique are again similar to the Gomori type of phosphatase method. Fixation is a problem with this technique; if unfixed cryostat or frozen sections are used, diffusion will occur. In formalin-fixed material (4°C for 24 h) loss of enzymes will occur, considerable in some tissues. It is recommended that if possible both fixed and unfixed sections are incubated and the results compared.

The section is incubated in a solution containing 0·125 per cent adenosine triphosphate (disodium salt) with 2 per cent lead nitrate and 2·5 per cent magnesium nitrate (activator) in a tris buffer pH 7·2. The enzyme in the section splits the phosphate from the ATP. A precipitate of lead phosphate occurs at the site of enzyme activity.

This is then converted to lead sulphide by immersing the section in a dilute solution of ammonium sulphide. The final result is a brownish black precipitate. Incubation is carried out at 37°C for 15 min to 2 h depending upon the tissue and method of preparation.

METHOD 99

Preparation of tissue for pre-fixation

Solutions required

(1) 4 per cent Formol calcium
(2) Gum sucrose
(3) Formaldehyde–gelatin mixture

Preparations for solutions

(1) *4 per cent formol calcium*

Formaldehyde	4 ml
Distilled water	96 ml
Calcium chloride	1 g

Further calcium chloride is added if necessary until pH reaches 7·0

(2) *Gum sucrose*

Gum acacia	2 g
Sucrose	60 g
Distilled water	200 ml

Allow to dissolve and store at 4°C

(3) *Formaldehyde–gelatin mixture*

1 per cent Gelatin	25 ml
2 per cent Formaldehyde	25 ml

Method

(1) Cut small block of fresh tissue
(2) Place in formol calcium solution precooled to 4°C overnight
(3) Blot dry, wash in tap water 2 min, blot dry
(4) Place in gum sucrose solution at 4°C for 24 h
(5) Blot dry
(6) Attach blocks to cryostat holder and freeze
(7) Section at 8–10 μm at —10°C
(8) Pick sections up on slides or coverslips precoated with formaldehyde–gelatin mixture; allow to dry before incubating

METHOD 100

Alkaline phosphatase: the Gomori Calcium method (1952) (modified) (metal precipitation)

Reagents required

(1) 2 per cent Sodium β-glycerophosphate
(2) 2 per cent Sodium veronal
(3) 2 per cent Calcium nitrate
(4) 1 per cent Magnesium chloride
(5) 2 per cent Cobalt nitrate
(6) Ammonium sulphide

Preparation of incubating medium

2 per cent Sodium β-glycerophosphate	2·5 ml
2 per cent Sodium veronal	2·5 ml
2 per cent Calcium nitrate	5·0 ml
1 per cent Magnesium chloride	0·25 ml
Distilled water	1·25 ml

The final pH of the incubating medium should be between 9·0 and 9·4.

Sections

Cryostat post-fixed
Cryostat pre-fixed
Freeze dried
Carefully processed paraffin sections
Frozen sections

Incubating method

(1) After suitable fixation, bring sections to water, incubate at 37°C for 45 min to 6 h
(2) Wash well in distilled water
(3) Repeat wash
(4) Treat section with 2 per cent cobalt nitrate, 3 min
(5) Wash well in distilled water
(6) Repeat wash
(7) Immerse sections in 1 per cent ammonium sulphide, 2 min
(8) Wash well in distilled water
(9) Counterstain in 2 per cent Methyl Green (chloroform extracted)
(10) Wash well in running tap water
(11) Mount in glycerin jelly

Results

Alkaline phosphatase activity: brownish black
Nuclei: green

Remarks

It is convenient to keep the stock solutions made up in batches of 20 ml

METHOD 101

Alkaline phosphatase: Azo Dye Coupling method (simultaneous coupling)

Reagents required

(1) 0·1 M Tris buffer stock solution (*see* page 328)
(2) Sodium α-naphthyl phosphate
(3) Diazonium salt (Fast Red TR)

Preparation of incubating medium

Sodium α-naphthyl phosphate	10 mg
0·1 M Tris buffer (stock solution), pH 10·0	10 ml
Diazonium salt (Fast Red TR)	10 mg

The final pH of the incubating medium should be between 9·0 and 9·4. The sodium α-naphthyl phosphate is dissolved in the buffer, the diazonium salt is added and the solution well mixed. The solution is then filtered and used immediately.

Sections

Cryostat post-fixed
Cryostat pre-fixed
Freeze dried
Carefully processed paraffin sections
Frozen sections

Incubating method

(1) After fixation, bring sections to water, incubate at room temperature for 10–60 min
(2) Wash in distilled water
(3) Counterstain in 2 per cent Methyl Green (chloroform extracted)
(4) Wash in running tap water
(5) Mount in glycerin jelly

Results

Alkaline phosphatase activity: reddish brown
Nuclei: green

Remarks

The final pH of incubating solution is about 9·2. If paraffin sections are used the incubating time will have to be extended.

METHOD 102

Alkaline phosphatase: Naphthol AS-BI method (simultaneous coupling with substituted naphthols)

Reagents required

Naphthol AS-BI phosphate
N:N′-Dimethyl formamide (DMF)
Sodium carbonate
Distilled water
Tris buffer (0·2 M) pH 8·3 (*see* p 328)

Solutions

Naphthol AS-BI stock solution

Naphthol AS-BI phosphate	25 mg
N:N′-Dimethyl formamide	10 ml
Distilled water	10 ml
Molar sodium carbonate	2–6 drops

The reagents are added in the above order, sufficient molar sodium carbonate is added until the pH is 8·0 then add:

Distilled water	300 ml
0·2 M Tris buffer, pH 8·3	180 ml

The solution, which is faintly opalescent, is stable for many months

Incubating solution

Stock naphthol AS-BI solution	10 ml
Fast Red TR	10 mg

Shake well, filter and use immediately

Sections

Cryostat post-fixed
Cryostat pre-fixed
Freeze dried
Carefully processed paraffin sections
Frozen sections

Suitable tissues for controls

Many tissues, including kidney and intestine

Incubating method

(1) After fixation and bringing sections to water, incubate at room temperature for 5–15 min

(2) Wash in water

(3) Counterstain in 2 per cent Methyl Green (chloroform extracted)

(4) Wash well in running tap water

(5) Mount in glycerin jelly

Results

Alkaline phosphatase activity: red
Nuclei: green

Remarks

This is a very reliable method that gives sharp localization of the enzyme. There are two points to watch in the technique.

(1) The addition of molar sodium carbonate. This changes the pH rapidly and care must be taken not to make the solution too alkaline.

(2) The reaction is fast. Care must be taken not to over-incubate.

METHOD 103

Acid phosphatase: the Gomori Lead method (metal precipitation)

Reagents required

(1) 0·5 M Veronal acetate buffer, pH 5·0 (*see* page 326)
(2) Sodium β-glycerophosphate
(3) Lead nitrate
(4) 1 per cent Ammonium sulphide

Preparation of incubating solution

(1) 0·5 M Veronal acetate buffer, pH 5·0	10 ml
(2) Sodium β-glycerophosphate	32 mg
(3) Lead nitrate	20 mg

The lead nitrate must be dissolved in the buffer before the β-glycerophosphate is added. The pH of the incubating medium should be approximately 5·0.

Sections

Cryostat post-fixed
Cryostat pre-fixed
Freeze dried
Frozen sections

Suitable tissues for controls

Intestine, liver and kidney

Incubating method

(1) Place sections in incubating medium at 37°C for $\frac{1}{2}$–2 h
(2) Wash in distilled water
(3) Immerse in 1 per cent ammonium sulphide (fresh), 2 min
(4) Wash well in distilled water
(5) Counterstain in either 2 per cent Methyl Green, or Mayer's Carmalum
(6) Wash in tap water
(7) Mount in glycerine jelly

Results

Acid phosphatase activity: black
Nuclei: green or red

METHOD 104

Acid phosphatase: Azo Dye Coupling method (simultaneous coupling)

Solutions required

(1) 0·1 M Acetate buffer, pH 5·0
(2) Sodium α-naphthyl phosphate
(3) Diazonium salt, Fast Garnet GBC

Preparation of incubating medium

Sodium α-naphthyl phosphate	10 mg
0·1 M Acetate buffer, pH 5·0	10 ml
Fast Garnet GBC	10 mg

The sodium α-naphthyl phosphate is dissolved in the buffer and the diazonium salt added. The solution is then filtered and used immediately.

Sections

Cryostat pre-fixed
Cryostat post-fixed
Freeze dried
Frozen sections

Suitable tissues for controls

Liver, kidney and intestine

Method

(1) Incubate at 37°C for 15–60 min
(2) Wash in distilled water
(3) Counterstain in 2 per cent Methyl Green (chloroform extracted)
(4) Wash in running tap water
(5) Mount in glycerin jelly

Results

Acid phosphatase activity: red
Nuclei: green

METHOD 105

Acid phosphatase: the Naphthol ASBI Phosphate method (Burstone, 1958; modified by Barka, 1960) (simultaneous coupling with substituted naphthols)

Reagents required

(1) Veronal acetate buffer (stock solution A)
(2) Distilled water
(3) Naphthol AS-BI phosphate
(4) N:N-Dimethyl formamide (DMF)
(5) Pararosanilin hydrochloride
(6) Hydrochloric acid
(7) Sodium nitrite
(8) 0·1 N Sodium hydroxide

Preparation of solutions

(1) *Substrate solution*

Naphthol AS-BI phosphate	50 mg
Dimethyl formamide	5 ml

(2) *Buffer solution*

Veronal acetate buffer stock A (*see* page 326)

(3) *Sodium nitrite*

Sodium nitrite	400 mg
Distilled water	10 ml

(4) *Pararosanilin stock* (*see* page 248)

(5) *Distilled water*

Preparation of incubating solution

Solution (1)	0·5 ml	
Solution (2)	2·5 ml	
Solution (3) } Solution (4) }	0·8 ml	{ 0·4 ml of solutions (3) and (4) mixed before adding to incubating solution
Solution (5)	6·5 ml	

It is necessary for the success of the technique that equal parts of solutions (3) and (4) are mixed together and allowed to stand for two minutes before being added to the incubating medium.

The final pH should be between 4·7–5·0; it is adjusted if necessary with 0·1 N NaOH.

Sections

Cryostat post-fixed
Cryostat pre-fixed
Freeze dried
Frozen sections

Suitable tissues for controls

Many tissues, including intestine, liver and kidney

Incubating method

(1) Incubate sections at 37°C for 15–60 min
(2) Wash in distilled water
(3) Counterstain in 2 per cent Methyl Green (chloroform extracted)
(4) Wash in running water
(5) Either (a) mount in glycerin jelly; or
(b) dehydrate rapidly through fresh alcohols to xylene and mount in DPX

Results

Acid phosphatase activity: red
Nuclei: green

Remarks

This is a reliable method giving sharp localization of the enzyme. There are three points to watch in the preparation of the incubating solution.

(1) That solution (3) (sodium nitrite) is fresh
(2) That the pH of the final incubating solution is correct
(3) That the solution is filtered

METHOD 106

Preparation of hexazotized pararosanilin (Davis & Ornstein, 1959)

Solution (1)

Pararosanilin hydrochloride	1 g
Distilled water	20 ml
Hydrochloric acid (conc)	5 ml

The pararosanilin is dissolved in the distilled water and the hydrochloric acid is added. The solution is heated gently, cooled, filtered and stored in a refrigerator.

Solution (2)

Sodium nitrite	2 g
Distilled water	50 ml

This solution will keep overnight at 4°C. I prefer, however, to make this solution fresh each time.

Solution for use

Solutions (1) and (2) in equal parts, allow to stand for 30 s until the solution becomes amber.

METHOD 107

5′-Nucleotidase: Lead method (Wachstein and Meisel, 1957)

Reagents required

(1) Adenosine-5-phosphate
(2) 0·2 M Tris buffer, pH 7·2
(3) 2 per cent Lead nitrate
(4) Magnesium sulphate

Preparation of incubating medium

1·25 per cent Adenosine-5-phosphate	4 ml
0·2 M Tris buffer, pH 7·2	4 ml
2 per cent Lead nitrate	0·6 ml
0·1 M Magnesium sulphate	1 ml
Distilled water	0·5 ml

Sections

Formol calcium 4°C fixed, free-floating
Cryostat sections cut directly into medium

Suitable tissues for controls

Liver, muscle and brain

Incubating method

(1) Incubating medium at 37°C for 30 min to 1 h
(2) Fix in formol saline if unfixed sections used
(3) Transfer sections with glass rod to distilled water
(4) Repeat wash in fresh distilled water
(5) 1 per cent Ammonium sulphide, 3 min
(6) Wash well in distilled water
(7) Repeat wash
(8) Mount on microscope slides and allow to dry partially in the usual way
(9) Mount in glycerin jelly

Result

5′-Nucleotidase: blackish brown deposits

Remarks

There is a considerable loss of enzyme activity with pre-fixed blocks, so the recommended method is to use cryostat sections of unfixed material.

METHOD 108

Glucose-6-phosphatase: Lead method (Wachstein and Meisel, 1956)

Reagents required

(1) Glucose-6-phosphate (potassium salt)
(2) Tris maleate, pH 6·7
(3) 2 per cent Lead nitrate
(4) Ammonium sulphide

Preparation of incubating medium

0·125 per cent Glucose-6-phosphate (aqueous)	4 ml
0·2 M Tris maleate, pH 6·7	4 ml
2 per cent Lead nitrate	0·6 ml
Distilled water	1·4 ml

Sections

Cryostat unfixed
Frozen sections unfixed

Suitable tissues for controls

Liver and small amounts of kidney

Incubating method

(1) Place fresh unfixed cryostat sections into incubating medium at 37°C for 5–20 min
(2) Wash well in distilled water, 2 changes, 2 min each
(3) Immerse sections in 1 per cent ammonium sulphide, 2 min
(4) Wash in distilled water
(5) Fix sections in 10 per cent formaldehyde, 15–30 min
(6) Wash in distilled water
(7) Mount in glycerin jelly

Result

Glucose-6-phosphatase activity: brownish black

Remarks

It is advisable to use sections 15 microns thick. Although less convenient, better results may be obtained by incubating the section free-floating.

METHOD 109

Adenosine triphosphatase: Lead method (Wachstein and Meisel, 1960)

Reagents required

(1) Adenosine triphosphate
(2) Tris buffer, pH 7·2
(3) 2 per cent Lead nitrate
(4) 2·5 per cent Magnesium nitrate
(5) Ammonium sulphide

Preparation of incubating medium

0·125 per cent Adenosine triphosphate	4 ml
Tris buffer	4 ml
2 per cent Lead nitrate	0·6 ml
2·5 per cent Magnesium nitrate	1 ml
Distilled water	0·4 ml

Sections

Cryostat pre-fixed
Cryostat unfixed
Frozen sections fixed

Suitable tissues for controls

Heart, skeletal muscle, kidney and prostate

Incubating method

(1) Incubate free-floating sections for 10–60 min at 37°C
(2) Wash in distilled water, 2 changes, 2 min each
(3) Immerse in 1 per cent ammonium sulphide, 2 min
(4) Wash in tap water, 2 min
(5) Mount in glycerin jelly

Results

Adenosine triphosphatase activity: brownish black deposit

Remarks

Check the pH of incubating medium before use. The wash after the sections are removed from the incubating medium should be rapid and with at least two changes.

REFERENCES

BARKA, T. (1960). *Nature, Lond.* **187,** 248
BURSTONE, M. S. (1958). *J. nat. Cancer Inst.* **21,** 523
— (1961). *J. Histochem. Cytochem.* **9,** 146
CHIQUOINE, A. D. (1954). *J. comp. Neurol.* **100,** 415
— (1955). *J. Histochem. Cytochem.* **3,** 471
DAVIS, B. J. and ORNSTEIN, L. (1959). *ibid.* **7,** 297
GOMORI, G. (1939). *Proc. Soc. exp. Biol., N. Y.* **42,** 23
— (1941). *Arch. Path.* **32,** 189
— (1951). *J. lab. clin. Med.* **37,** 520
— (1952a). *Int. Rev. Cytol.* **1,** 323
— (1952). *Microscopic Histochemistry,* Chicago University Press
GROGG, E. and PEARSE, A. G. E. (1952). *Nature, Lond.* **170,** 578
MENTON, M. L., JUNGE, J. and GREEN, M. H. (1944). *J. biol. Chem.* **153,** 471
PADYKULA, H. A. and HERMAN, E. (1955). *J. Histochem. Cytochem.* **3,** 170
PEARSE, A. G. E. (1960). *Histochemistry, Theoretical and Applied,* London: Churchill
— and REIS, J. L. (1952). *Biochem. J.* **50,** 534
RUTTENBERG, A. M. and SELIGMAN, A. M. (1955). *J. Histochem. Cytochem* **3,** 455
TAKAMATSU, H. (1939). *Trans. Soc. Path., Japan* **29,** 429
WACHSTEIN, M. and MEISEL, E. (1956). *J. Histochem. Cytochem.* **4,** 592
— — (1957). *Amer. J. clin. Path.* **27,** 13
— — (1960). *J. Histochem. Cytochem.* **8,** 387

16

Esterases

Esterases are enzymes which are capable of hydrolyzing esters. Therefore by definition the phosphatases dealt with in Chapter 15 are strictly esterases, since they hydrolyze phosphate esters. This chapter is devoted to those esterases which hydrolyze esters of carboxylic acids. Within this group there are many different types of esterases, acting upon a number of different substrates. Unfortunately there is considerable overlap between the different types of esterases, since many of the esterases are capable of hydrolyzing the same substrate to some extent. This makes a classification of esterases difficult to define. Any subdivision of esterases depends upon the application of enzyme inhibitors to the various enzyme methods. The most useful classification is based upon the differential inhibition.

Non-specific esterases

If the substrate is a simple ester such as α-naphthyl acetate the hydrolyzing enzyme is called a non-specific esterase. However, because of the considerable overlap in activity previously mentioned the more specific esterases such as cholinesterase are capable of hydrolyzing these simple esters. Non-specific esterases can be further subdivided into several different groups, according to the particular type of ester they hydrolyze most efficiently and according to the effect of organophosphate inhibitors.

The subdivision of non-specific esterases based on their most suitable substrate is:

(1) carboxyl esterases
(2) aryl esterases
(3) acetyl esterases.

Fortunately this approximate classification coincides neatly with the classification based on the effects of organophosphate inhibitors (*see below*).

Specific esterases

The most important specific esterases histochemically are the cholinesterases; these are of two types, acetyl cholinesterase ('true') and cholinesterase ('pseudo'). Acetyl cholinesterases are capable of hydrolyzing acetyl thiocholine, whereas cholinesterase will hydrolyze esters of choline other than acetyl thiocholine more rapidly. Both these enzymes are capable of hydrolyzing simple esters. Cholinesterases are differentiated from the non-specific esterases by their particular capacity to hydrolyze choline esters and by the fact that this capacity is destroyed by the action of the specific inhibitor eserine (10^{-5}M). Non-specific esterases are not inhibited by eserine.

Lipases

The term is generally applied to those esterases which have a particular facility for hydrolyzing long chain esters (i.e. those esters containing fatty acids with more than seven carbon atoms in the chain). There is, however, considerable overlap between the lipases and non-specific esterases since both are capable of hydrolyzing simple esters.

Inhibitors

The application of esterase inhibitors to the histochemical reactions has permitted a more accurate identification of various enzymes. The use of the specific inhibitor, eserine, in the identification of the cholinesterases and acetyl cholinesterases has already been mentioned. The most useful esterase inhibitors are the organophosphorus compounds such as di-isopropyl fluorophosphate (DFP) and diethyl p-nitrophenyl phosphate (E600). The esterases have been subdivided into so-called A, B and C esterases as described by Pearse (1972). The A esterases are resistant to a concentration of 1mM of E600 but sensitive to some other inhibitors, whereas B esterases are sensitive to E600 in a concentration as low as 10μM. The C esterases are resistant to most esterase inhibitors. The A, B and C esterases are resistant to the effects of eserine, but since the specific cholinesterases are also sensitive to low concentrations of E600 some authorities arbitrarily group them with the B esterases.

It is found that the carboxyl esterases are B esterases, the aryl esterases are A-type esterases, and the acetyl esterases are C-type esterases.

There are histochemical methods for the demonstration of each of the groups listed in Table 16.1. The following seven methods are given at the end of this chapter.

(1) α-Naphthyl Acetate method with Fast Blue B for non-specific esterases (*see* Method 110).

(2) α-Naphthyl Acetate method with hexazonium pararosanalin for non-specific esterases (*see* Method 111).

(3) Indoxyl Acetate method for non-specific esterases, E600-resistant esterases (*see* Method 112).

(4) Naphthol AS-LC Acetate method for non-specific esterase (*see* Method 113).

(5) Tween method for lipase (*see* Method 114).

(6) Myristoyl Choline for cholinesterases (*see* Method 115).

(7) Thiocholine method for acetyl cholinesterase (*see* Method 116).

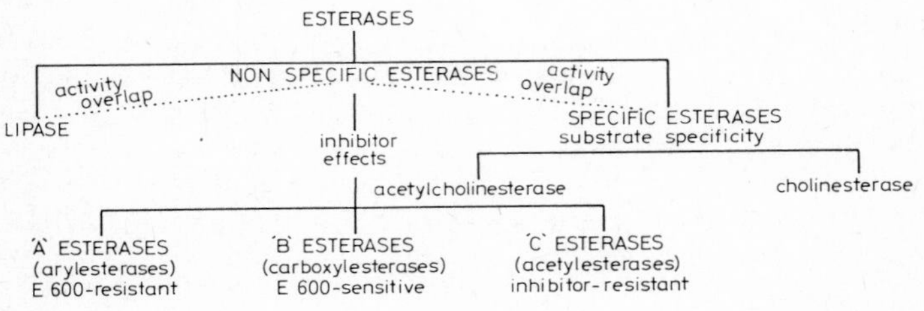

Figure 16.1 Histochemical classification of esterases.

HISTOCHEMICAL METHODS FOR THE DEMONSTRATION OF ESTERASES

Because of the wide range of activity of the various types of esterases, substrates such as α-naphthyl acetate, indoxyl acetates and substituted naphthol acetates can be used in the demonstration of A, B and C esterases as well as cholinesterases.

Non-specific esterases

α-Naphthyl Acetate method for non-specific esterase

This method will probably demonstrate all types of esterase activity. It is normally carried out at a pH of 7·4. It is an azo dye simultaneous coupling method which was first described by Nachlas and Seligman (1949). The authors suggested the use of β-naphthyl acetate as a substrate, and Diazo Blue B as a coupling agent. Gomori (1950) substituted α-naphthyl acetate for β-naphthyl acetate, pointing out that the azo dye produced with the latter was soluble in water, but that produced with α-naphthyl acetate was not. Localization of the enzyme is therefore more precise. The method can be carried out employing the diazonium salt Fast Blue B as the coupling

The α-naphthyl acetate is dissolved in the acetone and the phosphate buffer added and thoroughly mixed. The Fast Blue B is added and the solution filtered, and used immediately.

Sections

Cryostat post-fixed
Cryostat pre-fixed
Freeze dried
Carefully processed paraffin sections
Frozen sections

Suitable controls

Intestine, liver and kidney

Incubating method

(1) After suitable fixation, bring section down to water
(2) Place in incubating medium for 30 s to 15 min at room temperature
(3) Wash in running tap water — 3 min
(4) Counterstain in Mayer's Carmalum — 5 min
(5) Wash in running tap water — 3 min
(6) Mount in glycerine jelly

Results

Esterase activity: reddish brown
Nuclei: red

Remarks

The method works very rapidly with the cryostat sections, and tissues containing a lot of esterase need to be incubated for 1–2 min only.

METHOD 111

Non-specific esterase: α-Naphthyl Acetate method using hexazotized pararosanilin (Gomori, 1950; Davis and Ornstein, 1959)

Reagents required

(1) α-Naphthyl acetate
(2) 0·2 M Phosphate buffer (stock solution A)
(3) Distilled water
(4) Acetone
(5) Pararosanilin hydrochloride
(6) Hydrochloric acid
(7) Sodium nitrite

Preparation of solutions

(1) *Substrate solution*

α-Naphthyl acetate	50 mg
Acetone	5 ml

(2) *Buffer solution*

0·2 M Phosphate buffer, stock solution A (*see* page 327)

(3) *Sodium nitrite*

Sodium nitrite	400 mg
Distilled water	10 ml

(4) *Pararosanilin-HCl stock*

Pararosanilin hydrochloride	2 g
2 N-Hydrochloric acid	50 ml

Heat gently, cool to room temperature and filter.

(5) *Distilled water*

Preparation of incubating medium

Solution (1)	0·25 ml	
Solution (2)	7·25 ml	
Solution (3) Solution (4)	0·8 ml	0·4 ml of solution (3) and (4) are mixed before adding to incubating solution.
Solution (5)	2·5 ml	

It is important that equal parts of solutions (3) and (4) are mixed together before adding to the incubating medium. Adjust pH to 7·4 if necessary with solution (2).

Sections

Cryostat post-fixed
Cryostat pre-fixed
Freeze dried
Carefully processed paraffin sections
Frozen sections

Suitable controls

Intestine, liver and kidney

Incubating method

(1) After suitable fixation, bring sections to water
(2) Incubate at 37°C for 2–20 min
(3) Wash in running water

(4) Counterstain in 2 per cent Methyl Green (chloroform extracted)
(5) Wash well in tap water
(6) Dehydrate rapidly through fresh alcohol to xylene and mount

Results

Esterase: reddish brown
Nuclei: green

METHOD 112

Non-specific esterase: Indoxyl Acetate method (Holt, 1954)

Reagents required

(1) 5-Bromo-4-chloro-indoxyl acetate
(2) Ethanol
(3) 0·2 M Tris buffer, pH 7·2
(4) Potassium ferricyanide
(5) Potassium ferrocyanide
(6) Calcium chloride
(7) Distilled water

Preparation of incubating medium

5 Bromo-4-chloro-indoxyl acetate	1 mg
Ethanol	0·1 ml
Tris buffer (0·2 M), pH 7·2 (*see* page 328)	2 ml
Potassium ferricyanide (0·05 M) (1·6 per cent)	17 mg
Potassium ferrocyanide (0·05 M) (2·1 per cent)	21 mg
Calcium chloride (0·1 M) (2·1 per cent)	11 mg
Distilled water	7·9 ml

The 5-bromo-4-chloro-indoxyl acetate is dissolved in the ethanol and the buffer is then added. The remaining chemicals are dissolved in the distilled water and the solution is mixed. It is important that the solution is freshly prepared.

Sections

Cryostat post-fixed
Cryostat pre-fixed
Freeze dried
Frozen sections
Carefully processed paraffin sections

Suitable controls

Kidney, liver and intestine

Incubating method

(1) After suitable fixation, bring sections to water
(2) Incubate at 37°C for 15–60 min
(3) Rinse in tap water
(4) Counterstain in Mayer's Carmalum for 5 min
(5) Rinse in tap water
(6) Mount in glycerin jelly or
(7) Dehydrate through graded alcohols to xylene
(8) Mount in DPX

Results

Esterase activity: blue
Nuclei: red

METHOD 113

Non-specific esterase: Naphthol AS-LC Acetate method (Gomori, 1952; Burstone, 1957)

Reagents required

(1) Naphthol AS-LC acetate
(2) Dimethyl formamide (DMF)
(3) Ethyl cellulose
(4) Tris buffer, pH 7·1
(5) Distilled water
(6) Fast Garnet GBC

Preparation of incubating medium

Naphthol AS-LC acetate	5 mg
Dimethyl formamide	0·4 ml
Ethyl cellulose	1·0 ml
Tris buffer, pH 7·1	2·0 ml
Distilled water	6·6 ml
Fast Garnet GBC	10 mg

The substrate naphthol AS-LC acetate is dissolved in solutions (2) and (3). The remaining solutions are added, the Fast Garnet GBC last; the solution is well mixed, filtered and used immediately.

Sections

Cryostat pre-fixed
Cryostat post-fixed
Frozen sections

Suitable control sections

Intestine, liver and kidney

Incubating method

(1) After suitable fixation, bring sections down to water
(2) Place in incubating medium at 20°C for 10–30 min
(3) Rinse in tap water
(4) Counterstain in 2 per cent Methyl Green or haematoxylin
(5) Wash in tap water
(6) Mount in glycerin jelly

Results

Esterase activity: reddish brown
Nuclei: green or deep blue

Remarks

The above technique is suitable for formalin-fixed frozen sections (cryostat, etc.). If the method is to be applied to paraffin-embedded material, *see* text.

METHOD 114

Lipase: Tween method (Gomori, 1952)

Reagents required

(1) Tween 40, 60 or 80 (Tween 80 is considered to be a more specific substrate for 'true' lipase)
(2) Tris buffer, pH 7·2
(3) Calcium chloride
(4) Thymol
(5) Lead nitrate
(6) Ammonium sulphide
(7) Distilled water

Preparation of solutions

Solution (1)

Tris buffer, pH 7·2 (*see* buffer tables, page 328)

Solution (2)

Tween 40, 60 or 80	5 g
Tris buffer, pH 7·2	100 ml
Thymol	1 crystal

Solution (3)

Calcium chloride	200 mg
Distilled water	10 ml

Solution (4)

Lead nitrate	1 g
Distilled water	50 ml

Preparation of incubating medium

Solution (1)	9 ml
Solution (2)	0·6 ml
Solution (3)	0·3 ml

Section

Formalin-fixed free-floating
Cryostat pre-fixed
Paraffin sections

Suitable controls

Pancreas, liver and adrenal gland

Incubating method

(1) After suitable fixation, bring sections to water
(2) Incubate at 37°C for 2–8 h. If paraffin sections, leave for 24 h
(3) Rinse sections in 3 changes of distilled water
(4) Place sections in pre-heated lead nitrate solution at 55°C for 10 min
(5) Rinse sections in distilled water for 2 min
(6) Wash in tap water for 10 min
(7) Place sections in 1 per cent ammonium sulphide for 3 min
(8) Rinse in distilled water
(9) Wash in tap water
(10) Counterstain in Mayer's Carmalum for 5 min
(11) Wash in tap water for 1 min
(12) Mount in glycerin jelly

Results

Lipase activity: yellow brown-black
Nuclei: red

Remarks

With this technique, it is advisable to have a control section which is processed through the whole technique, except that the incubating medium lacks Tween. Paraffin sections according to Gomori should be fixed in acetone. Formalin-fixed, frozen sections work well.

METHOD 115

Cholinesterase: Myristoyl Choline method (Gomori, 1948)

Reagents required

(1) Myristoyl choline
(2) 0·1 M Veronal acetate buffer, pH 7·6
(3) Cobalt acetate
(4) Calcium chloride
(5) Magnesium chloride
(6) Manganese chloride
(7) Distilled water
(8) Ammonium sulphide
(9) Thymol

Preparation of solutions

Solution (1)

Cobalt acetate	400 mg
Distilled water	80 ml
0·1 M Veronal acetate, pH 7·6 (*see* page 328)	20 ml
Magnesium chloride	1 mg
Calcium chloride	1 mg
Manganese chloride	1 mg
Thymol	1 crystal

Solution (2)

Myristoyl choline	70 mg
Distilled water	10 ml
Thymol	1 crystal

This solution is stored at 4°C

Incubating medium

Solution (1) (at 37°C)	10 ml
Solution (2)	0·2 ml

Sections

Cryostat pre-fixed
Formalin-fixed free-floating
Cryostat post-fixed
Paraffin sections

Suitable controls

Rat diaphragm, skeletal muscle and heart muscle

Incubating method

(1) Bring suitably fixed sections to water
(2) Incubate at 37°C for 1–4 h; if paraffin sections, 2–16 h
(3) Wash in distilled water, 1 min
(4) Wash in tap water, 2 min
(5) Place sections in 2 per cent ammonium sulphide, 3 min
(6) Wash in tap water, 5 min
(7) Counterstain if required in 0·05 per cent eosin, 30 s
(8) Wash in tap water
(9) Mount in glycerin jelly

Results

Cholinesterase activity: dark brown to black

Remarks

If this method is being used regularly, it is advisable to store solution (1) at 37°C. This method almost certainly demonstrates some non-specific esterase as well and this can be confirmed by the use of inhibitors.

METHOD 116

Cholinesterase: Thiocholine method (Gerebtzoff, 1959)

Reagents required

(1) Acetylthiocholine iodide or butyrylthiocholine iodide
(2) 0·1 M Acetate buffer, various pH, 5·0–6·2
(3) Cupric sulphate
(4) Glycine
(5) Distilled water
(6) Ammonium sulphide

Preparation of solutions

Solution (1)

0·1 M Acetate buffer, pH 5·0–6·2 (*see* page 326)

Solution (2)

Acetylcholine iodide	15 mg
Cupric sulphate	7 mg
Distilled water	1·4 ml

This solution is centrifuged at 4,000 r.p.m. for 15 min and the supernatant used

Solution (3)

Glycine	375 mg
Distilled water	10 ml

Solution (4)

Cupric sulphate	250 mg
Distilled water	10 ml

Solution (5)

Distilled water

Preparation of incubating medium

Solution (1)	5 ml
Solution (2)	0·8 ml
Solution (3)	0·2 ml
Solution (4)	0·2 ml
Solution (5)	3·8 ml

The pH of the incubating medium is varied according to the tissue and the amount of activity expected in the tissues. Gerebtzoff (1959) states 'tissues with high cholinesterase activity are incubated at pH 5·0 and other tissues at 6·2'.

Sections

Cryostat pre-fixed
Formalin-fixed free-floating
Cryostat post-fixed
Paraffin sections

Suitable controls

Heart muscle, brain and skeletal muscle

Incubating method

(1) Incubate sections at 37°C for 10–90 min
(2) Rinse in two changes of distilled water
(3) Treat sections with 2 per cent ammonium sulphide for 2 min
(4) Wash well in distilled water
(5) Counterstain if required
(6) Wash in tap water
(7) Mount in glycerin jelly

Results

Cholinesterase activity: brown

Remarks

All the stock solutions will keep in a refrigerator. It is a reproduceable method that works best with free-floating sections.

REFERENCES

Barrnett, R. J. and Seligman, A. M. (1951). *Science, N.Y.* **114,** 579
Burstone, M. S. (1957). *J. nat. Cancer Inst.* **18,** 167
Davis, B. J. and Ornstein, L. (1959). *J. Histochem. Cytochem.* **7,** 297
Gerebtzoff, M. A. (1959). *Cholinesterases*, Oxford: Pergamon
Gomori, G. (1945). *Proc. Soc. exp. Biol., N.Y.* **58,** 362
— (1948). *ibid.* **68,** 354
— (1950). *J. lab. clin. Med.* **35,** 802
— (1952). *Microscopical Histochemistry*, Chicago University Press
Holt, S. J. (1954). *Proc. roy. Soc., Series B* **142,** 160
— and Withers, R. F. J. (1952). *Nature, Lond.* **170,** 1012
Koelle, G. B. and Friedenwald, J. S. (1949). *Proc. Soc. exp. Biol., N.Y.* **70,** 617
Nachlas, M. M. and Seligman, A. M. (1949). *J. nat. Cancer Inst.* **9,** 415
Pearse, A. G. E. (1953). *J. Path. Bact.* **66,** 331
— (1972). *Histochemistry, Theoretical and Applied*, 3rd Edn., Vol. 2, London: Churchill Livingstone

17

Oxidoreductases
I. Oxidases

The oxidoreductases comprise a number of enzymes sharing the ability to oxidize substrates, either by catalyzing the reaction between the substrate and atmospheric oxygen ('oxidases'), or by removing hydrogen from the substrate and transferring it to a hydrogen acceptor system ('dehydrogenases').

The oxidases are found in most animal and plant tissues, and most contain iron or copper. They are distinguished from dehydrogenases by the fact that they are unable to function anaerobically (Davenport, 1960).

The oxidases demonstrable histochemically can be divided into:—

(1) Cytochrome oxidase	(iron- and copper-containing) *See* Method 121
(2) Peroxidases	(iron-containing) *See* Method 117
(3) DOPA oxidase	(copper-containing) *See* Methods 118, 119
(4) Monoamine oxidase	(copper co-factor) *See* Method 120

The enzyme catalase is also regarded as an oxidative enzyme and can be demonstrated histochemically; unfortunately the specificity of the methods devised so far is open to doubt.

Cytochrome oxidase

This enzyme is found in many tissues, being particularly rich in kidney, liver and muscle. It is closely attached to cell mitochondria, and recent work has shown that it contains both haem groups and copper atoms (Lemberg, 1969). Cytochrome oxidase and other cytochromes are concerned in the main oxidation pathway. Cytochrome oxidase (otherwise known as cytochrome A_3) is thought to have cytochrome C as its substrate.

The nomenclature of cytochromes and cytochrome oxidase is confusing; cytochrome oxidase has also been called indophenol oxidase.

Peroxidases

These enzymes break down peroxides; a special type of peroxidase is catalase which breaks down hydrogen peroxide. Peroxidases are found in leucocytes, haemoglobin, and also in spleen and liver.

DOPA oxidase

This enzyme is also known as tyrosinase and catechol oxidase. It catalyzes the oxidation of tyrosine to dihydroxyphenylalanine (DOPA) and the final oxidations of DOPA to the melanin pigments. It is also capable of oxidizing diphenol compounds such as catechol and adrenalin. The method is used as a means of identifying cells capable of producing melanin, particularly in the malignant tumour of melanocytes, malignant melanoma.

Monoamine oxidase

This enzyme acts mainly on short chain monoamines, although some diamines are also attacked. Monoamine oxidase acts particularly rapidly on tyramine and dopamine (Weiner, 1960), but also is involved in the breakdown of adrenalin and 5-hydroxytryptamine to their respective breakdown products.

Monoamine oxidase is found in small concentrations in many tissues but is present in larger quantities in liver and kidney.

HISTOCHEMICAL METHODS

Cytochrome oxidase

This important enzyme has been demonstrated biochemically for many years. The first histochemical method was introduced by Graff (1916). A number of techniques are now available for the demonstration of cytochrome oxidase including the nadi-type of reaction, as modified by Nachlas, Crawford, Goldstein and Seligman (1958), and the metal chelation methods of Burstone (1959, 1960). The Burstone technique given on page 276 has the advantage of producing an intense colour reaction and is considered more specific than the original nadi-type techniques. The cytochrome oxidase in the section couples with the 1-hydroxy-2-naphthoic acid to form a naphthol compound which in turn couples with a free radical amine (from N-phenyl-para-phenylene diamine). This secondary reaction product is then chelated to cobalt ions. Other methods available include the Thiazol Blue method of Thiele (1967) and the modified nadi-type reaction of Seligman *et al.* (1968) which uses 3,3′ diaminobenzidine (DAB).

Peroxidase

The demonstration of peroxidases in tissue sections is often difficult to perform and not very specific. Many different peroxidase enzymes are present in tissues. The majority of suitable substrates for peroxidases give a weakly coloured reaction product upon oxidation. The most popular type of method to demonstrate peroxidases was the benzidine method, in which the benzidine is oxidized to a blue-brown colour. Benzidine is now recognized as a carcinogenic substrate and as a result of this, benzidine substitutes are being employed in histochemistry. For the demonstration of peroxidases,

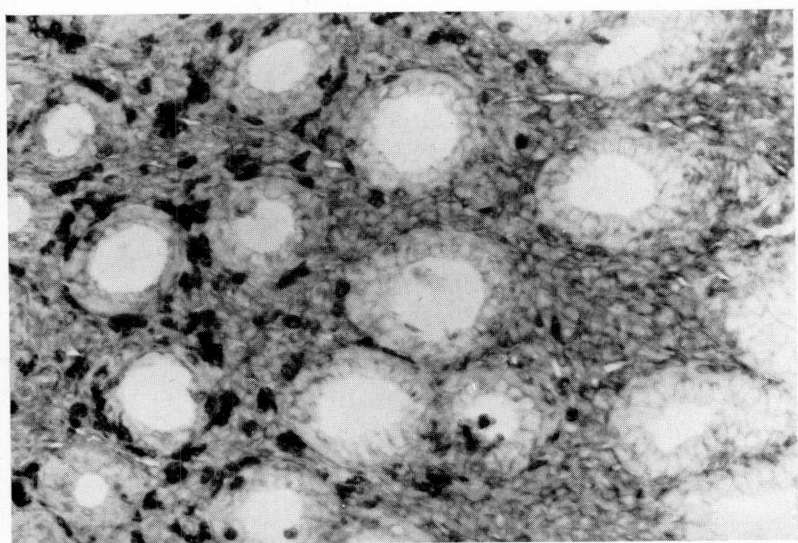

Figure 17.1 Human colon—distribution of peroxidase in leucocytes and macrophages in lamina propria shown by DAB technique. (× *325*)

(Reduced to two-thirds in reproduction)

3,3′-diaminobenzidine (DAB) introduced by Graham and Karnovsky (1966) gives excellent results (*See Figure 17.1*) in this laboratory and is given as Method 117, page 272. An alternative means of demonstration is by the leuco-dye methods introduced by Lison (1936).

DOPA oxidase (tyrosinase)

The first histochemical method for the demonstration of DOPA oxidase was that by Bloch (1917), subsequently modified by Laidlow and Blackberg (1932). Becker, Draver and Thatcher (1935) introduced a further modification applicable to blocks for paraffin sectioning. This latter method is simple and reproduceable, and is given as Method 119 on page 274. The basis of the reaction is that dihydroxy-phenylalanine (DOPA) in the incubating medium is oxidized by tyrosinase (DOPA oxidase) in the section. The oxidation produces a brownish-black pigment which is found in cells producing melanin. Control sections are carried through the method (minus the DOPA) to exclude preformed melanin.

However recent work (Okun 1967, and Okun *et al.* 1969, 1970) has shown that peroxidase is capable of catalyzing the oxidation of tyrosine and DOPA, so the specificity of DOPA oxidase methods is in some doubt.

Monoamine oxidase

Histochemical methods for the demonstration of monoamine oxidase (MAO) date back to the method of Oster and Schlossman (1942) with their aldehyde-PAS method. The first technique involving the use of tetrazolium salts was published by Francis (1953). In this method, tyramine was used as the substrate and neotetrazolium as the tetrazolium salt. Glenner, Burtner and Brown (1957) introduced a method in which they used tryptamine as the substrate and nitro-blue tetrazolium (NBT) as the tetrazolium salt. This method gives a reliable and reproduceable result and is the one recommended.

The theory of the reaction is not fully understood, but the monoamine oxidase in the section oxidizes tryptamine in the incubating medium. The product of this oxidation then reduces the tetrazolium salt to produce a formazan deposit.

In the technique given at the end of this chapter (Method 120), tetra-nitro-blue tetrazolium (TNBT) is used instead of NBT. This gives better localization of the enzyme. The incubation must be carried out on unfixed sections at 37°C for approximately 45 minutes. Activity is strong in heart muscle, kidney and many other tissues.

METHOD 117

DAB technique for peroxidase (Graham and Karnovsky, 1966)

Reagents required

(1) 3,3′ Diaminobenzidine tetrahydrochloride
(2) Tris-HCl buffer, pH 7·6
(3) 1 per cent Hydrogen peroxide

Preparation of incubating solution

3,3′ Diaminobenzidine tetrahydrochloride	5 mg
Tris-HCl buffer (pH 7·6)	10 ml
1 per cent hydrogen peroxide	1·2 ml

Sections

Fixation is important. Graham and Karnovsky (1966) utilized two different fixatives in a mixture, *ie* 5 per cent glutaraldehyde and formaldehyde (from paraformaldehyde) in cacodylate buffer (*see* Pearse (1972). Tissues should be prefixed in this solution, or possibly in formol calcium (*see Remarks*).

Suitable controls

Red blood cells

Incubating method

(1) Rinse fixed sections in distilled water
(2) Place in incubating medium for 5 min
(3) Wash well in distilled water
(4) Counterstain in 2 per cent Methyl Green (chloroform washed) for 5 min
(5) Wash well in distilled water
(6) Dehydrate through graded alcohols to xylene
(7) Mount in DPX

Results

Peroxidase activity: brown granules
Nuclei: green

Remarks

This technique was originally described as a suitable method for electron microscopy and for this fixation is critical. For optical microscopy the fixation is less important but best results are obtained by using the gluteraldehyde–formaldehyde mixture.

METHOD 118

DOPA oxidase (tyrosinase): DOPA reaction (Becker *et al.*, 1935)

Reagents required

(1) D.L.3:4-Dihydroxyphenylalanine (DOPA)
(2) Phosphate buffer, pH 7·4
(3) Formol saline

Preparation of incubating solution

D.L.3:4-Dihydroxyphenylalanine	100 mg
0·1 M Phosphate buffer, pH 7·4 (*see* page 328)	100 ml

Sections

The method is carried out on small blocks of tissue. See next method for modification for frozen sections.

Suitable control sections

Skin

Method

(1) Fix small pieces of tissue in 10 per cent formol saline at room temperature	4 h
(2) Cut thin slices (3mm) from surface of blocks, wash in tap water	3 min
(3) Place slices in incubating medium at 37°C	1 h
(4) Place slices in fresh incubating medium at 37°C	overnight
(5) Wash the pieces of tissue in running tap water	5 min
(6) Fix blocks in 10 per cent formol saline	overnight

(7) Dehydrate blocks through alcohol to chloroform, then wax
(8) Cut paraffin sections 8 microns thick
(9) Dewax and take down to water
(10) Counterstain in Mayer's Carmalum, if required
(11) Dehydrate through graded alcohols to xylene and mount in DPX

Results

DOPA oxidase: blackish brown granules

METHOD 119

DOPA oxidase (tyrosinase): DOPA reaction (Becker *et al.*, 1935) (Modified)

Reagents Required

(1) D.L.3:4-Dihydroxyphenylalanine (DOPA)
(2) 0·1 M Phosphate buffer, pH 7·4
(3) Formol saline

Preparation of incubating medium

D.L.3:4-Dihydroxyphenylalanine	100 mg
0·1 M Phosphate buffer, pH 7·4 (*see* page 328)	100 ml

Sections

Cryostat post-fixed (formalin)
Cryostat pre- fixed (formalin)
Frozen sections (formalin)

Suitable control sections

Skin

Method

(1) Wash fixed frozen sections briefly in distilled water
(2) Place sections in incubating solution at 37°C for 45 min
(3) Transfer sections to fresh incubating solution at 37°C for approximately 2–4 h
(4) Wash in running tap water, 5 min
(5) Counterstain if required in Mayer's Carmalum
(6) Wash in tap water
(7) Dehydrate through graded alcohols to xylene and mount in DPX

Result

DOPA oxidase: brownish black
Nuclei: red

METHOD 120

Monoamine oxidase: Tetrazolium method (Glenner *et al.*, 1957)

Reagents required

(1) Tryptamine hydrochloride
(2) Sodium sulphate
(3) Tetranitro-blue tetrazolium
(4) 0·1 M Phosphate buffer, pH 7·6
(5) Distilled water
(6) 10 per cent Formol saline

Incubating solution

Tryptamine hydrochloride	25 mg
Sodium sulphate	4 mg
Tetranitro-blue tetrazolium	5 mg
0·1 M Phosphate buffer, pH 7·6 (*see* page 328)	5 ml
Distilled water	15 ml

Sections

Cryostat unfixed, 15–20 microns thick

Suitable control sections

Heart muscle, liver and kidney

Method

(1)	Place sections in incubating medium at 37°C	45 min
(2)	Wash in running tap water	2 min
(3)	Place sections in 10 per cent formol saline	30 min
(4)	Wash well in tap water	2 min
(5)	Mount in glycerin jelly	

Result

Monoamine oxidase activity: bluish black

Remarks

This is a very reliable technique giving reproduceable results.

METHOD 121

Cytochrome oxidase: Metal Chelation (Burstone, 1959)

Reagents required

(1) 1-Hydroxy-2-naphthoic acid
(2) N-Phenyl-*p*-phenylenediamine
(3) Absolute alcohol
(4) Distilled water
(5) Tris buffer, 0·2 M, pH 7·4
(6) Cobalt acetate

Preparation of incubating solutions

Solution (1)

1-Hydroxy-2-naphthoic acid	10 mg
N-Phenyl-*p*-phenylenediamine	10 mg
Absolute alcohol	0·5 ml
Distilled water	35 ml
0·2 M Tris buffer, pH 7·4 (*see* page 328)	15 ml

The first two reagents are dissolved in the absolute alcohol and then the distilled water and the buffer are added.

Solution (2)

Cobalt acetate	500 g
Formaldehyde, conc.	5 ml
Distilled water	45 ml

Sections

Unfixed cryostat sections

Suitable control sections

Liver and kidney

Incubating method

(1) Place sections into incubating solution for 15 min–2 h

(2) Transfer sections directly to 1 per cent cobalt acetate, solution (2), for 1 h

(3) Wash in distilled water

(4) Mount in glycerin jelly

Result

Cytochrome oxidase activity: blue-black

REFERENCES

BECKER, S. W., DRAVER, L. L. and THATCHER, H. (1935). *Arch. Dermat. Syph.* **31,** 190

BLOCH, B. (1917). *Arch. Dermat. Syph.* **124,** 129

BURSTONE, M. S. (1959). *J. Histochem. Cytochem.* **7,** 112

DAVENPORT, H. A. (1960). *Histological and Histochemical Technic*, Philadelphia: Saunders

FRANCIS, C. M. (1953). *Nature, Lond.* **171,** 701

GLENNER, G. G., BURTNER, H. J. and BROWN, G. W. (1957). *J. Histochem. Cytochem.* **5,** 591

GRAFF, S. (1916). *Zeutbl. Path.* **27,** 318

GRAHAM, R. C., Jr. and KARNOVSKY, M. J. (1966). *J. Histochem. Cytochem.* **14,** 291

LAIDLAW, G. F. and BLACKBERG, S. N. (1932). *Am. J. Path.* **8,** 491

LEMBERG, M. R. (1969). *Physiol. Rev.* **49,** 48

LISON, L. (1938). *Beitr. Path. Anat. allg. Path.* **101,** 94

NACHLAS, M. M., CRAWFORD, D. T., GOLDSTEIN, T. P. and SELIGMAN. (1958). *J. Histochem. Cytochem.* **6,** 445

OKUN, M. R. (1967). *J. invest. Derm.* **48,** 424

— EDELSTEIN, L., OR N., HAMADA, G. and DONNELAN, B. (1970). *J. invest. Derm.* **55,** 1

OSTER, K. A. and SCHLOSSMAN, N. C. (1942). *J. cell. comp. Physiol.* **20,** 373

PEARSE, A. G. E. (1972). *Histochemistry, Theoretical and Applied*, London: Churchill Livingstone

SELIGMAN, A. M., KARNOVSKY, M. J., WASSERKRUG, H. L. and HANKER, J. S. (1968). *J. Cell. Biol.* **38,** 1

THIELE, H. J. (1967). *Acta histochem.* **26,** 373

WEINER, N. (1960). *Archs Biochem. Biophys.* **91,** 182

18

Oxidoreductases II. Dehydrogenases

The dehydrogenases are enzymes which have the ability to remove hydrogen from the substrate and transfer it to another substance. The substance which acts as a hydrogen acceptor is either nicotinamide adenine dinucleotide (NAD), or nicotinamide adenine dinucleotide phosphate (NADP), or a flavoprotein. NAD and NADP are also known as co-enzymes 1 and 2 respectively (*see* Table 18.1); when they have accepted the hydrogen released by the action of the dehydrogenase they are known as reduced NAD and NADP, signified as NADH and NADPH (*see* Table 18.1).

TABLE 18.1

Co-enzymes

Chemical name	*Standard abbreviations*	*Previously known as*	*Also known as*
Nicotinamide adenine dinucleotide	NAD	DPN	Co-enzyme 1
Nicotinamide adenine dinucleotide reduced	NADH	DPNH	Co-enzyme 1 reduced
Nicotinamide adenine dinucleotide phosphate	NADP	TPN	Co-enzyme 2
Nicotinamide adenine dinucleotide phosphate reduced	NADPH	TPNH	Co-enzyme 2 reduced

In some instances the dehydrogenase itself can act as a hydrogen acceptor, and is then reduced by flavoproteins in a subsequent reaction.

Because of the ability of dehydrogenases to remove hydrogen from the substrate, they can be regarded as being oxidative in action. Nevertheless, they are more flexible than the oxidases discussed in Chapter 17 because dehydrogenases can function anaerobically whereas oxidases can only act where atmospheric oxygen is available.

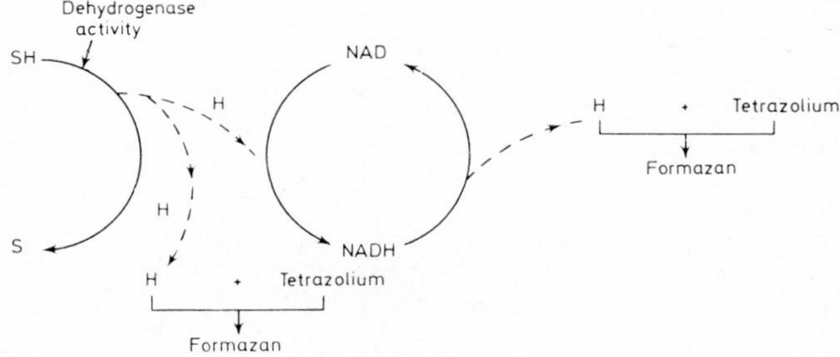

Figure 18.1 SH is the substrate, and S the oxidized substrate. Normally the hydrogen released is accepted by a hydrogen acceptor such as NAD or NADP before combining with the tetrazolium. Where the dehydrogenase itself can act as hydrogen acceptor (e.g. succinate dehydrogenase), no other hydrogen acceptor system is necessary.

Some of the dehydrogenases which can be demonstrated histochemically, with the reactions which they catalyze, are listed in Table 18.2.

TABLE 18.2

Dehydrogenase	*Reaction catalyzed*
Succinate dehydrogenase	Succinate ⟶ fumarate
Lactate dehydrogenase	Lactate ⟶ pyruvate
Malate dehydrogenase	Malate ⟶ oxaloacetate
Isocitrate dehydrogenase	Isocitrate ⟶ oxalosuccinate
Glutamate dehydrogenase	Glutamate ⟶ ketoglutarate
Glucose-6-phosphate dehydrogenase	Glucose-6-phosphate ⟶ 6 phosphoglucononolactone
Alcohol dehydrogenase	ethanol ⟶ acetaldehyde
NAD diaphorase	NADH ⟶ NAD^+
NADP diaphorase	NADPH ⟶ $NADP^+$

The 'diaphorases' are dehydrogenases which catalyze the dehydrogenation of the reduced forms of NAD and NADP, i.e. they catalyze the reactions

$$NADH \longrightarrow NAD^+ + H$$
$$NADPH \longrightarrow NADP^+ + H$$

Demonstration of dehydrogenases

Dehydrogenase activity is demonstrated histochemically using tetrazolium salts. These salts, which are almost colourless and are water-soluble, are able to accept the hydrogen released from the substrate by the enzyme action. Tetrazolium salts which have been reduced in this way produce an insoluble, highly coloured, microcrystalline deposit of a formazan compound. In histochemical reactions the conditions of the method have to be carefully controlled for the successful production and accurate localization of the formazan deposit (*see Figure 18.2*).

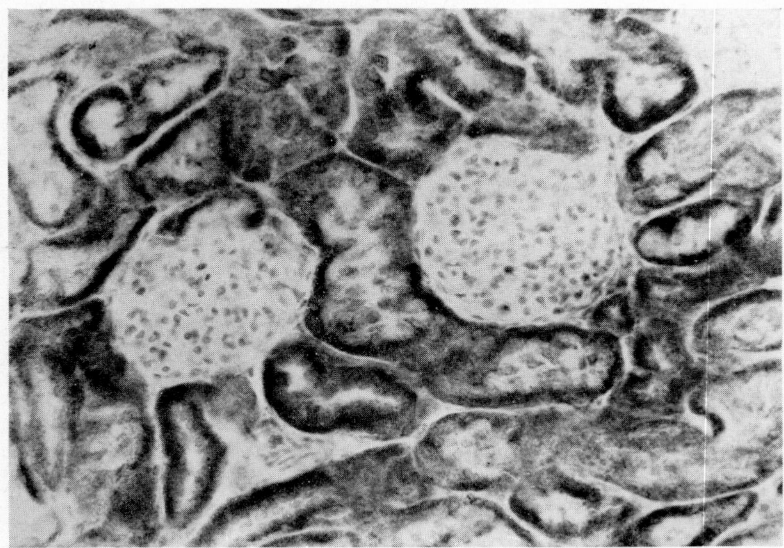

Figure 18.2 Rat kidney—distribution of succinate dehydrogenase by the MTT technique. (× *325*)

(Reduced to two-thirds in reproduction)

An unfixed frozen section is incubated in a medium containing the specific substrate, the tetrazolium salt, buffer, the co-enzyme (if required), and any activators or chelators necessary.

Types of tetrazolium salts

In the development of histochemistry many types of tetrazolium salts have been used for a number of techniques. They are most commonly used in the field of oxidase and dehydrogenase histochemistry.

They may be divided into two groups, the monotetrazolium salts and the ditetrazolium salts. A great deal of work has been devoted to tetrazolium salts to make them suitable for histochemical procedures. At the present time, salts from each of the two groups are in routine use for dehydrogenase methods.

Ditetrazolium chloride-nitro-BT (NBT) was introduced into dehydrogenase histochemistry by Nachlas, Tsou, Sousa, Cheng and Seligman (1957) for the demonstration of succinic dehydrogenase. The formazan produced with this salt is highly coloured, microcrystalline and insoluble in lipid; thus deposits of formazan may be seen in areas of lipid.

The salt of the monotetrazolium group is 3(4:5-dimethyl thiazolyl-2):5-diphenyl tetrazolium bromide (MTT). This monotetrazole was introduced by Pearse (1957). The formazan produced with this salt is immediately chelated to cobalt ions, which are present in the incubating medium. The final formazan deposit is deeply coloured and finely granular. It is soluble in fat deposits. Using this tetrazolium salt, Scarpelli, Hess and Pearse (1958) and Hess, Scarpelli and Pearse (1958) and Pearse (1972) described methods for a number of dehydrogenase enzymes.

There has been a great deal of theoretical consideration given to the choice of the tetrazolium salt in relation to reductability, substantivity, solubility, production of formazans and the size of the formazan deposits. For detailed discussions on these topics readers are referred to Pearse (1972).

HISTOCHEMICAL METHODS

Succinate dehydrogenases: MTT technique

Succinate dehydrogenase in the section releases hydrogen from the substrate (sodium succinate). The hydrogen reduces the tetrazolium salt to form a formazan which is then chelated with cobalt ions to form a coloured insoluble granular deposit (*see Figure 18.2*). For the histochemical demonstration of succinate dehydrogenase no co-enzyme is required since the enzyme itself acts as a hydrogen acceptor.

Succinate dehydrogenase: NBT technique

Succinate dehydrogenase in the section releases hydrogen from the succinate. This reduces the nitro-BT to form a water-insoluble coloured formazan. Again no co-enzyme is required.

Lactate dehydrogenase: NBT or MTT techniques

Lactate dehydrogenase in the section releases hydrogen from the lactate in the incubating medium. NAD is required as a hydrogen acceptor before the tetrazolium salt can be converted into a formazan.

Other dehydrogenase methods

Other dehydrogenase methods work on the principles outlined above. A list of the enzymes and details of the preparation of the incubating media will be found in the Methods section at the end of this chapter. Table 18.4 also shows which enzymes require the presence of a hydrogen acceptor in the form of a co-enzyme.

NAD and NADP diaphorases: MTT technique

The NAD and NADP diaphorases oxidize NADH and NADPH to NAD and NADP. The hydrogen passes to the tetrazolium salt which then chelates with the cobalt to form a formazan deposit at the site of activity.

PREPARATION OF SECTIONS AND INCUBATING METHODS FOR DEHYDROGENASE TECHNIQUES

Sections for the demonstration of dehydrogenase enzymes should be prepared from fresh unfixed material. Fixation of any sort will destroy all dehydrogenase activity except a small amount of enzyme firmly bound in the cytoplasm. Cryostat sections are recommended. The material should be frozen by one of the techniques described in Chapter 5. The sections are incubated unfixed at 37°C for 30–40 min. After incubation, the sections are transferred to formol saline to stop the reaction and to fix the section. They are then counter-stained in 2 per cent Methyl Green (chloroform-washed) or Mayer's Carmalum.

Histochemical demonstration

As briefly discussed in the text, the dehydrogenases may be demonstrated by using suitable tetrazolium salts. The two salts of choice are the monotetrazolium MTT and the ditetrazolium NBT. For convenience these tetrazolium salts can be prepared as stock solutions in suitable buffers along with chelating agents (if used) and activators. The various substrates can also be pre-prepared as stock substrate solutions. The reagents are dissolved in distilled water and neutralized. Details of these stock solutions are given in Tables 18.3 and 18.4; both types of solution keep well at —20°C. Suitable controls, particularly specific enzyme inhibitors, should be used whenever possible.

*Demonstration of dehydrogenase activity using MTT**

(1) Preparation of stock substrate solutions with pH adjusted to 7·0

TABLE 18.3

Substrate	*Chemical*	*Conc.* (M)	*Amount of substance*	*Vol. of water* (ml)	*Neutralization*	*Final vol.* (ml)
Succinate	Sodium succinate	2.5	6·75 g	8	0·05 ml N-HCl approx.	10
Malate	Sodium hydrogen malate	1	1·55 g	8	0·9 ml 40% NaOH	10
Isocitrate	DL-Isocitric acid (trisodium salt)	1	0·27 g	0·8	0·1 ml 1 N-HCl approx.	1·0
Glutamate	L-Glutamic acid (Na salt) Monohydrate	1	1·87 g	8	0·05 ml N-HCl	10
Glucose-6 phosphate	Glucose-6-phosphate (Disodium salt)	1	0·30 g	0·8	0·06 ml N-HCl	1·0
α-Glycero-phosphate	Sodium α-glycero-phosphate	1	3·15 g	8	0·7 ml N-HCl	10
Alcohol	Absolute alcohol	1	0·58 ml	8	1 drop stock tris buffer, pH 10·4	10
Lactate	Sodium DL-lactate	1	1·25 ml	8·75	—	10
β-Hydroxy butyrate	DL-β-Hydroxy butyric acid (Na salt)	1	1·27 g	8	0·15 ml N-HCl	10

(2) Preparation of buffer (*see* Page 328)

(3) Preparation of tetrazolium stock solution

MTT (1 mg per 1 ml distilled water)	2·5 ml
Tris buffer, pH 7·4	2·5 ml
0·5 M Cobalt chloride	0·5 ml
0·05 Magnesium chloride	1·0 ml
Distilled water	2·5 ml

The pH is checked and adjusted to 7·0, if necessary, using either stock tris buffer (*see* page 328) or N-hydrochloric acid. The stock solution is kept frozen and is stable for many months if stored in this manner.

(4) Preparation of incubating media for volume of 1 ml

TABLE 18.4

Enzyme to be demonstrated	*Vol. of stock tetrazolium solution* (ml)	*Vol. of substrate stock soln.* (ml)	*Vol. of distilled water* (ml)	*Co-enzyme* 2 mg	*Menaphthone*
NAD Diaphorase	0·9	Nil	0·1	NADH	Nil
NADP Diaphorase	0·9	Nil	0·1	NADPH	Nil
Succinic dehydrogenase	0·9	0·1	Nil	Nil	Nil
α-Glycerophosphate dehydrogenase	0·9	0·1	Nil	Nil	Sat. in stock soln.
Lactate dehydrogenase	0·9	0·1	Nil	NAD	Nil
Malate dehydrogenase	0·9	0·1	Nil	NAD	Nil
Glucose-6-phosphate dehydrogenase	0·9	0·1	Nil	NADP	Nil
Isocitrate dehydrogenase	0·9	0·1	Nil	NAD	Nil
β-Hydroxybutyrate dehydrogenase	0·9	0·1	Nil	NAD	Nil
Glutamic dehydrogenase	0·9	0·1	Nil	NAD	Nil
Alcohol dehydrogenase	0·9	0·1	Nil	NAD	Nil

The co-enzymes are added just before use. The pH should be checked and adjusted to 7·0–7·1 with 0·1 N-HCl or stock tris buffer.

* 3(4: 5-Dimethyl thiazolyl-2)5-diphenyl tetrazolium bromide

Note that in the methods for the diaphorases, the respective co-enzymes are the substrates for the reaction.

Demonstration of dehydrogenase activity using NBT (nitro-blue tetrazolium)

(1) Preparation of stock substrate solution (*see* Table 18.3, page 238)

(2) Preparation of stock buffer solution (*see* page 328)

(3) Preparation of stock tetrazolium solution (Pearse, 1972)

NBT 4 mg/ml	2·5 ml
0·2 M Tris or phosphate buffer (pH 7·4)	2·5 ml (*see* page 328)
0·05 M Magnesium chloride	1·0 ml
Distilled water	3·0 ml

Check pH of solution and adjust to 7·0 if necessary, using stock buffer or 0·2 M HCl. If stored at —20°C, the stock tetrazolium solution is stable for 3 months.

This stock tetrazolium solution is used with the various substrate solutions, as shown in Table 18.3, for the demonstration of most of the standard dehydrogenase enzymes. Nitro-blue tetrazolium is also used in the demonstration of more exotic dehydrogenases such as prostaglandin dehydrogenase and choline dehydrogenase.

PRACTICAL DEMONSTRATION OF DEHYDROGENASES

The methods detailed below illustrate the techniques of dehydrogenase histochemistry. The same techniques can be applied to the dehydrogenases listed in Table 18.4 by simply substituting the specific substrate solutions, with the addition or substitution of the correct co-enzyme if needed. Either MTT or NBT can be used with any of the enzymes listed in Table 18.4.

METHOD 122

Succinate dehydrogenase: (Pearse, 1972)

Reagents required

(1) 3(4:5-Dimethyl thiazolyl-2)5-diphenyl tetrazolium bromide (MTT) *or* nitro-blue tetrazolium (NBT)

(2) Tris buffer, pH 7·4

(3) Cobalt chloride (if MTT is used)

(4) Sodium succinate

(5) Formol saline

(6) Methyl Green

(7) 0·05 M Magnesium chloride

Preparation of solutions (*see* also Table 18.3)

(1) *Succinate substrate solution*

Sodium succinate	6·75 g
Distilled water	8·0 ml
N-Hydrochloric acid	0·05 ml

The sodium succinate is dissolved in the distilled water, the N-hydrochloric acid is added and the solution tested for pH. It is adjusted to 7·1, if necessary, and the total volume made up to 10 ml. The solution keeps well when frozen.

(2) Stock MTT or NBT tetrazolium solutions (*see* pages 283, 284)

(3) 10 per cent Formol saline

(4) 2 per cent Methyl Green (chloroform extracted) (*see* page 322)

Incubating medium

Stock tetrazolium solution	0·9 ml	(*see* Table 18.3)
Succinate substrate solution	0·1 ml	

Sections

Cryostat unfixed
Frozen unfixed

Suitable control sections

Kidney, liver

Incubating method

(1) Cover sections with incubating medium at 37°C, 30 min–1 h	
(2) Transfer sections to formol saline	10–15 min
(3) Wash well in tap water	2 min
(4) Counterstain in 2 per cent Methyl Green	5 min
(5) Rinse in tap water	
(6) Mount in glycerin jelly	

Result

Succinate dehydrogenase: black formazan deposit
Nuclei: green

Remarks

The preparation is stable for a limited period of time (i.e. about 3 months). To prolong the period of storage it is recommended that the sections be kept at 4°C.

Note. In the diaphorase methods which follow, the NADH and NADPH are referred to as 'co-enzymes'; it is important to realize that in this instance they are acting as the substrates.

METHOD 123

Glucose-6-phosphate dehydrogenase: (Pearse, 1972)

Reagents required

(1) 3(4:5-Dimethyl thiazolyl-2)5-diphenyl tetrazolium bromide (MTT) *or* nitro-blue tetrazolium (NBT)
(2) Tris buffer, pH 7·4
(3) Cobalt chloride (if MTT is used)
(4) Glucose-6-phosphate (disodium salt)
(5) Formol saline
(6) 2 per cent Methyl Green
(7) Nicotinamide adenine dinucleotide phosphate (NADP)
(8) 0·5 M Magnesium chloride

Preparation of solutions

(1) *Glucose-6-phosphate substrate solution* (*see* Table 18.3)

Glucose-6-phosphate (disodium salt)	304 mg
Distilled water	0·8 ml
N-Hydrochloric acid	0·06 ml

The glucose-6-phosphate is dissolved in the distilled water, the pH is adjusted with N-hydrochloric acid to 7·1. The total volume is then made up to 1 ml. The solution should be kept frozen until used.

(2) Stock MTT or NBT tetrazolium solution (*see* page 283)
(3) 10 per cent Formol saline
(4) 2 per cent Methyl Green (chloroform-extracted) (*see* page 322)

Preparation of incubating medium

Stock tetrazolium solution	0·9 ml
Glucose-6-phosphate substrate solution	0·1 ml
Co-enzyme NADP	2 mg

The NADP is added to the 1 ml of the medium. The pH is checked and adjusted, if necessary, with N-HCl or Tris buffer to pH 7·1.

Sections

Cryostat unfixed
Frozen unfixed

Suitable control sections

Kidney, liver

Incubating method

(1)	Cover sections with incubating medium at 37°C	30 min–1h
(2)	Place sections in 10 per cent formol saline	10–15 min
(3)	Wash well in tap water	2 min
(4)	Counterstain in 2 per cent Methyl Green	5 min
(5)	Wash in tap water	
(6)	Mount in glycerin jelly	

Result

Glucose-6-phosphate dehydrogenase: black formazan deposit with MTT Nuclei: green

METHOD 124

NADH diaphorase: MTT method (Pearse, 1972)

Reagents required

(1) 3(4:5-Dimethyl thiazolyl-2)5-diphenyl tetrazolium bromide (MTT)
(2) Tris buffer, pH 7·4
(3) Cobalt chloride
(4) NADH
(5) Formol saline
(6) Methyl Green
(7) Distilled water
(8) 0·05 Magnesium chloride

Preparation of solutions

(1) Stock MTT tetrazolium solution (*see* page 283)
(2) Co-enzyme NADH
(3) 10 per cent Formol saline
(4) 2 per cent Methyl Green (chloroform extracted)
See page 322

Preparation of incubating medium

Stock tetrazolium (MTT) solution	0·9 ml
Distilled water	0·1 ml
Co-enzyme: NADH	2·0 mg

The co-enzyme is added to the 1 ml of the medium. The pH is checked and adjusted if necessary with N-HCl or stock buffer (*see* page 328) to pH 7·1.

Sections

Cryostat unfixed
Frozen unfixed

Suitable control sections

Kidney, liver

Incubating method

(1)	Cover section with incubating medium at 37°C	30–40 min
(2)	Place sections in 10 per cent formol saline	15 min
(3)	Wash well in tap water	5 min
(4)	Counterstain in 2 per cent Methyl Green	5 min
(5)	Wash in tap water	
(6)	Mount in glycerin jelly	

Results

NADH diaphorase: black formazan deposit
Nuclei: green

METHOD 125

NADPH diaphorase using NBT (Pearse, 1972)

Reagents required

(1) Nitro-blue tetrazolium (NBT)
(2) Tris or phosphate buffer pH 7·4
(3) 0·05 M Magnesium chloride
(4) NADPH
(5) 0·1 N Hydrochloric acid
(6) Distilled water

Preparation of solutions

(1) Stock NBT tetrazolium solution (*see* page 284)
(2) Co-enzyme NADPH 2 mg
(3) 10 per cent formol saline

Preparation of incubating medium

Stock tetrazolium solution	0·9 ml
Distilled water	0·1 ml
NADPH	2·0 mg

The co-enzyme is added just before use, check pH and adjust to 7·1 if necessary, with N-HCl or stock buffer as necessary.

Sections

Cryostat unfixed

Suitable control sections

Kidney, liver

Incubating method

(1) Cover section with incubating medium, place at 37°C for 30–60 min
(2) Place sections in 10 per cent formol saline 10–15 min
(3) Rinse well in distilled water
(4) Dehydrate through graded alcohols to xylene
(5) Mount in synthetic resin, i.e. DPX

Results

Enzyme activity: purple formazan deposit.

REFERENCES

HESS, R., SCARPELLI, D. G. and PEARSE, A. G. E. (1958). *Nature, Lond.* **181,** 1531

NACHLAS, M. M., TSOU, K. C., SOUSA, E., CHENG, C. S. and SELIGMAN, A. M. (1957). *J. Histochem. Cytochem.* **5,** 420

PEARSE, A. G. E. (1957). *ibid.* **5,** 515

— (1972). *Histochemistry, Theoretical and Applied,* Vol. 2. London: Churchill Livingstone

SCARPELLI, D. G., HESS, R. and PEARSE, A. G. E. (1958). *J. Biophys. biochem. Cytol.* **4,** 747

19

Miscellaneous Techniques

In this chapter a number of techniques are described. The methods discussed are usually from a group of enzymes whose demonstration as an entity are outside the scope of this book, but single methods such as Leucine Aminopeptidase from the peptidases and Phosphorylase from the glycosyltransferases are amongst the most common of enzyme techniques applied to sections. Microincineration is also briefly considered, mainly in regard to its application to pigments and minerals. The enzyme methods described at the end of the chapter are (1) Leucine Aminopeptidase; (2) Sulphatase; (3) Phosphorylase; (4) β-Glucuronidase.

Leucine aminopeptidase (LAP)

This enzyme is frequently found in animal tissues. It is able to act on peptides and will also hydrolyze free amino groups. LAP can be inhibited with potassium cyanide or ethylene diamine tetra-acetic acid (EDTA) when used in 10 mM solutions (Burstone and Folk, 1956). In their paper, these authors also recommended freeze drying with double embedding as the processing method of choice. Good results may be obtained with this technique or by using cryostat sections. Nachlas, Crawford and Seligman, (1957) reported that, if cryostat sections were dried at 37°C for 30 min before use, less diffusion of the enzyme was observed (*see Figure 19.1*)

There are two types of methods available for the demonstration of this enzyme. They are: (1) the Metal Chelation Diazo-Coupling method (Nachlas, Crawford and Seligman, 1957; Method 126); and (2) the Diazo-Coupling method (Burstone and Folk, 1956).

Sulphatase

This hydrolytic enzyme, so termed because it hydrolyzes sulphuric esters, is not easy to demonstrate in human material. Sulphatases may be divided into five groups (Pearse, 1972): (1) arylsulphatase;

(2) sterol sulphatase; (3) glucosulphatase; (4) chondrosulphatase; and (5) myrosulphatase.

Arylsulphatase is the only one which may be demonstrated by histochemical means. Glucosulphatase and chondrosulphatase are not found in higher animals (Fromageot 1950). Arylsulphatase is divided biochemically into three different enzymes which are termed A, B and C (Roy, 1953, 1954; Dodgson, Spencer and Wynn, 1956). These different sulphatases cannot be separated histochemically. Two types of method are available for the demonstration of arylsulphatase: the Post-Coupling method of Ruttenberg, Cohen and Seligman (1952) or the substituted naphthol method, using naphthol AS sulphate and pararosanilin hydrochloride (Methods 127 and 128, respectively).

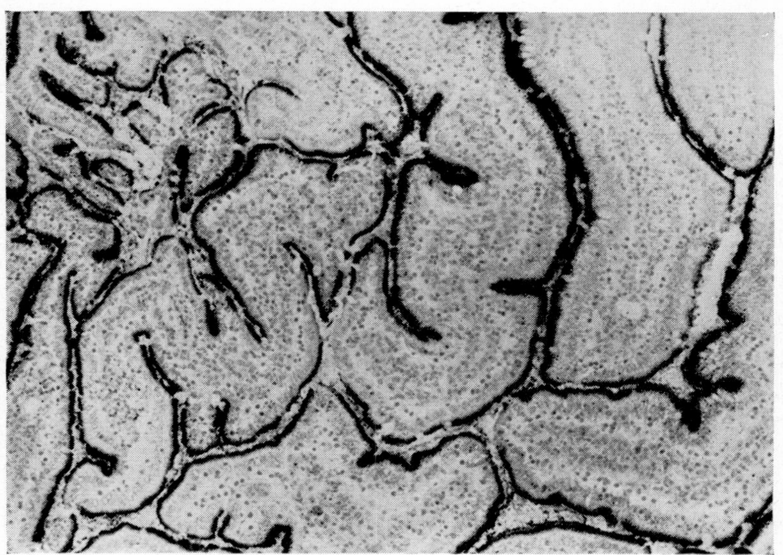

Figure 19.1 Rat intestine. Leucine aminopeptidase method. (× *150*)
(Reduced to six-tenths in reproduction)

Phosphorylase

This enzyme is involved in glycogen synthesis and can be demonstrated by a number of techniques. Fresh frozen sections must be used and these transferred directly into the incubating medium. The first satisfactory method was published by Takeuchi and Kuriaki (1955). Method 129 is a modification of the Takeuchi and Kuriaki method by Eränkö and Palkama (1961). Lake (1970) introduced a technique that omitted the use of insulin; this method gives excellent results on human muscle biopsies but as Lake states the method is not so reliable when applied to rat tissue. Lake (1974) produced a further modification in which glycogen and alcohol were not included. Amylase was substituted for the glycogen as the acceptor molecule. This method produces a strong reddish brown colouration and works very well on human liver biopsies, but is no better than his 1970 method when applied to human muscle biopsies (*see Figure 19.2*). Both the phosphorylase techniques are reproduceable, although a little practice is required to obtain consistently good results.

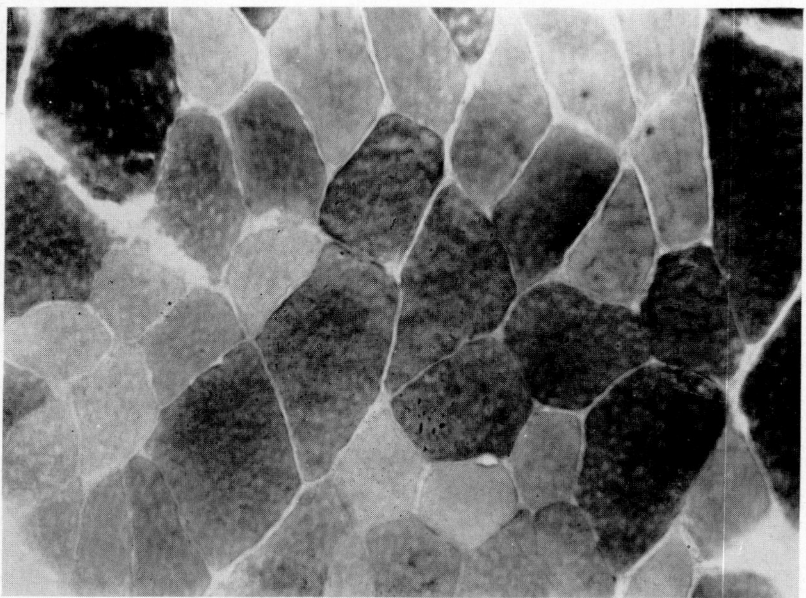

Figure 19.2 Rat striated muscle—differentiation of fibre types by Phosphorylase method. (× *80*)

β-Glucuronidase

This enzyme, which is widespread in mammalian tissues, hydrolyzes the esters of glucuronic acid. The enzyme is most commonly found in spleen, liver and kidney. The precise role it plays is not yet fully understood.

Methods for the demonstration of this enzyme have caused a great deal of controversy in recent years, in regard to localization of the enzyme, and even to whether the enzyme is actually being demonstrated at all. Three techniques are employed at present: (1) Azo Dye method (Seligman *et al.*, 1954); (2) Ferric Hydroquinoline method (Fishman and Baker, 1956); (3) Naphthol AS method (Pugh and Walker, 1961; Hayashi, Nakajima and Fishman, 1964).

The recommended method is the Naphthol AS technique first developed by Pugh and Walker (1961). They used a substituted naphthol, naphthol AS-LC glucuronide which they prepared themselves. Following this paper came one by Hayashi, Nakajima and Fishman, (1964), who used naphthol AS-BI glucuronide (*see Figure 19.3*). The localization of the enzyme using these substituted naphthols is far superior than with the first two methods.

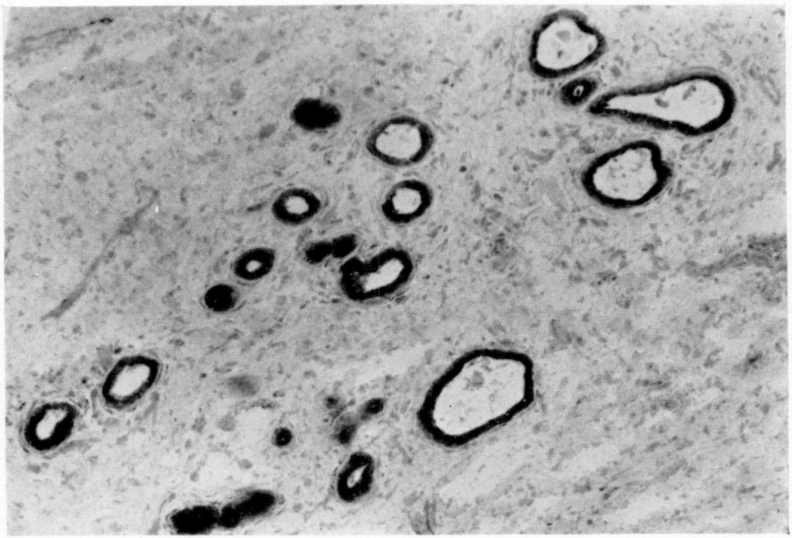

Figure 19.3 Human breast—distribution of β-glucuronidase in breast duct epithelium shown by simultaneous coupling method. (× *126*)

(Reduced to two-thirds in reproduction)

Microincineration

This technique is useful for confirming the presence of a number of substances. After incineration, iron appears a yellowish red colour and silicates can be seen by their crystalline structure when viewed with a polarizing microscope. Magnesium and calcium form a white ash.

HISTOCHEMICAL METHODS

Incubating method for leucine aminopeptidase

Incubation is normally carried out at 37°C for times varying between 15 minutes and two hours, depending upon the tissue. It is preferable to use sections about 5 microns thick. The reaction takes place when leucine aminopeptidase in the section splits β-naphthylamine from the substrate, L-leucyl-4-methoxy-β-naphthylamine. The β-naphthylamine then combines with the diazonium salt Fast Blue B to produce an insoluble azo dye. After rinsing in saline, the sections are treated with dilute copper sulphate. The copper ions chelate with the azo dye. The final result is a purplish red deposit at the site of enzyme activity. Small intestine, large intestine and kidney make excellent controls.

Post-Coupling method for arylsulphatase

This technique, which employs 6-benzoyl-2-naphthyl sulphate as the substrate, was introduced by Ruttenberg, Cohen and Seligman (1952) after earlier work by Seligman *et al.* (1949). The specificity of this method is open to doubt as with any sulphatase method.

The sulphatase enzyme in the section splits 6-benzoyl-2-naphthyl from the substrate. This is then coupled with Fast Blue B salt to form an insoluble azo dye which may be red (monocoupling) or blue (dicoupling), or a mixture of both. The red coupling, according to Pearse (1960), is lipid soluble and hence the localization is open to doubt. Incubation is normally carried out at pH 5·0 at 37°C for 2–16 h before coupling with Fast Blue B. The method gives best results when applied to pre-fixed frozen sections.

Simultaneous Coupling for sulphatase

The technique given was described by Woohsmann and Hartrodt (1965), and later modified by Wachtler and Pearse (1966). The substrate used is naphthol AS sulphate, prepared as described by Woohsmann and Hartrodt (1965). Sulphatase activity in the section splits the substrate to produce α-naphthol. The released naphthol then combines with hexazonium pararosanilin to form an insoluble azo dye. The localization obtained by this method is far superior to that of the previous technique. Best results are obtained using pre-fixed cryostat sections with incubation at 37°C for 30 min to 2 h.

Iodine method for phosphorylase

The substrate used is glucose-1-phosphate. This is converted into a polysaccharide by the action of the phosphorylase. It is necessary to add water-soluble glycogen to the medium in order to initiate the reaction. The polysaccharide is then treated with iodine to form a dark brown reaction product. Adenosine-5-phosphate and insulin may be included in the medium as activators for the enzyme.

Simultaneous Coupling method for β-glucuronidase

The first naphthol compound used as a substrate for the method was synthesized by Pugh and Walker (1961). The substrate they employed, naphthol AS-LC glucuronide, was never produced commercially. However, Hayashi, Nakajima and Fishman (1964) synthesized naphthol AS-BI glucuronide from acetobromoethyl glucuronate and the potassium salt of naphthol AS-BI. The chemical reaction is basically similar to that of other methods using substituted naphthols. The β-glucuronidase in the section splits the substrate, releasing naphthol AS-BI. The diazonium salt in the incubating medium combines with the naphthol to give an insoluble azo dye at the site of enzyme activity. Hexazonium pararosanilin is recommended as the coupling agent. Hayashi, Nakajima and Fishman found that 0·3 ml per 10 ml of incubating solution gave the most satisfactory result.

The method gives the best result when employed on cryostat sections of pre-fixed material, i.e. formol calcium at 4°C, followed by gum sucrose before sectioning (*see* Method 99). Incubation is carried out at 37°C for 20 min to 3 h, depending upon the tissue and species. The final pH of the incubating medium should be between 4·6 and 5·5. Hayashi, Nakajima and Fishman recommended pH 5·2.

Preparation of tissue for microincineration

Microincineration is used for the demonstration of minerals. Freeze drying is the preparative method of choice, in order to cause little alteration of the mineral site or content. If it is not possible to use freeze dried material, tissue should be fixed in 10 per cent buffered formol saline, or in alcohol, to prevent loss of water-soluble substances. Two sections must always be used, one stained in the normal way to act as a control.

Sections for the microincineration technique are placed in a muffle furnace and heated to temperatures up to 650°C. At temperatures between 400°C and 650°C, inorganic tissue components are turned to ash. After incineration, the slide is cooled to room temperature, a coverslip is gently placed over the section and it is then viewed under the microscope. For details of the microincineration techniques, *see* Method 132.

METHOD 126

Leucine aminopeptidase: (Nachlas, Crawford and Seligman 1957)

Reagents required

(1) L-Leucyl-4-methoxy β-naphthylamide
(2) Ethyl alcohol
(3) Distilled water
(4) 0·1 M Acetate buffer
(5) Potassium cyanide
(6) Copper sulphate
(7) Sodium chloride
(8) Fast Blue B salt

Preparation of solutions

(1) *Substrate solution*

L-Leucyl-4-methoxy β-naphthylamide	4 mg
Ethyl alcohol	0·1 ml
Distilled water	4·9 ml

Owing to the low solubility of the substrate in water, it should first be dissolved in alcohol.

(2) *Sodium chloride 0·85 per cent*

Sodium chloride	425 mg
Distilled water	50 ml

(3) *Copper sulphate 0·1 M*

Copper sulphate	798 mg
Distilled water	50 ml

(4) *Potassium cyanide*

Potassium cyanide	65 mg
Distilled water	50 ml

(5) *0·1* M *Acetate buffer, pH 6·5. See* page 327

Incubating medium

Substrate solution	0·5 ml
0·1 M Acetate buffer, pH 6·5	5 ml
0·85 per cent Sodium chloride	4 ml
Potassium cyanide	0·5 ml
Fast Blue B salt	5 mg

Sections

Cryostat pre-fixed
Cryostat post-fixed
Freeze dried sections

Suitable control sections

Large intestine, small intestine, and kidney

Incubating method

(1)	Place sections in incubating medium	15 min–2h
(2)	Rinse in saline, solution (2)	2 min
(3)	Immerse in copper sulphate, solution (3)	2 min
(4)	Rinse sections in saline	2 min
(5)	Dehydrate through graded alcohols to xylene	
(6)	Mount in DPX	

Results

LAP activity: red

Remarks

Sections may be counterstained in 2 per cent Methyl Green if required.

L-Leucyl-β-naphthylamide may be employed as the substrate, but with results inferior to those obtained with the substrate in the above technique.

METHOD 127

Arylsulphatase: Post-Coupling method (Ruttenberg, Cohen and Seligman, 1952)

Reagents required

(1) 6-Benzoyl-2-naphthyl sulphate
(2) Sodium chloride
(3) 0·5 M Acetate buffer, pH 6·1
(4) 0·05 M Phosphate buffer, pH 7·6
(5) Fast Blue B salt
(6) Distilled water

Preparation of solutions

(1) *0·85 per cent Sodium chloride*

Sodium chloride	850 mg
Distilled water	100 ml

(2) *1 per cent Sodium chloride*

Sodium chloride	1 g
Distilled water	100 ml

(3) *2 per cent Sodium chloride*

Sodium chloride	2 g
Distilled water	100 ml

(4) *Buffer*

0·1 M Acetate buffer, *see* page 326

(5) *Substrate solution*

6-Benzoyl-2-naphthyl sulphate	25 mg
0·85 per cent hot sodium chloride, solution (1)	80 ml
Acetate buffer, pH 6·1, solution (4)	20 ml
Sodium chloride	2·6 g

If fixed frozen sections are used, the 2·6 g of sodium chloride may be omitted.

(6) *Solution Fast Blue B*

Fast Blue B	50 mg
0·05 M Phosphate buffer, pH 7·6	50 ml

Sections

Human material must be fresh frozen sections. Rat and mouse may be 10 per cent neutral formalin-fixed, then frozen sections.

Suitable control sections

Kidney, liver of rat

Incubating method

(1) Place all sections in 0·85 per cent sodium chloride, solution (1) — 1 min
(2) Transfer sections to 1 per cent sodium chloride, solution (2) — 1 min
(3) Transfer sections to 2 per cent sodium chloride, solution (3) — 1 min
(4) Place sections in substrate solution, solution (5) — 2–20 h
(5) Transfer sections to 2 per cent sodium chloride, solution (3) — 1 min
(6) Transfer sections to 1 per cent sodium chloride, solution (2) — 1 min
(7) Transfer sections to 0·85 per cent sodium chloride, solution (1) — 1 min

(Last three steps (5, 6, 7), for unfixed frozen sections *only* at 4°C)

(8) Wash fixed section only in distilled water at 4°C — 1 min
(9) Transfer sections to Fast Blue B, solution (6), 4°C — 5 min
(10) Wash sections in 0·85 per cent sodium chloride at 4°C — 5 min
(11) Mount in glycerin jelly

Results

Arylsulphatase: red to blue

Remarks

The sections should be examined immediately. They are stable for about 10 days if stored at 4°C.

METHOD 128

Arylsulphatase: Naphthol AS Sulphate method (Woohsmann and Hartrodt, 1965) modified (Wächtler and Pearse, 1966)

Reagents required

(1) Naphthol AS sulphate (potassium salt)
(2) Sodium chloride
(3) 0·2 M Acetate buffer stock 'A' solution
(4) Sodium nitrite
(5) Pararosanilin hydrochloride

Preparation of solutions

(1) *Buffer stock solution*
0·2 M Acetate buffer stock 'A' solution (page 326)

(2) *Sodium chloride (0·85 per cent)*

Sodium chloride	850 mg
Distilled water	100 ml

(3) *Naphthol AS sulphate*

Naphthol AS sulphate (potassium salt)	20 mg
Sodium chloride, solution (2)	8 ml
Acetate buffer, solution (1)	2 ml

(4) *Hexazonium pararosanilin*

Pararosanilin hydrochloride	0·3 ml	(*see page* 248)
Fresh 4 per cent sodium nitrite	0·3 ml	

Preparation of incubating solution

Solution (3)	10 ml
Sodium chloride	260 mg
Solution (4)	0·6 ml

The final pH of this solution should be adjusted to between 6 and 7 and the solution filtered before use.

Sections

Pre-fixed cryostat sections

Control sections

This technique has not been found to give a positive result with mammalian tissues, but the intestine of the marine snail and of the Amphioxus give strong results.

Incubating method

(1) Place sections into incubating medium at 37°C ½ to 2 h
(2) Wash well in distilled water
(3) Counterstain in 2 per cent Methyl Green if required
(4) Wash in running tap water for 30 s
(5) Dehydrate through graded alcohols to xylene
(6) Mount in DPX

Result

Arylsulphatase: red
Nuclei: green

METHOD 129

Phosphorylase: Iodine method (Takeuchi and Kuriaki, 1955; modified Eränkö and Palkama, 1961)

Reagents required

(1) Glucose-1-phosphate
(2) Adenosine-5-phosphate
(3) Glycogen
(4) Sodium fluoride
(5) Polyvinyl pyrrolidone
(6) Insulin 40 I.U.
(7) Ethyl alcohol
(8) 0·1 M Acetate buffer, pH 5·9
(9) Sucrose
(10) Gram's iodine
(11) Glycerol

Preparation of solutions

(1) *0·32* M *Sucrose*

Sucrose	11 g
Distilled water	100 ml

(2) *Gram's iodine sucrose*

Iodine	330 mg
Potassium iodide	660 mg
Sucrose	11 g
Distilled water	100 ml

(3) *40 per cent Alcohol*

Ethyl alcohol	40 ml
Distilled water	60 ml

(4) *Acetate buffer,* pH *5·9*
See page 326

(5) *Incubating solution*

Glucose-1-phosphate	100 mg
Adenosine-5-phosphate	10 mg
Glycogen	7 mg
Sodium fluoride	180 mg
Polyvinyl pyrrolidone	900 mg
Insulin 40 I.U.	1 drop
Absolute alcohol	2 ml
Acetate buffer, pH 5·9	10 ml

Sections

Unfixed cryostat sections

Suitable control tissues

Muscle and liver

Incubating method

(1) Place sections immediately they are cut into the incubating medium, at 37°C	15 min—3 h
(2) Allow sections to dry	
(3) Transfer sections to 40 per cent alcohol, solution (3)	2 min
(4) Allow sections to dry	
(5) Transfer sections to sucrose solution, solution (1)	5 min
(6) Place sections in iodine-sucrose, solution (2)	5 min
(7) Mount sections in glycerol–iodine mixture 4:1	

Remarks

In the author's experience the method works best when the fresh sections are placed *immediately* into the incubating medium without drying.

METHOD 130

Phosphorylase (Lake, 1970)

Reagents required

(1) Magnesium chloride
(2) Glucose-1-phosphate (dipotassium salt)
(3) Glycogen
(4) Adenosine-5-triphosphate
(5) Sodium fluoride
(6) Ethyl alcohol
(7) Polyvinyl-pyrrolidone
(8) Acetate buffer
(9) Lugol's iodine
(10) Glycerol

Preparation of incubating solution

0·1 M Acetate buffer, pH 5·9	10 ml	(*see* page 326)
0·1 M Magnesium chloride	1 ml	
Glucose-1-phosphate (dipotassium salt)	100 mg	
Glycogen (rabbit or oyster)	2 mg	
Adenosine-5-triphosphate	5 mg	
Sodium fluoride	180 mg	
Ethyl alcohol	2 ml	
Polyvinyl pyrrolidone	900 mg	

Add the reagents in the order listed and use unfiltered. It is convenient to prepare the above solutions and freeze at —20°C until required.

Sections

Unfixed cryostat sections

Suitable control sections

Muscle, liver

Incubating method

(1) Place fresh unfixed cryostat sections in incubating medium for 1 h at 37°C
(2) Rinse in 40 per cent alcohol 5 s
(3) Air dry rapidly
(4) Fix sections in absolute alcohol 3 min
(5) Air dry
(6) Place in Lugol's iodine 1 part, distilled water 30 parts 5 min
(7) Mount in Lugol's iodine 1 part, glycerol 9 parts

Results

Phosphorylase activi y: bluish black

Remarks

Fading takes place fairly rapidly, colouration can be brought back by repeating stages 6 and 7.

METHOD 131

β-Glucuronidase: Naphthol AS-BI method (Hayashi, Nakajima and Fishman, 1964)

Reagents required

(1) Naphthol AS-BI glucuronide

(2) Acetate buffer, pH 5.0
(3) Sodium bicarbonate
(4) Sodium nitrite
(5) Hexazonium pararosanilin
(6) Distilled water
(7) 1 N sodium hydroxide

Preparation of solutions

(1) *Sodium bicarbonate*

Sodium bicarbonate	210 mg
Distilled water	50 ml

(2) *Substrate solution*

Naphthol AS-BI glucuronide	14 mg
Solution (1), sodium bicarbonate	0.6 ml
0·1 M Acetate buffer, pH 5.0	50 ml

(3) *Hexazonium pararosanilin solution*
See Method 106, page 248

Pararosanilin hydrochloride	0.3 ml
*4 per cent Sodium nitrite	0.3 ml

(4) *Incubating solution*

Substrate solution, solution (2)	5 ml
Hexazonium pararosanilin, solution (3)	0.3 ml
Distilled water	5 ml

The pararosanilin is added just before use, and the pH of the solution adjusted with 1N NaOH to 5·2.

Sections

Pre-fixed cryostat sections (*see* Method 5)

Suitable control sections

Liver and kidney

Incubating method

(1) Place sections in incubating medium at 37°C	20–40 min
(2) Wash well in distilled water	2 min
(3) Counterstain in 2 per cent Methyl Green (chloroform-washed)	4 min
(4) Wash rapidly in tap water	
(5) Dehydrate through graded alcohols to xylene	
(6) Mount in DPX	

* This solution must be freshly prepared.

Results

Glucuronidase activity: red
Nuclei: green

Remarks

(1) The pH of the incubating solution should be between 5·0 and 5·3
(2) The sodium nitrite should be freshly prepared
(3) The localization obtained with this technique is good

METHOD 132

Minerals: Microincineration

Equipment required

Muffle furnace or a thermostatically controlled heater up to 700°C

Preparation of tissue

(1) Freeze dried if possible (*see* Chapter 6 for techniques)
(2) 10 per cent Buffered formalin-fixed, paraffin-embedded sections
(3) Absolute alcohol-fixed, paraffin-embedded material

Technique

(1) Process material by one of the above methods
(2) Cut paraffin sections 3–5 microns thick, attach well to slides
(3) Place test section in furnace at 70°C for 10 min
(4) Increase heat gradually (50°C at time) till 650°C is reached
(5) Leave temperature at 650°C for 20 min
(6) Switch off current and allow temperature to drop
(7) Mount with coverslip containing drop of glycerin, or mount dry
(8) Examine by microscopy—dark field illumination, ultraviolet, polarized light, etc.

REFERENCES

BURSTONE, M. S. and FOLK, J. E. (1956). *J. Histochem. Cytochem.* **4,** 217
DODGSON, K. S., SPENCER, B. and WYNN, C. H. (1956). *Biochem. J.* **62,** 500
ERÄNKÖ, O. and PALKAMA, A. (1961). *J. Histochem. Cytochem.* **9,** 585
FISHMAN, W. H. and BAKER, J. R. (1956). *ibid.,* **4,** 570

REFERENCES

FROMAGEOT, C. (1950). *The Enzymes, Chemistry and Mechanism of Action*, Vol. 1, Part 1, New York: Academic Press

HAYASHI, M., NAKAJIMA, J. and FISHMAN, W. H. (1964). *J. Histochem. Cytochem.* **12,** 293

LAKE, B. D. (1970). *Histochemical. J.* **2,** 441

— (1974). *Proc. Ro. Microsc. Soc.* **9** part **2,** 113

NACHLAS, M. M., CRAWFORD, D. T., and SELIGMAN, A. M. (1957). *ibid.* **5,** 264

PEARSE, A. G. E. (1972). *Histochemistry, Theoretical and Applied*, Vol. 2, London: Churchill Livingstone

PUGH, D. and WALKER, P. G. (1961). *J. Histochem. Cytochem.* **9,** 105

ROY, A. B. (1953). *Biochem. J.* **53,** 12

— (1954). *ibid.* **57,** 465

RUTTENBERG, A. M., COHEN, R. B. and SELIGMAN, A. M. (1952). *Science, N.Y.* **116,** 539

SELIGMAN, A. M., NACHLAS, M. M., MANHEIMER, L. H., FRIEDMAN, O. M. and WOLF, G. (1949). *Ann. Surg.* **130,** 333

— TSOU, N. L., RUTTENBERG. S. H. and COHEN, R. B. (1954). *J. Histochem. Cytochem.* **2,** 209

TAKEUCHI, T. and KURIAKI, H. (1955). *ibid.* **3,** 153

WACHTLER, K., and PEARSE, A. G. E. (1966). *Z. Zellforsch. mikrosk. Anat.* **69,** 326

WOOHSMAN, H. and HARTRODT, W. (1965). *Histochemie* **4,** 366

20

Ultra-histochemistry

One of the most rapidly expanding fields in histochemistry is ultra-histochemistry. This is the application of histochemical methods for the demonstration of enzymes and other substances to electron microscopy. This enables an accurate localization of these substances within cytoplasmic organelles. The problems which face the histochemist and electron microscopist are manifold.

In histochemical techniques using light microscopy, the aim is to produce a visible coloured end product, well localized to the site of the substance being demonstrated, therefore preferably insoluble. In ultra-histochemistry the aim must be to produce a well localized end product which is detectable by electron microscopy; therefore the most important property of the reaction product is that it must be electron-dense. It is fortunate that some of the methods used in light microscopy histochemistry result in the formation of a reaction product which, in addition to being coloured and insoluble, is also adequately electron-dense. Such methods have required very little modification before being applicable to electron microscopy. Nevertheless, there are considerable limitations to most techniques because of the fundamental differences in the preparation of tissue for histochemistry and for electron microscopy. One of the major problems is that of fixation.

FIXATION

Most of the fixatives which are used in electron microscopy will remove or damage the chemical substance which is to be demonstrated by histochemical means. Osmium tetroxide, which is used in electron microscopy both as a fixative and as a 'stain', will destroy enzyme activity. Conversely, the fixatives which are used in histochemistry because they cause so little chemical damage, rarely permit adequate ultrastructural preservation. The result is that although the substance can be satisfactorily demonstrated, the localization and ultrastructural preservation is so poor that the technique is often worthless. Formol calcium, which is one of the most satisfactory fixatives for enzyme histochemistry, fails to preserve the ultrastructural integrity of the tissue. The ideal fixative for ultrastructural histochemistry should:

(a) preserve and localize the substance to be demonstrated;
(b) preserve the ultrastructure of the tissue;
(c) protect the reaction product from dehydration, embedding, and the effects of the vacuum and the electron beam.

Unfortunately no such ideal fixative exists, and a compromise combination of two fixatives has to be used in succession. The aldehyde fixatives, glutaraldehyde and fresh paraformaldehyde, do not totally destroy enzymes and can be used as the first fixative. After this first fixation the histochemical technique can be performed, and the tissue post-fixed in osmium tetroxide prior to resin-embedding and thin sectioning. This treatment with osmium tetroxide is also an integral part of some of the methods, rendering the reaction product more electron-dense. For the first fixative paraformaldehyde is preferable to glutaraldehyde since it causes marginally less enzyme loss; the greatest saving of enzyme activity occurs in the acid phosphatase methods.

SECTIONS FOR ELECTRON CYTOCHEMISTRY

For conventional electron microscopy, thin sections are required to obtain maximum information from the tissue. Sections produced for light microscopy are unusable from two points of view; firstly they are too thick, but more importantly they would be damaged in the electron beam. To resolve these problems tissues for electron microscopy are embedded in resins. These allow ultrathin sections to be cut and the resin protects the tissue in the electron beam.

In electron microscopy, as in paraffin-embedding, fixation is an important stage as the quality of the final picture depends very much upon the choice of fixative, the rapid transfer of fresh tissue into fixative, and the size of the tissue block. A suitable size of tissue block for electron microscopy is $1 mm^3$ or smaller. In morphological electron microscopy the fixatives of choice are aldehyde fixatives, usually glutaraldehyde or formaldehyde, and then osmium tetroxide. Both the aldehydes and osmium tetroxide act as crosslinking agents by forming chemical bonds with cell substance. The aldehydes are more effective as crosslinking agents for proteins, and osmium preserves phospholipids well; phospholipids are not well fixed by glutaraldehyde. Cell cytoplasm appears to be better preserved by glutaraldehyde. To utilize the advantages of both fixatives, they are normally used in sequence—primary fixation taking place in glutaraldehyde for 4 hours, followed by secondary fixation in osmium tetroxide for 1 hour. Both fixatives are used in buffer solutions at a pH of 7·2–7·4 and at 4°C. Following suitable fixation the small blocks of tissue are dehydrated and embedded in the resin of choice, which may be methacrylates, the epoxy resins or the polyester resins. The epoxy resin, Epon, is frequently used for electron cytochemistry. The embedding of the tissue in the resins allows the production of ultrathin sections of 500–600 Å thick. These are cut on an ultramicrotome with a glass or diamond knife. For the morphological electron microscopist this thickness is ideal for it gives a high resolution with a correctly adjusted microscope and a well contrasted section.

In electron cytochemistry the standard techniques, briefly outlined above, have to be altered to allow for the demonstration of the cytochemical substance. Sections in which enzymes or other chemical substances are to be demonstrated must be treated in a considerably different manner.

Fixation, which is so important for morphological structure, can destroy the enzymes, as will the standard processing techniques. Also the freezing techniques required for some methods may considerably damage the morphological picture.

The thin sections produced from the resin-embedded material are unsuitable for the application of ultra-histochemistry, for if the chemical substances have withstood the fixation and processing, the reagents are unable to penetrate the resin surrounding the tissue. To overcome this, histochemical methods can be employed on:—

(1) frozen sections
(2) very small blocks of tissue, fixed or unfixed
(3) tissue sections produced on a tissue chopper or vibratome,

before the tissue section or block is embedded in resin. These techniques, whilst allowing for the histochemical demonstration of chemical substances, may greatly reduce the accuracy of preservation of ultrastructural detail.

Frozen sections

The tissue is frozen rapidly and sectioned in the cryostat at 40 μm. The histochemical method is then applied to the section, before fixing and processing into resin. 500 Å resin-embedded sections of the cryostat sections are then cut. These unfixed cryostat sections are technically very difficult to handle and some diffusion of enzyme and reaction product does occur. To minimise these two problems the block of tissue can be fixed in formol calcium before freezing. This also has two drawbacks; the damage caused by freezing of fixed tissue is greater than that of unfixed tissue, and also the initial fixation reduces the amount of enzyme activity. The fresh tissue block, 4 mm^3, is fixed in buffered aldehyde fixative, either glutaraldehyde or paraformaldehyde. After washing in buffer, thick sections, 35–40-micron sections, are cut after suitable freezing. The thick section is then incubated in the histochemical medium and subsequently post-fixed in osmium tetroxide. Finally the sections are dehydrated and embedded.

Small tissue blocks

Small blocks approximately 1 mm^3 are cut from the fresh tissue and are incubated in the histochemical incubating medium before being processed to resin for thin sectioning. The main problem with this technique is the generally poor penetration of the incubating medium into what is a comparatively thick piece of tissue.

Sections produced on tissue chopper or vibratome

Using this technique sections only 40 μm thick can be cut from fresh tissue. The vibratome is a device which uses a rapidly vibrating razor blade to produce these tissue sections. The sections are then incubated in the histochemical medium, before resin embedding and ultramicrotomy. This is a useful method since there is none of the architectural artefact which can be a problem with frozen sections, and there are few problems resulting from poor penetration of the histochemical incubating medium.

A number of centres are working on techniques of cryo-ultramicrotomy, that is, the production of ultrathin sections from frozen tissue blocks. The technical problems of cutting ultrathin sections at —180°C, and picking the sections up on grids without damage, are immense. If these problems can be solved, and histochemical methods can be successfully applied to the ultrathin sections then this will be a considerable advance in electron cytochemistry technique.

ENZYME DEMONSTRATION

If an enzyme acts upon a specific substrate and produces an electron-dense reaction product, or a product which can subsequently be made electron-dense, it can be seen with the electron microscope. Electron histochemistry has developed mainly from the standard methods of histochemistry. In addition to the problems discussed in relation to fixation, consideration must be given to the problems involved in producing suitable sections for the histochemical reaction to be carried out. Fixation, whilst easing the technical problems, reduces the amount of enzyme activity, and depending upon the fixative used, can produce only moderate morphological preservation.

The classical *metal precipitation techniques* of Gomori for the demonstration of phosphatases have been the starting point for many of the cytochemical methods developed for the electron microscope. The resultant reaction products with both the acid and the alkaline phosphatases are insoluble and highly electron-dense. There are a number of problems associated with these methods at the electron microscope level, including diffusion of the primary reaction product. Also, lead is always liable to be adsorbed non-specifically on free tissues surfaces, giving false positive results. Even with adequate control sections this problem cannot always be resolved.

The *osmiophilic polymer generation principle* (Hanker, Anderson and Bloom, 1971) is becoming increasingly used in electron cytochemistry. Hanker and his colleagues (1971) suggested that metal ions produced as the result of a cytochemical reaction should be used as a catalyst to produce an osmiophilic polymer. The secondary metal, osmium, is attached to the sites where osmiophilic polymer has been bound by the action of the primary metal catalyst (Pearse, 1972). Karnovsky (1965) and Graham and Karnovsky (1966) used diaminobenzidine (DAB) as a substrate for demonstrating the peroxidases. The reaction product produced by the oxidation of DAB is osmiophilic. Diaminobenzidine (DAB) is an ideal monomer from which the osmiophilic polymer can be produced. The osmiophilic polymer generation technique is being applied to the demonstration of hydrolytic enzymes and dehydrogenases. The technique is also used to convert cupric ferrocyanide (produced in methods to demonstrate the cholinesterases) to sulphide and to attach this product to osmium.

ULTRASTRUCTURAL DEMONSTRATION OF SOME COMMON ENZYMES

Alkaline phosphatase

Most of the methods for alkaline phosphatase are based on the metal precipitation technique of Gomori. The most common substrate used is sodium β-glycerophosphate, although other substrates e.g. cytidine monophosphate, have been suggested. A number of metal salts, mainly lead salts, have been used, as well as Gomori's original calcium–cobalt combination. The method given at the end of this chapter uses sodium β-glycerophosphate as substrate, and lead citrate as the metal salt. Other methods have used a calcium–lead combination (Reale, 1962) and lead nitrate (Hugon and Borgers, 1966).

Many methods exist for the demonstration of some of the specific alkaline phosphatases, including the adenosine triphosphatases (ATPase). Readers are referred to Pearse (1972) for details of the methods.

Acid phosphatase

Again Gomori's metal precipitation technique forms the cornerstone of the methods for the ultrastructural demonstration of acid phosphatase, and the modification of Holt and Hicks (1961) has been widely used. The method given at the end of this chapter is based on the osmium bridging technique discussed previously, and was devised by Hanker and his colleagues (1971). The substrate used is DDNTP (di-dicyclohexylammonium 2-naphthylthiol phosphate). This method gives rather better localization than the metal precipitation techniques.

Esterases

Many methods have been proposed for the demonstration of both non-specific esterases and the cholinesterases. Many of the methods for cholinesterase are based upon the thiocholine–copper–ferrocyanide method introduced by Karnovsky (1964). A modification using thiocholine—copper–lead was introduced by Kasa and Csillik (1966, 1968) and gives particularly fine localization. For a critical account of the many methods available, readers are referred to Pearse (1972).

Aryl sulphatase

Aryl sulphatase can be demonstrated by methods which use various organic sulphates as substrates, and lead or barium ions as the capture agent. One such method, that published by Hopsu-Havu *et al.* (1967), incorporates barium ions and has 2-hydroxy-5 nitrophenyl sulphate (*p*-nitrocatechol sulphate, 'NCS') as substrate; the method is given at the end of this chapter.

Other enzymes

Methods exist for the ultrastructural demonstration of many other enzymes, including the dehydrogenases, cytochrome oxidase, carbonic anhydrase, β-glucuronidase and some peptidases. The reader is referred to Pearse (1972).

Other substances

Carbohydrates

Glycogen is the most often demonstrated substance. It is well preserved after glutaraldehyde fixation. It appears to stain strongly with lead ions, and following periodic acid oxidation, glycogen granules are clearly seen (Perry, 1967). They can be removed by treatment with diastase. Acid mucosubstances are not easily demonstrated at the E.M. level. The most suitable method is the ruthenium red technique of Pihl *et al.* (1968).

Lipids

A major problem is to keep any lipid substance in E.M. sections after fixation and resin embedding. Following glutaraldehyde fixation alone, lipids are not present. Glutaraldehyde followed by osmium tetroxide preserves phospholipid membranes and some lipid droplets will appear complete.

Nucleic acids

These are well preserved after glutaraldehyde and osmium fixation and can be demonstrated by modifications of the classical Feulgen technique, alkaline silver solutions being used in place of Schiff's reagent. Adams, Bayliss and Weller (1965) used a periodic acid-silver diamine technique to demonstrate DNA. The standard methods of extraction using enzymes or acids can be used as suitable control methods.

Proteins

These are well preserved after glutaraldehyde fixation and a number of methods exist to demonstrate the various protein end-groups. These are again modifications of the methods used with the light microscope. These include methods for tyrosine, tryptophan, histidine and carboxyl groups.

METHOD 133

Alkaline phosphatase: Lead Citrate method (Mayahara *et al.*, 1967)

Reagents required

(1) Glutaraldehyde
(2) 0·1 M Cacodylate buffer, pH 7·4
(3) Sucrose
(4) Sodium β-glycerophosphate
(5) Magnesium sulphate
(6) Alkaline lead citrate solution
(7) 0·2 M Tris buffer, pH 8·5

(3) Epon tends to be hygroscopic and all containers and solutions should be covered to prevent the uptake of water.

REFERENCES

ADAMS, C. W. M., BAYLISS, O. B. and WELLER, R. O. (1965). *J. Histochem. Cytochem,* **13,** 694

GRAHAM, R. C. and KARNOVSKY, M. J. (1966). *J. Histochem. Cytochem.* **14,** 291

HANKER, J. S., ANDERSON, W. E. and BLOOM, F. E. (1971). *Science, N.Y.* **175,** 991

HOLT, S. J. and HICKS, R. M. (1961). *J. Biophys. biochem. Cytol.* **11,** 47

HOPSU-HAVU, V. K., ARSTILA, A., HELMINEN, H. J.,KALIMO, H. O. and GLENNER, G. G. (1967). *Histochemie* **8,** 54

HUGON, J. and BORGERS, M. (1966). *J. Histochem. Cytochem.* **14,** 429

KARNOVSKY, M. J. (1964). *J. Cell Biol.* **23,** 217

— (1965). *J. Cell Biol.* **27,** 137A

KASA, P. and CSILLIK, B. (1966). *J. Neurochem.* **13,** 1345

— — (1969). *Histochemie* **12,** 175

LUFT, J. H. (1961). *J. Biophys. biochem. Cytol.* **9,** 409

MAYAHARA, H., HIRANO, H., SAITO, T. and OGAWA, K. (1967). *Histochemie* **11,** 88

PEARSE, A. G. E. (1972). *Histochemistry, Theoretical and Applied*, Vol. 2, 3rd Edn., Edinburgh and London: Churchill Livingstone

Further Reading

PEARSE, A. G. E. (1972). *Histochemistry, Theoretical and Applied*, Vol. 2, 3rd Edn., Edinburgh and London: Churchill Livingstone

Appendix I

LIST OF METHODS

Appendix II

PREPARATION OF DYES AND MOUNTING MEDIA

Aqueous mounting media

Glycerin jelly (1)

Gelatine	15 g
Distilled water	100 ml
Glycerol	100 ml

Dissolve the gelatine in distilled water with moderate heating, then add the glycerol and mix the solution well. Filter through glass wool whilst hot. Store the bulk supply in a refrigerator.

Glycerin jelly (2) (Carleton, H. M. and Leach, E. H. (1938). *Histological Technique,* 2nd Edn., London: Oxford University Press)

Gelatine	10 g
Distilled water	60 ml
Glycerol	70 ml
Phenol crystals	250 mg

Prepare the solution in the manner described above. Glycerin jelly (1) is recommended for use when methods demonstrating dehydrogenases are to be mounted.

Apathys Medium (modified by Lillie, R. D. and Ashburn, L. L. (1943). *Arch Path.* **36,** 432)

Gum arabic	50 g
Cane sugar	50 g
Distilled water	100 ml
Thymol	100 mg

The cane sugar and gum arabic are dissolved in the distilled water by heating to 60°C.

Nuclear stains

2 per cent Methyl Green (chloroform-washed)

Methyl Green	2 g
Distilled water	100 ml

The Methyl Green is dissolved in the distilled water (slight heat may be necessary). The solution is poured into a separating funnel with an equal quantity of chloroform and the mixture is well shaken. The extraction with chloroform continues until the chloroform is colourless. The solution is then heated to 60°C to evaporate residual chloroform.

1 per cent Methyl Green (Barka, T. and Anderson, P. J. (1963). *Histochemistry Theory, Practice and Bibliography*, New York: Hoeber)

Methyl Green	1 g
Phosphate buffer, pH 4·0	100 ml

Coles haematoxylin

Haematoxylin	1·5 g
Warm distilled water	250 ml
1 per cent Iodine in 95 per cent alcohol	50 ml
Ammonium alum (sat. soln)	700 ml

The haematoxylin is dissolved in the distilled water and the iodine solution added, this solution is well mixed and the ammonium alum added. The solution is then brought to the boil, cooled and stored in a dark place. The solution must be filtered before use.

Scotts tap water

Sodium bicarbonate	3·5 g
Magnesium sulphate	20 g
Tap water	1000 ml

Appendix III

DIAZONIUM SALTS

The salts listed below are the more commonly used ones. The numbering system is that used by Pearse (PEARSE, A. G. E. (1960) *Histochemistry, Theoretical and Applied*, London: Churchill) Not all the salts listed by Pearse are given here.

Diazonium Salts

No.	*Preferred Common Name*	*Colour Index No.*
1	Fast Red A.L.	37275
2	Fast Blue R.R.	37155
3	Fast Red G.G.	37035
4	Fast Red 3G (3GL)	37040
6	Fast Blue B	37235
7	Fast Red R.C.	37120
8	Fast Red B	37125
9	Fast Red T.R.	37085
10	Fast Scarlet R	37130
16	Fast Red R.L.	37100
17	Fast Black K.	37190
18	Fast Garnet G.B.C.	37210
19	Fast Red I.T.R.	37150
20	Fast Violet B	37165
22	Fast Black B	37245
—	Fast Dark Blue R	37195
—	Fast Blue B.B.	37175

Appendix IV

BUFFER TABLES AND PREPARATION OF MOLAR AND NORMAL SOLUTIONS

Preparation of one litre of a molar solution

(1) Calculate the gram molecular weight (using atomic weights) of the solute
(2) Weigh out one gram molecule of the solute
(3) Measure out 1000 ml of distilled water
(4) Dissolve the solute in a small quantity of the water
(5) Add the remaining distilled water, to make the solution up to one litre

For solutions of different molarity: e.g. 2M and 0·1M

2 M solution = 2 × gram molecular wt in 1000 ml water
0·1 M solution = 0·1 × gram molecular wt in 1000 ml water

For example:

Sodium β-glycerophosphate
Molecular weight of sodium β-glycerophosphate = 315·13
Molar solution (M) = 315·13 g in 1000 ml distilled water
0·1 M = 31·513 g in 1000 ml distilled water.

The chemical is dissolved in a small quantity of the water and the volume is made up to one litre.

Preparation of molar solutions of liquids

(1) Calculate the molecular weight of the liquid
(2) Find the liquid's (a) valency
(b) specific gravity
(c) concentration

(3) Using the formula:
No. of ml of liquid per 1000 ml of distilled water =

$$\frac{\text{molecular weight}}{\text{valency} \times \text{specific gravity} \times \text{concn}}$$

Substitute the values found in (2) to the formula to find the volume of liquid required to make up a molar solution.

(4) Measure out the required volume of liquid and make up to 1000 ml by adding distilled water.

For solutions of different molarity adjustments have to be made to the volume of liquid used.

For example:

For a 2M solution, the volume required for a 1M solution has to be doubled, then made up to a litre with distilled water.

For an 0·1M solution the volume required for a 1M solution has to be divided by 10, then made up to a litre with distilled water.

Preparation of normal solutions

A normal solution contains one gram molecular weight of the substance, divided by the hydrogen equivalent of the substance.

For example:

(a) Sodium hydroxide, NaOH

Molecular weight of sodium hydroxide = 40·0. Valency = 1.

Normal solution = 40·0 g in 1000 ml distilled water divided by 1

= 4·0 g in 100 ml distilled water.

(b) For liquids, the following formula may be used:

ml of fluid per 1000 ml of distilled water

$$= \frac{\text{mol. wt}}{\text{valency} \times \text{specific gravity} \times \text{concn}}$$

For example: Hydrochloric acid, HCl

Valency 1, specific gravity 1·18, concn. 36 per cent, mol. wt 36·4

$$\frac{36{\cdot}4}{1 \times 1{\cdot}18 \times 0{\cdot}36} = 85{\cdot}6 \text{ ml}$$

N HCl = 85·6 ml HCl + 914·4 ml distilled water.

For example: Sulphuric acid, H_2SO_4

Valency 3, specific gravity 1·835, concn. 98 per cent mol. wt 98·08

$$\frac{98{\cdot}08}{2 \times 1{\cdot}835 \times 0{\cdot}98} = 29{\cdot}1 \text{ ml}$$

N $H_2S_2O_4$ = 29·1 ml H_2SO_4 + 970·9 ml distilled water

0·1 N H_2SO_4 = 2·91 ml H_2SO_4 + 997·09 ml distilled water.

BUFFER TABLE 1

Buffer	*Molarity*	*Preparation*	pH *Range*										
			3·6	3·8	4·0	4·2	4·4	4·6	4·8	5·0	5·2	5·4	5·6
1. Acetate Buffer													
A. Sodium acetate (anhydrous) (Mol. wt 82)	0·2 M	1·64 g in 100 ml	3·7	6·0	9·0	13·2	19·5	24·5	30·0	35·2	39·5	41·2	45·2
B. Acetic acid	0·2 M	1·2 ml in 100 ml	46·3	44	41·0	36·8	30·5	25·5	20·0	14·8	10·5	8·8	4·8
Distilled water			50·0	50	50	50	50	50	50	50	50	50	50
2. Veronal Acetate													
A. Sodium acetate (trihydrate) (Mol. wt 136) Sodium barbitone (Mol. wt 206)		1·94 g and 2·94 g in 100 ml	5	5	5	5	5	5	5	5	5	5	—
B. Hydrochloric acid	0·1 N	0·84 ml in 100 ml	14·0	13·0	12·5	12·0	11·0	10·0	9·5	9·0	8·5	8·0	—
Distilled water			4	5	5·5	6	7	8	8·5	9·0	9·5	10·0	—
3. Citrate–Citric acid													
A. Sodium citrate (Mol. wt 294)	0·1 M	3·57 g in 100 ml	13·0	15	17	18·5	22	24·5	27·0	29·5	32·0	34·0	36·3
B. Citric acid (Mol. wt 210)	0·1 M	2·10 g in 100 ml	37·0	35·0	33·0	31·5	28	25·5	23·0	20·5	18	16·0	13·7
Distilled water			50	50	50	50	50	50	50	50	50	50	50
4. Phosphate–Citrate													
A. Disodium hydrogen orthophosphate (Mol. wt 142)	0·2 M	2·83 g in 100 ml	32·2	35·5	38·5	41·4	44·1	46·7	49·3	51·5	53·6	55·7	58·0
B. Citric acid (Mol. wt 210)	0·1 M	2·10 g in 100 ml	67·8	64·5	61·5	58·6	55·9	53·3	50·7	48·5	46·4	44·3	42·0
Distilled water			—	—	—	—	—	—	—	—	—	—	—

BUFFER TABLE 2

Buffer	*Molarity*	*Preparation*	pH *Range*										
			5·2	5·4	5·6	5·8	6·0	6·2	6·4	6·6	6·8	7·0	7·2
1. *Phosphate*													
A. Sodium dihydrogen orthophosphate NaH_2PO_4 (Mol. wt 156)	0·2 M	3·12 g in 100 ml	—	—	—	46·0	43·8	40·7	36·7	31·2	25·5	19·5	14·0
B. Disodium hydrogen orthophosphate Na_2HPO_4 (Mol. wt. 142)	0·2 M	2·83 g in 100 ml	—	—	—	4·0	6·2	9·3	13·3	18·8	24·5	30·5	36·0
Distilled water			—	—	—	50	50	50	50	50	50	50	50
2. *Phosphate–Citrate*													
A. Disodium hydrogen orthophosphate Na_2HPO_4 (Mol. wt 142)	0·2 M	2·83 g in 100 ml	53·6	55·7	58·0	60·4	63·1	66·1	69·2	72·7	77·2	82·3	86·9
B. Citric acid (Mol. wt 210)	0·1 M	2·101 g in 100 ml	46·4	44·3	42·0	39·6	36·9	33·9	30·8	27·3	22·8	17·7	13·1
Distilled water			—	—	—	—	—	—	—	—	—	—	—
3. *Tris–Maleate*													
A. (1) Tris* (Mol. wt 121)		2·42 g } in											
(2) Maleic acid (Mol. wt 116)	0·2 M	2·32 g } 100 ml	25	25	25	25	25	25	25	25	25	25	25
B. Sodium hydroxide (Mol. wt 40)	0·2 M	0·8 g in 100 ml	3·5	5·4	7·7	10·2	13·0	15·7	19·5	21·2	22·5	24·0	25·5
Distilled water			71·5	69·6	67·3	64·8	62·0	59·3	55·5	53·8	52·5	51·0	49·5
4. *Veronal Acetate*													
A. (1) Sodium acetate (trihydrate) $3H_2O$ (Mol. wt 136)		1·94 g } in											
(2) Sodium barbitone (Mol. wt 206)		2·94 g } 100 ml	—	5·0	—	—	—	5·0	—	—	5·0	5·0	5·0
B. Hydrochloric acid	0·1 N	0·85 ml in 100 ml	—	8·0	—	—	—	7·0	—	—	6·5	6·0	5·5
Distilled water		—	—	10	—	—	—	11	—	—	11·5	12	12·5

* 2-Amino-2-(hydroxy-methyl)-propane- 1 : 3 diol

BUFFER TABLE 3

Buffer	Molarity	Preparation	pH *Range* 7·4	7·6	7·8	8·0	8·2	8·4	8·6	8·8	9·0	9·2	9·4
1. *Phosphate*	0·1 M												
A. Sodium dihydrogen orthophosphate NaH_2PO_4 (Mol. wt 156)	0·2 M	2·75 g in 100 ml	9·5	6·5	4·2	2·6	—	—	—	—	—	—	—
B. Disodium hydrogen phosphate Na_2HPO_4 (Mol. wt 142)	0·1 M	2·83 g in 100 ml	40·5	43·5	45·8	47·4	—	—	—	—	—	—	—
Distilled water			50·0	50·0	50·0	50·0	—	—	—	—	—	—	—
2. *Phosphate–Citrate*													
A. Disodium hydrogen phosphate Na_2HPO_4 (Mol. wt 142)	0·2 M	2·83 g in 100 ml	90·8	93·6	95·7	97·2	—	—	—	—	—	—	—
B. Citric acid (Mol. wt 210)	0·1 M	2·101 g in 100 ml	9·2	6·4	4·3	2·8	—	—	—	—	—	—	—
Distilled water			—	—	—	—	—	—	—	—	—	—	—
3. *Veronal Acetate*													
A. (1) Sodium acetate, (trihydrate) $3H_2O$ (Mol. wt 136)	—	1·94 g } in 100 ml	5	5	—	5	5	—	5	—	—	5	—
(2) Sodium barbitone (Mol. wt 206)	—	2·94 g } in 100 ml											
B. Hydrochloric acid	0·1 N	0·85 ml in 100 ml	5	4	—	3	2	—	0·75	—	—	0·25	—
Distilled water			13	14	—	15	16	—	17·25	—	—	17·75	—
4. *Tris–Maleate*													
A. (1) Tris* (Mol. wt 121)	0·2 M	2·42 g } in 100 ml	25·0	25·0	25·0	25·0	25·0	25·0	25·0	—	—	—	—
(2) Maleic acid (Mol. wt 116)		2·32 g } in 100 ml											
B. Sodium hydroxide (Mol. wt 40)	0·2 M	0·8 g in 100 ml	27·0	28·0	31·7	34·5	37·5	40·5	43·2	—	—	—	—
Distilled water			48·0	47·0	43·3	40·5	37·5	34·5	31·8	—	—	—	—
5. *Tris–HCl*†													
A. Tris* (Mol. wt 121)	0·2 M	2·42 g in 100 ml	25·0	25·0	25·0	25·0	25·0	25·0	25·0	—	25·0	—	—
Hydrochloric acid	0·1 N	0·85 ml in 100 ml	42·5	37·5	32·5	27·5	22·5	17·5	12·5	—	5·0	—	—
Distilled water			32·5	37·5	42·5	47·5	52·5	57·5	62·5	—	70·0	—	—

* 2-Amino-2-(hydroxy-methyl)-propane-1: 3-diol
† For Tris-HCl buffer pH 7·2 add 25 ml Tris stock + 47·5 ml 0·1N HCl and 27·5 ml distilled water

Appendix V

SOME SOURCES OF SUPPLY FOR THE CHEMICALS AND REAGENTS USED IN THE METHODS GIVEN IN THIS BOOK

Chemicals	*Sources*
Acetyl Thiocholine Iodide	L; KL; Si
Acid Fuchsin	L; S; BDH; HW
Acridine Orange	L; S; Si; BDH
Acrolein	BDH
Adenosine-5-Diphosphate	L; KL; Si; B
Adenosine-5-Triphosphate	L; KL; Si; B
Alcian Blue	L; S; BDH; HW
Alloxan	KL; Si; BDH
Aluminium Chloride	KL; BDH; HW
Aluminium Hydroxide	KL; BDH; HW
2-Amino-2 (Hydroxy-methyl) 1:3-Propanediol	KL; Si; BDH; HW
Ammonia Solution	KL; BDH; HW
Ammonium Sulphide	KL; BDH; HW
Arcton 22	ICI
Azure A	L; S
Barbitone Sodium	L; KL; BDH; HW
Basic Fuchsin	L; Si; HW
Benzidine	KL*
Benzidine Dihyrochloride	KL; L
6-Benzoyl-2-Naphthyl Sulphate	KL; Si
Bromine Water	BDH; HW
5-Bromo-4-Chloro-Indoxyl Acetate	L; Si
Butyryl Thiocholine Iodide	L; KL; Si
Calcium Carbonate	KL; BDH; HW
Calcium Chloride	L; KL; BDH; HW
Carmine	L; BDH; HW
Celloidin	L; S; BDH; HW
Charcoal (activated)	L; Si; BDH; HW
Chrome Alum	L; BDH; HW

* Carcinogenic

Chemicals	*Sources*
Chromium Trioxide	KL; BDH; HW
Citric Acid	L; KL; BDH; HW
Cobalt Acetate	Si; BDH; HW
Cobalt Chloride	KL; BDH; HW
Cobalt Nitrate	KL; BDH; HW
Congo Red	L; S; BDH; HW
Cupric Acetate	KL; BDH; HW
Cupric Sulphate	KL; Si; BDH; HW
DDSA (Dodecenyl Succinate Anhydride)	TAAB
Deoxyribonuclease	L; KL; Si; B
3 3′ Diaminobenzidine Tetrahydrochloride	KL; KK
Di-Dicyclohexylammonium-2-Naphthylthiol-phosphate	Polaron
Digitonin	L; KL; Si; B
2:2-Dihydroxy-6:6-Dinaphthyl Disulphide (DDD)	KL; Si; BDH
Dihydroxyphenylalanine (DOPA)	L; KL; Si; BDH
N:N-Dimethyl Formamide (DMF)	L; KL; Si; BDH
N:N-Dimethyl-m-Phenylenediamine Dihydrochloride	EK
N:N-Dimethyl-p-Phenylenediamine Hydrochloride	EK; Si
3(4:5-Dimethyl Thiazolyl-2)25-Diphenyl Tetrazolium Bromide (MTT)	KL; Si; NBC
Dinitro-Fluoro-Benzine	BDH
Dioxan	KL
DMP 30 2,4,6 Tri (Dimethyl-Amino Methyl Phenol)	TAAB
Eosin	L; KL; BDH; HW
Epon 812	TAAB
Ethyl Cellulose	BDH; HW
N-Ethyl Maleimide	KL; Si
Ethylenediamine Tetra-Acetic Acid (Disodium)	L; KL; BDH; HW
Fast Blue B	L; S; Si; ICI
Fast Garnet GBC	L; S; Si; ICI
Fast Red B	L; S; HW; ICI
Fast Red TR	L; S; KL; ICI
Ferric Ammonium Sulphate	BDH; HW
Ferric Chloride	S; BDH; HW; ICI
Formaldehyde Solution	L; KL; BDH; HW
Freon 22	ICI
Gallocyanin	L; S; BDH; HW
Gelatin	L; Si
Giemsa's Stain	L; S; BDH; HW
Glucose-1-Phosphate	KL; Si; BDH; HW
Glucose-6-Phosphate (K salt)	KL; Si; B
Glucose-6-Phosphate (Sodium salt)	KL; Si; B
Gum Acacia	BDH; HW
L-Glutamic Acid (sodium salt)	KL; Si; BDH
Glutaraldehyde	KL; Si

Chemicals	*Sources*
Glycerin	L; Si; BDH
Glycogen	Si; BDH; HW
H-acid (8 Amino-1 Naphthol-3-6-Disulphonic Acid)	BDH
Hexamine (Methenamine)	BDH; HW
Hyaluronidase (testicular)	KL; Si; BDH
Hydrogen Peroxide	BDH; HW
DL-3-Hydroxy Butyric Acid (sodium salt)	KL; BDH
2-Hydroxy-3-Naphthaldehyde	Sig; Polaron
2-Hydroxy-3-Naphthoic Acid Hydrazide	KL
2-Hydroxy-5-Nitrophenyl Sulphate (p-Nitrocatechol Sulphate)	KL
Insulin	Si
Iodine	L; KL; BDH; HW
Isocitric Acid (trisodium salt)	KL; Si; NBC
Isopropanol	KL; Si; BDH; HW
Lead Nitrate	KL; BDH; HW
L-Leucyl-4-Methoxy-3-Naphthylamide	KL; Si
L-Leucyl-3-Naphthylamide	KL; Si
Lithium Carbonate	L; KL; BDH; HW
Magnesium Chloride	KL; Si; BDH; HW
Magnesium Nitrate	KL; BDH; HW
Magnesium Sulphate	KL; Si; BDH; HW
Maleic Acid	KL; Si; BDH; HW
Manganese Chloride	KL; Si; BDH; HW
Mayer's Carmalum	L; S; BDH; HW
Mercuric Chloride	L; KL; BDH; HW
Mercuric Sulphate	BDH; HW
Mercury Orange	S; KL; Si; NBC
Methyl Green	L; S; BDH; HW
Methyl Nadic Anhydride (MNA)	TAAB
Methyl Violet	L; S; BDH; HW
3(4:5-Dimethyl Thiazolyl-2) 5-Diphenyl Tetrazolium Bromide (MTT)	KL; Si; NBC
Myristoyl Choline Chloride	KL; Si
Naphthochrome Green B	L; S
α-Naphthol	L; KL; Si
α-Naphthol Acetate	L; KL; Si
Naphthol AS-BI Phosphate	KL; Si; NBC
Naphthol AS-BI Glucuronide	KL; Si; NBC
Naphthol AS-CL Phosphate	KL; Si; NBC
Naphthol AS-LC Acetate	KL; Si; NBC
Naphthol AS Sulphate (potassium salt)	KL; Si; NBC
1:2-Naphthoquinone-4-Sulphonic Acid	KL; Si; NBC
α-Naphthyl Phosphate	KL; Si; HW; NBC
α-Naphthylamine	BDH; HW
Neutral Red	L; S; BDH; HW
Nicotinamide-Adenine Dinucleotide (NAD)	Si; B; BDH; NBC
Nicotinamide-Adenine Dinucleotide reduced (NADH)	Si; B; BDH; NBC

Chemicals	*Sources*
Nicotinamide-Adenine Dinucleotide Phosphate (NADP)	Si; B; BDH; NBC
Nicotinamide-Adenine Dinucleotide Phosphate reduced (NADPH)	Si; B; BDH; NBC
Nile Blue	L; S; BDH; HW
Ninhydrin	BDH
Nitro Blue Tetrazolium (NBT)	KL; Si; NBC
Oil Red O	L; S; BDH; HW
Osmium Tetroxide	L; S; JM
Patent Blue V	L; S; BDH; HW
Paraformaldehyde	KL; BDH; HW
Paraldehyde	BDH; HW
Pararosanilin Hydrochloride	L; S; BDH
Perchloric Acid	BDH; HW
Periodic Acid	L; S; BDH; HW
N-Phenyl Phenylene Diamine	KL
Phosphoric Oxide	BDH; HW
Picric Acid	L; S; BDH; HW
Polyvinyl Pyrrolidone	KL; BDH; HW; NBC
Potassium Bicarbonate	BDH; HW
Potassium Carbonate	BDH; HW
Potassium Chloride	BDH; HW
Potassium Cyanide	BDH; HW
Potassium Dichromate	BDH; HW
Potassium Ferricyanide	BDH; HW
Potassium Ferrocyanide	BDH; HW
Potassium Hydroxide	BDH; HW
Potassium Metabisulphite	BDH; HW
Potassium Perchlorate	BDH; HW
Propionic Acid	KL; BDH; HW
Propylene Oxide	TAAB
Pyridine	BDH; HW
Pyronin Y	L; S; BDH
Ribonuclease	KL; Si; B
Rubeanic Acid	KL; HW
S-Acid (8-Amino-1-Naphthol-5-Sulphonic Acid)	EK
Sialidase (Neuraminidase) ex. V. Cholerae	KL; Si
Silver Nitrate	L; S; BDH; HW
Sodium Acetate	BDH; HW
Sodium Alizarin Sulphonate (Alizarin Red S)	L; S; BDH; HW
Sodium Bicarbonate	BDH; HW
Sodium Cacodylate	BDH; HW
Sodium Chloride	BDH; HW
Sodium Cyanide	BDH; HW
Sodium Fluoride	BDH; HW
Sodium β-Glycerophosphate	L: Si; BDH; HW
Sodium Hydroxide	BDH; HW
Sodium Hydrogen Malate	BDH; HW
Sodium Hypochlorite	BDH; HW
Sodium Iodate	BDH; HW

Chemicals	*Sources*
Sodium DL-lactate	BDH; HW
Sodium Metabisulphite	BDH; HW
Sodium Nitrite	BDH; HW
Sodium Nitroprusside	BDH; HW
Sodium Dihydrogen Orthophosphate	BDH; HW
Disodium Hydrogen Orthophosphate	BDH; HW
Sodium Rhodizonate	KK; KL
Sodium Succinate	BDH; HW
Sodium Sulphate	BDH; HW
Sodium Tetraborate	BDH; HW
Sodium Thiosulphate	BDH; HW
Solochrome Azurine	L; S
Sucrose	BDH; HW
Sudan Black B	BDH; HW
Tetra Nitro-Blue Tetrazolium (TNBT)	L; KL; Si; BDH
Thiocarbohydrazide	KL
Thioflavine T	L; BDH; HW
Thionyl Chloride	L; BDH; HW
Thymol	BDH; HW
Titanous Chloride	KL; BDH
Trichloroacetic Acid	BDH; HW
Triethyl Phosphate	L; S; BDH; HW
Tryptamine Hydrochloride	BDH
Tweens, 40,60,80	KL; Si
Uranyl Nitrate	BDH; HW
Urea	BDH; HW
Zinc (powdered)	

B

Boehringer Corporation (London) Ltd.,
Bell Lane, Lewes, East Sussex,
BN17 1LG

BDH

British Drug Houses Ltd.,
Laboratory Chemicals Division,
Poole, Dorset.

EK

Eastman Kodak Ltd.,
Kirby,
Liverpool, Lancs.
and

Eastman Organic Chemicals,
Eastman Kodak Company,
Rochester, NY 14650,
USA.

KL

Koch-Light Ltd.,
Colnbrook, Bucks.

L

Raymond A. Lamb,
6 Sunbeam Road,
London NW10 6JL.

NBC

Agent
Micro-Bio Laboratories,
46 Pembridge Road,
London, W11.

Nutritional Biochemicals
Corporation,
Cleveland 28,
Ohio, USA.

HW

Hopkin and Williams Ltd.,
Freshwater Road,
Chadwell Heath,
Essex.

ICI

Imperial Chemical Industries Ltd.,
PO Box 19,
Templar House,
81–87 High Holborn,
London.

JM

Johnson Matthey,
73–83 Hatton Garden,
London EC1.

KK

Agents,
K & K Laboratories
Kodak Ltd.,
Kirby, Liverpool,
Lancs.

K and K Laboratories Inc.,
121 Express Street,
Engineers Hill,
Plainview,
New York 11803,
USA.

Polaron

Polaron Equipment Ltd.,
4 Shakespeare Road,
Finchley,
London N3 1XH.

S

Searle Scientific Ltd.,
Coronation Road,
Cresswick Industrial Estate,
High Wycombe,
Bucks.

Si

Sigma (London) Chemical Company,
Norbiton Station Yard,
Kingston-Upon-Thames,
Surrey KT2 7BH.
and
Sigma
PO 14508,
St. Joseph 63178,
Missouri, USA.

TAAB

Taab Laboratories,
52 Kidmore End Road,
Emmer Green,
Reading.

Index